International Issues in Early Intervention
Series editor: Michael J. Guralnick

ISEI

Interdisciplinary Clinical Assessment of Young Children with Developmental Disabilities

A book series from the
International Society on Early Intervention

ISEI

Interdisciplinary Clinical Assessment of Young Children with Developmental Disabilities

edited by

Michael J. Guralnick, Ph.D.
University of Washington
Seattle

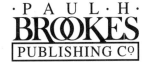

·P A U L·H·
BROOKES
PUBLISHING CO

Baltimore • London • Toronto • Sydney

Paul H. Brookes Publishing Co.
Post Office Box 10624
Baltimore, Maryland 21285-0624

www.brookespublishing.com

Typeset by Barton Matheson Willse and Worthington, Baltimore, Maryland.
Manufactured in the United States of America by
The Maple Press Co., York, Pennsylvania.

All of the vignettes in this book are composites based on the authors' actual
experiences. In all instances, names have been changed; in some instances, identifying
details have been altered to protect confidentiality.

Library of Congress Cataloging-in-Publication Data

Interdisciplinary clinical assessment of young children with developmental disabilities/
edited by Michael J. Guralnick.
    p.   cm.—(International issues in early intervention)
Includes bibliographical references and index.
ISBN 1-55766-450-1 (hardcover)
    1. Developmentally disabled children.   2. Medical care—Needs assessment.
3. Developmentally disabled children—Care.   4. Developmental disabilities.
I. Guralnick, Michael J. II. Series.
    [DNLM: 1. Developmental Disabilities.   2. Needs Assessment—Child,
Preschool.   3. Needs Assessment—Infant.   4. Patient Care Team.
WS 350.6 I588 2000]
RJ135 .I547 2000
618.92'8588—dc21

                                          99-045303

British Library Cataloguing in Publication data are available from the British Library.

Contents

About the Editor

Michael J. Guralnick, Ph.D., is Director of the Center on Human Development and Disability (CHDD) and Professor of Psychology and Pediatrics at the University of Washington, Seattle. Comprising both a University Affiliated Program and a Mental Retardation and Developmental Disabilities Research Center, CHDD is one of the largest interdisciplinary research and training centers in the United States, addressing issues directly related to developmental disabilities. More than 600 faculty and staff members and doctoral and post-doctoral students operate within the four CHDD buildings on the campus of the University of Washington and in community sites to conduct basic and applied research, to provide clinical services to individuals and their families, to provide interdisciplinary clinical and research training, and to provide technical assistance and outreach training to practitioners and community agencies.

Dr. Guralnick has directed research and development projects in the fields of early childhood intervention, inclusion, peer relationships, and pediatric education. He has published more than 100 articles and book chapters (including 6 edited volumes). Dr. Guralnick's publications have appeared in a diverse group of well-respected journals, including *Child Development*, *Pediatrics*, *American Journal on Mental Retardation*, *Journal of Early Intervention*, *Developmental Psychology*, *Journal of Developmental and Behavioral Pediatrics*, *Journal of Applied Developmental Psychology*, and *Development and Psychopathology*. He currently directs a major research project supported by the National Institute of Child Health and Human Development designed to determine the effectiveness of a comprehensive early intervention program in promoting the peer-related social competence of young children with developmental delays.

Dr. Guralnick received the 1994 Research Award from the American Association on Mental Retardation and the 1997 Distinguished Research Award from The Arc of the United States. He is a past president of the American Association of University Affiliated Programs and the Council for Exceptional Children's Division for Early Childhood, and he is a former chair of the Mental Retardation and Developmental Disabilities Research Center Directors. He is currently Chair of the International Society on Early Intervention and is President-Elect of the Academy on Mental Retardation.

Contributors

Giorgio Albertini, M.D.
Director
Child, Adult, Aging Development
Center Silvana Paolini Angelucci
Via della Pisana, 235
Casa de Cura San Raffaele
Professor, Child Neurology, Psychiatry,
and Geriatrics
University Tor Vergata
00163, Rome, Italy

Susan J. Astley, Ph.D.
FAS/FAE Clinic, Clinical
Training Unit
University Affiliated Program
Center on Human Development
and Disability
Assistant Professor
Departments of Epidemiology
and Pediatrics
University of Washington
Division of Genetics and Development
Children's Hospital and Regional
Medical Center
CH-47, Box 359300
Seattle, WA 98105

Eva Björk-Åkesson, Ph.D.
Professor of Education
Department of Social Sciences
Malardalen University, Box 883
S-72123 Vasteres, Sweden

Patricia Brandt, Ph.D.
Professor
Department of Family and Child Nursing
University of Washington, Box 357262
Seattle, WA 98195

Amy G. Breiger, Ph.D.
Psychology, Clinical Training Unit
University Affiliated Program
Center on Human Development
and Disability
Clinical Instructor
Department of Psychiatry and
Behavioral Sciences
University of Washington, Box 357920
Seattle, WA 98195

Carla A. Brooks, M.A., C.C.C.
Speech-Language Pathologist
Children's Hospital and Regional
Medical Center
4800 Sand Point Way NE
Seattle, Washington 98105

Sandra G.B. Clarren, Ph.D.
FAS/FAE Clinic, Clinical
Training Unit
University Affiliated Program
Center on Human Development
and Disability
Professional Staff
Department of Pediatrics
University of Washington
Seattle, WA 98195

Sterling K. Clarren, M.D.
FAS/FAE Clinic, Clinical
Training Unit
University Affiliated Program
Center on Human Development
and Disability
Robert A. Aldrich Professor
Department of Pediatrics
University of Washington
Division of Genetics and Development
Children's Hospital and Regional
Medical Center
CH-47, Box 359300
Seattle, WA 98105

Truman E. Coggins, Ph.D.
Speech/Language Pathology
(Discipline Leader)
Clinical Training Unit, University
Affiliated Program
Center on Human Development
and Disability
Associate Professor
Department of Speech and
Hearing Sciences
University of Washington, Box 357920
Seattle, WA 98195

Douglas S. Cook, Ph.D.
Social Work (Discipline Leader)
Clinical Training Unit, University
  Affiliated Program
Center on Human Development
  and Disability
Clinical Assistant Professor
School of Social Work
University of Washington, Box 357920
Seattle, WA 98195

Nuhad D. Dinno, M.D.
Pediatrics, Clinical Training Unit
University Affiliated Program
Center on Human Development
  and Disability
Clinical Professor
Department of Pediatrics
University of Washington, Box 357920
Seattle, WA 98195

Theresse Douglass,
  A.R.N.P., Ph.D.
Nursing, Clinical Training Unit
University Affiliated Program
Center on Human Development
  and Disability
University of Washington, Box 357920
Seattle, WA 98195

Richard C. Folsom, Ph.D.
Audiology (Discipline Leader)
Clinical Training Unit, University
  Affiliated Program
Center on Human Development
  and Disability
Professor
Department of Speech and
  Hearing Sciences
University of Washington, Box 357920
Seattle, WA 98195

Janet Garretson, M.S.W.
Pediatric Genetics, University
  Affiliated Program
Social Worker, PKU Clinic
Center on Human Development
  and Disability
University of Washington, Box 357920
Seattle, WA 98195

Mats Granlund, Ph.D.
Associate Professor in Psychology
ALA Research Foundation
Sibyllegat 7
Mälardalen University
S-72123 Vasteres, Sweden

Anne Hay, Ph.D.
Psychology, Clinical Training Unit
University Affiliated Program
Center on Human Development
  and Disability
University of Washington, Box 357920
Seattle, WA 98195

Janie Heffernan, M.S., R.D.
Pediatric Genetics, University
  Affiliated Program
Nutritionist, PKU Clinic
Center on Human Development
  and Disability
University of Washington, Box 357920
Seattle, WA 98195

Vanja A. Holm, M.D.
Pediatrics, Clinical Training Unit
University Affiliated Program
Center on Human Development
  and Disability
Associate Professor Emeritus
Department of Pediatrics
University of Washington, Box 357920
Seattle, WA 98195

Gail Kieckhefer, A.R.N.P.,
  CS-PNP, Ph.D.
Associate Professor
Department of Family and
  Child Nursing
University of Washington, Box 357262
Seattle, WA 98195

Elena Kozhevnikova, Ph.D.
Director
St. Petersburg Early
  Intervention Institute
Chaikovskogo, 73
St. Petersburg, Russia 191123

Anne Leavitt, M.D.
Pediatrics, Clinical Training Unit
University Affiliated Program
Center on Human Development
  and Disability
Clinical Assistant Professor
Department of Pediatrics
University of Washington, Box 357920
Seattle, WA 98195

**Betty L. Lucas, M.P.H.,
  R.D., C.D.**
Nutrition, Clinical Training Unit
University Affiliated Program
Center on Human Development
  and Disability
Lecturer
Department of Family and
  Child Nursing
University of Washington, Box 357920
Seattle, WA 98195

**Diane Magyary, M.N.,
  A.R.N.P., Ph.D.**
Professor
Department of Psychosocial and
  Community Health
University of Washington, Box 357263
Seattle, WA 98195

Heather Carmichael Olson, Ph.D.
FAS/FAE Clinic, University
  Affiliated Program
Research Assistant Professor
Department of Psychiatry and
  Behavioral Sciences
University of Washington, Box 375925
Seattle, WA 98195

Julie A. Osterling, Ph.D.
Associate Director, Autism Program
University Affiliated Program
Center on Human Development
  and Disability
Research Associate
Department of Psychology
University of Washington
Seattle, WA 98195

Peggy L. Pipes, M.P.H.
Nutrition, Clinical Training Unit
University Affiliated Program
Center on Human Development
  and Disability
Lecturer Emeritus
Department of Family and
  Child Nursing
University of Washington, Box 357262
Seattle, WA 98195

Salvatore Rubino, M.D.
Medical Director
Casa di Cura San Raffaele
00163 Rome, Italy

David T. Scott, Ph.D.
Psychology (Discipline Leader)
Clinical Training Unit, University
  Affiliated Program
Center on Human Development
  and Disability
Associate Professor
Department of Psychiatry and
  Behavioral Sciences
University of Washington, Box 357920
Seattle, WA 98195

Rune J. Simeonsson, Ph.D.
Professor
School of Education
Research Professor
Department of Psychology
Frank Porter Graham Child
  Development Center
University of North Carolina at
  Chapel Hill
Chapel Hill, NC 27599

**Katherine B. Stewart, M.S.,
  OTR/L**
Clinical Associate Professor
School of Occupational Therapy and
  Physical Therapy
University of Puget Sound
1550 N. Warner Avenue
Tacoma, WA 98416

William Eric Strong, M.S.
Speech-Language Pathology,
   Clinical Training Unit
University Affiliated Program
Center on Human Development
   and Disability
Speech-Language Pathologist
Department of Speech and
   Hearing Sciences
University of Washington, Box 354875
Seattle, WA 98195

Marcia W. Swanson, M.P.H., P.T.
Physical Therapy, Clinical
   Training Unit
University Affiliated Program
Center on Human Development and
   Disability
Lecturer
Department of Rehabilitation Medicine
University of Washington, Box 357920
Seattle, WA 98195

**Mary E. Tatarka, Ph.D., P.T.
(deceased)**
Physical Therapy, Clinical
   Training Unit
University Affiliated Program
Center on Human Development
   and Disability
University of Washington, Box 357920
Seattle, WA 98195

Geralyn Timler, M.S.
Speech-Language Pathology, Clinical
   Training Unit
Department of Speech and
   Hearing Sciences
University of Washington
Seattle, WA 98105

Cristine M. Trahms, M.S.
Nutrition (Discipline Leader)
Clinical Training Unit, University
   Affiliated Program
Center on Human Development and
   Disability
Lecturer
Department of Pediatrics
University of Washington, Box 357920
Seattle, WA 98195

Alan S. Unis, M.D.
Autism Program, University
   Affiliated Program
Center on Human Development and
   Disability
Associate Professor
Department of Psychiatry and
   Behavioral Sciences
Division of Psychiatric Neurosciences
University of Washington, Box 356560
Seattle, WA 98195

**Kathleen A. Washington,
Ph.D., P.T.**
Physical Therapy (Discipline Leader)
Clinical Training Unit, University
   Affiliated Program
Center on Human Development
   and Disability
Clinical Assistant Professor
Department of Rehabilitation Medicine
University of Washington, Box 357920
Seattle, WA 98195

Renee Watling, M.S.
College of Education
University of Washington, Box 353600
Seattle, WA 98195

Susan Wendel, M.S., OTR
Occupational Therapy (Discipline
   Leader)
Clinical Training Unit, University
   Affiliated Program
Center on Human Development and
   Disability
Clinical Faculty
Department of Rehabilitation Medicine
University of Washington, Box 357920
Seattle, WA 98195

Joan C. Zerzan, M.S., R.D.
Pediatric Dietitian
Food and Nutrition Services,
   Clinical Training Unit
University Affiliated Program
Center on Human Development
   and Disability
University of Washington, Box 357920
Seattle, WA 98195

Preface

Interdisciplinary clinical assessment is a central component of the larger system of services and supports for young children at risk for or with established developmental disabilities. Parents of young children generally initiate this process when developmental concerns arise, and it often results in a recommendation for a comprehensive early intervention program. Even for children enrolled in early intervention, the interdisciplinary clinical assessment process is often called upon when unexpected or unusual developmental patterns occur or when disagreements emerge as to what is the most appropriate course of action.

Effective interdisciplinary teams not only recognize their role in the early intervention system but also develop a close working relationship that evolves over time with other team members (see Section I). Interdisciplinary collaboration has proven to be a challenge in virtually every circumstance, yet it remains essential in ensuring that young children and their families receive the best care possible.

In this volume, the contributors in Sections II and III collectively represent many years of interdisciplinary clinical experience as part of the University Affiliated Program at the University of Washington, Seattle. Some of the members of the various interdisciplinary teams have participated in this process for the vast majority of their long and distinguished careers. Others are relative newcomers and have learned their trade through an initial apprenticeship, followed by extensive practice.

As such, the primary purpose of *Interdisciplinary Clinical Assessment of Young Children with Developmental Disabilities* is to facilitate the process of involving and assimilating new members of an interdisciplinary assessment team or facilitating the establishment of an entirely new team. Students or trainees in the field of developmental disabilities may find this volume especially helpful. Accordingly, discipline-specific information and techniques in the context of interdisciplinary practice are provided (Section II), as are case studies designed to illustrate the details and dynamic nature of the interactions that take place (Section III). Every effort was made to articulate the thought processes, specific expertise, diverse interests, and ways in which teams collaborate. Yet the book's authors are under no illusion that any volume can truly capture the subtleties and variations of a complex interactional process. It is hoped, however, that these subtleties and variations will be easier to detect as a result of this volume.

Interdisciplinary clinical assessments have been practiced widely not only in the United States but in many other nations as well. Despite some universal features, this process must, of course, be adapted to and consistent with each country's historical and prevailing conditions. Cultural perspectives and the value system associated with young children—particularly those with disabilities—as well as political and economic circumstances are only some of the factors that influence this process. Section IV offers a summary of inter-disciplinary clinical assessment from countries with very different approaches to help us look globally at the issues addressed in this inaugural volume in the International Issues in Early Intervention series. This important series, con-ceived by the International Society on Early Intervention (ISEI; see http://depts.washington.edu/isei), will help to advance the practice of early interven-tion by providing a forum for sharing information from a global advantage. It is fitting to begin the series with a topic as critical as assessment.

Acknowledgments

I wish to thank the many people who have made *Interdisciplinary Clinical Assessment of Young Children with Developmental Disabilities* possible. I am deeply indebted to the many contributors to the volume who have worked so hard to communicate their thinking. This is particularly true for those clinicians who are part of the University Affiliated Program's Clinical Training Unit. Over a period of 2 years, we held monthly lunch meetings that became well known for their lively discussions of the interdisciplinary process. Although perhaps not aiding our digestion, this volume has immeasurably benefited from these exchanges.

Moreover, this volume simply could not have been completed without the expert editorial assistance of Carolyn Hamby. Through her diligent efforts, this volume has achieved a level of quality even we had not anticipated.

Finally, I wish to thank Paul H. Brookes Publishing Co. for its fine editorial and production work, as well as its ongoing support of the International Society on Early Intervention.

To Vanja A. Holm,
for her pioneering and insightful contributions
to the interdisciplinary clinical process

International Issues in Early Intervention
Series editor: Michael J. Guralnick

ISEI

Interdisciplinary Clinical Assessment of Young Children with Developmental Disabilities

Section I

OVERVIEW

Chapter 1

Interdisciplinary Team Assessment for Young Children

Purposes and Processes

Michael J. Guralnick

The interdisciplinary team assessment of young children with possible developmental delays or of those with established developmental disabilities constitutes a critical component of the larger system of services and supports for children and their families during the early childhood years. The importance of gaining insights from many disciplines with respect to a child's development and how it unfolds in the context of family and community life is well recognized. After all, child development, health, and early intervention professionals agree that an ecological-developmental perspective that considers the influence of numerous biosocial factors is essential both to understand development and to design interventions that benefit children and families (Belsky, 1984; Bronfenbrenner, 1979; Guralnick, 1997; Sameroff, 1993).

Many factors are, of course, involved in carrying out an effective interdisciplinary team assessment. At a minimum, the specific purposes and associated interdisciplinary processes must be designed to address the initial concerns that families present to the team as well as those that arise as the process unfolds. Often parents are referred to an interdisciplinary team for assessment because of their own concerns about their child's development. Sometimes these concerns are highly specific, perhaps relating to their child's cognitive or motor development. In other instances, the problems are more difficult for caregivers to articulate, reflecting a general sense that something is not quite right or a lingering fear that the child's development has been compromised by a medical condition (e.g., prematurity and low birth weight, maternal diabetes). Occasionally, certain issues are raised by the family physician or a child care professional or perhaps even a close relative. Increasingly, however, interdisciplinary teams are also asked to become involved with children who have well-established developmental delays but are now exhibiting unanticipated difficulties. Concerns about unusually slow progress, even when early intervention services are being provided, or the appearance of behavior problems are common. Finally, interdisciplinary teams often form specialized groups within the larger team to address specific disorders such as phenylketonuria (PKU) or matters such as feeding difficulties.

As might be expected, the diversity of child, family, and community circumstances likely to be encountered by an interdisciplinary team is considerable. Biologically based conditions that can adversely affect development, including genetic disorders and congenital infections, are numerous and complex (Lipkin, 1996). Conservative estimates suggest that as many as 1 million children in the United States from birth through 5 years of age can be identified as having significant disabilities (see Bowe, 1995). Moreover, the extraordinary vulnerability of young children to developmental difficulties in contemporary society has been well documented (Baumeister & Woodley-Zanthos, 1996; Guralnick, 1998; Hanson & Carta, 1995). Conditions associated with poverty, the risks of adolescent parenting, the impact of prenatal illicit drug or alcohol exposure, and concerns related to parental mental health conditions and limited intellectual abilities are among the risk factors that increasingly challenge a child's development as well as community service and support systems. Often environmental and biological risk factors co-occur, as in the case of many children born prematurely at low birth weights. The number of children facing other forms of multiple risks, either due to the combination of environmental risk and disability factors or the co-occurrence of multiple problems for children with established disabilities (e.g., cognitive delay, epilepsy), is increasing as well. When one adds to these circumstances the cultural diversity of the families seeking services and the variability in resources found in home communities, it is apparent that all concerned face extraordinary challenges in developing a meaningful set of recommendations and programs.

CONTEXT OF THE INTERDISCIPLINARY PROCESS

The hallmark of an interdisciplinary team is its ability to integrate and synthesize information from numerous disciplines through an interactive, group decision-making process (Garner, 1994a; Rokusek, 1995). Yet, it is important to note at the outset the parameters within which this interactive process unfolds. In particular, this is an expensive undertaking, one that not only requires the involvement of professionals from many different disciplines but also a staff to coordinate and schedule assessments and to help organize relevant information. In addition, there is the investment of time from the family, the child, and perhaps community professionals. Moreover, families may be required to travel considerable distances in order to locate a team with adequate resources to meet their needs. As a consequence, most interdisciplinary assessment teams try to complete the entire process within 1 or 2 days. Although vital questions can be addressed during this time, numerous other issues are often raised that must be considered in reevaluations or as part of another component of the service and support system for children and families. Clearly, both the advantages and the limitations of the interdisciplinary team approach must be recognized, and they are discussed throughout this volume.

Interdisciplinary team assessments are most valuable if they contribute information to help the child and family in the larger home community context. By including community professionals as much as possible either in the process itself or through extensive communications, the team's recommendations are more likely to be implemented effectively and to be realistic. Early intervention systems vary dramatically from community to community, and this fact must be recognized as part of the team's deliberations and recommendations. Similarly, interdisciplinary assessment teams must work closely with other teams in the service system, particularly those involved in developing individualized family service plans (IFSPs) for infants and toddlers and individualized education programs (IEPs) for preschool-age children.

The composition, scope of effort, and location of interdisciplinary assessment teams can vary considerably as well. However, this book emphasizes the operation of comprehensive interdisciplinary teams, often located at major medical centers and universities. These teams are similar in many respects to the child development teams addressing the concerns of children with developmental disabilities or those at risk for developmental delays as described by the seminal work of Holm and McCartin (1978). Nevertheless, it is anticipated that the discussions in this book that focus on comprehensive interdisciplinary teams, including both disciplinary assessments and the interdisciplinary process, can be readily applied to a range of interdisciplinary teams.

PURPOSE OF INTERDISCIPLINARY TEAM ASSESSMENTS

The overarching purpose of the interdisciplinary team assessment of young children is to develop plans and recommendations, including locating community resources to meet the identified needs of the child and family. To accomplish this, the interdisciplinary team assessment process should yield at least five outcomes. First, it is essential to establish the child's developmental and health patterns and to profile family functioning in a community context.

This outcome is achieved through assessments by representatives of disciplines considered relevant to the presenting concerns. In essence, this process begins by ensuring that team members from each discipline are able to gather information and to understand thoroughly, in relation to their domains of expertise, child and family functioning. These discipline assessments that establish patterns of strength and concern form the core of a more complex process that integrates and reconciles this material.

A second outcome is to determine areas in which additional information is needed. This is an important feature of the clinical assessment because, as described previously, the process is time limited. Even with reasonably good records or history taking, the nature of the information that can be gathered is nevertheless limited by the assessments that occur during a restricted time period. Moreover, additional issues may arise during the course of the assessment that require information to be obtained at a later time. This point highlights that the team's conclusions and recommendations will vary considerably in terms of their degree of certainty. Accurately estimating this degree of certainty, communicating it effectively to the family, and formulating a strategy for obtaining additional information to increase the degree of certainty are all expected outcomes of the interdisciplinary team assessment.

Third, if necessary, the interdisciplinary team assessment will need to help establish a diagnosis or at least provide the probable source or sources of the child's difficulties. This diagnostic process can occur at many levels. At minimum, the team can provide a classification diagnosis in which a category is assigned that best fits the child's developmental profile. Terms such as developmental delay, autism spectrum disorder, or cerebral palsy constitute such categorical diagnoses. Standard classification systems, such as the *Diagnostic and Statistical Manual of Mental Disorders, Fourth Edition* (American Psychiatric Association, 1994), are often used for this purpose. When no clear biological markers are available to assist in determining a categorical diagnosis, as is often the case, the team must engage in the generally difficult task of integrating the diverse disciplinary information to achieve a reasonable level of agreement. It is essential, however, that the child's individual developmental profile and the variability inherent in any classification system be communicated adequately to parents. Oversimplifying the diagnostic findings, especially regarding young children, can be misleading and can redirect the family's focus from the rich and diverse patterns of their child's behavior.

At another level, the team tries to determine an etiology as part of the diagnostic process. With the development of more sophisticated genetic testing, the source of a developmental delay, for example, such as that associated with fragile X syndrome, can be confidently established. Other nongenetic, biologically based etiologies are often more tenuous, but a team can reasonably identify the likely source or sources of the child's major problems. In the same way, environmental etiologies or influences are examined by the team. The nature of the parent–child relationship, possible abuse or neglect, related chronic health conditions, or the mental health status of the parents are all important contributors to identifying either a specific etiology or gaining insight into the source or sources of the problem.

Despite the often uncertain nature of the diagnostic outcome, it is a critical feature of the interdisciplinary team process. Establishing a diagnosis may help link families to specific parent support groups, determine eligibility for services, provide a focus for the team's recommendations, facilitate anticipatory guidance for families, and supply parents with some deeper understanding of the nature of their child's problem despite frequent difficulties in working through a diagnosis. It also may have family planning implications.

Fourth, the interdisciplinary team assessment is expected to provide recommendations and suggestions for intervention. From both a disciplinary and an interdisciplinary perspective, perhaps the most valuable feature of the process is the recommendations that result. In some instances, recommendations will be quite specific, focusing on interventions such as prescribing a diet for a child with PKU, recommending a specific program to facilitate a child's language development, or encouraging the family to seek a particular community service. In other instances, the recommendations will be quite general, such as suggesting that the child be enrolled in therapeutic child care or an intensive early intervention program or explaining how to locate a qualified physical therapist in the community. The advice should, of course, respond to the concerns that originally prompted the assessment but may well go beyond those issues as the situation dictates.

The interdisciplinary team assessment recommendations in many ways are the starting point for a new intervention program. The interventions themselves generally are not carried out by team members, although some team members or groups within teams do elect to provide longer-term management, at least for some issues. Discussions with the family and community providers are essential to determine whether the team wishes to take a management role.

Finally, an outcome of the interdisciplinary team assessment is often to establish a framework for more detailed, intervention-oriented assessments. The global nature of many of the assessments comprising the interdisciplinary team approach, although valuable for addressing the issues that brought families to the team, is typically only the first stage in an extended undertaking of disciplinary- and interdisciplinary-based assessments and early interventions. For example, for children newly identified as exhibiting developmental delays that require intervention services, additional steps designed to gather information uniquely suited for intervention often occur in the context of the community early intervention service system. Community teams providing assessments that assist in the creation of IFSPs and IEPs are also interdisciplinary in their composition. Information from the initial interdisciplinary assessment team can focus and refine these community team intervention-oriented assessments. This final expected result of the interdisciplinary team emphasizes its role in the continuum of early intervention services and supports.

PROCESS OF INTERDISCIPLINARY TEAM ASSESSMENTS

For these five outcomes to occur in an accurate and sensitive fashion, a coherent and systematic process governing the interdisciplinary team assessment must be in place. A considerable burden is placed on the team to gather past and current information in a timely, sensitive, and accurate manner; to integrate it effectively; to be prepared to alter the plan and make rapid decisions; and to communicate effectively with families throughout the entire assessment. The critical features of this process described by Holm and McCartin (1978) remain applicable today and are discussed in this section as five sequential steps. Specific case examples utilizing this process can be found in Section III.

In the first step of the interdisciplinary team process, referred to as the Preliminary Conference (Step 1), an initial team leader or service coordinator is chosen by clinic intake staff based on the nature of the problems identified in the referral and the availability of team members. Relying on initial information about the child and telephone contacts with the family, issues of concern and the disciplines that should be involved are then tentatively selected by the team leader. Additional information from school, community professionals, or families also is requested at this time.

Following the receipt of new information (e.g., family questionnaires, school service data, clinic forms), a Preassessment Conference (Step 2) is convened in which the tentatively identified team members evaluate this information, determine any other issues of concern, and finalize the assessment plans and disciplines that will participate. This course of action is then shared with the family; if they agree, the formal assessment is scheduled.

This formal assessment begins with the Disciplinary Assessments (Step 3), whereby individual disciplines conduct an evaluation within the scope of their expertise and within the context of the concerns identified in the previous two steps. Some types of information are collected routinely by each discipline, but disciplinary assessments are also uniquely tailored to the circumstances presented by each child and family. When appropriate, especially to reduce redundancy in the assessment, two or more disciplines may see the child or the family at one time. In establishing the schedule of disciplinary assessments, particular attention is devoted to ensure that the child will experience minimal fatigue or boredom from what clearly is a demanding process. At this step, every effort is made to strike a balance between an ideal schedule from the child's and family's perspective and the practical demands of a busy clinic program.

Following the assessments, each discipline provides a Discipline Summary (Step 4) organized in a series of notes with respect to test scores, observations, decision points, and new information or new issues that may have arisen in the course of the assessment. Informal contact among team members also occurs during this period as ideas are formulated, often complementing the informal exchanges that have occurred during the previous disciplinary assessment process. As teams gain experience and confidence working with one another, these informal contacts become more useful and facilitate the remainder of the process. In any event, this step concludes with each discipline's having developed a set of tentative recommendations that will be shared with the team and family.

The fifth and final step is the Integration of Disciplinary Information and Recommendations. It is here, in face-to-face meetings with all involved, that the original and newly emerging issues are addressed from the perspectives of all disciplines. Under the guidance of the team leader, disciplinary summaries are presented, information is synthesized, new problems are considered, and a final set of conclusions and recommendations—with all reasonable qualifications—is presented to families. This, of course, is the most challenging part of the interdisciplinary team assessment, demanding that the team displays its most sophisticated level of interpersonal, clinical, and communicative skills.

It is important to point out that these five steps are an idealized version of the actual process. In practice, many steps overlap. As noted previously, the process is a dynamic one, with disciplines exchanging information at points other than the final step of the assessment. This dynamic quality often changes the nature and type of assessments, raising new issues that must be dealt with in a timely and flexible manner.

PRINCIPLES OF INTERDISCIPLINARY TEAM ASSESSMENT

The purposes and processes of the interdisciplinary team assessment are governed by what might best be referred to as a set of principles. These principles are intended to represent late 20th century values and practices in the general fields of child development, early intervention, and developmental disabilities. It is these principles that provide guidance for the behavior of team members toward one another, the way in which assessments are conducted, the type of relationships established with the family and with community providers, and the team members' understanding of the child as a developing individual. The following discussion provides a number of such guidelines for the attitudes and actions of the team. This list is certainly not exhaustive, but it highlights the many underlying issues faced by interdisciplinary team assessment members and how late 20th century values and practices can influence the entire enterprise.

Ecological Validity of Assessments

Standardized formats are required in many assessment situations, and information gained from these assessments is correlated with important developmental and behavior patterns that occur in everyday activities. Yet, many test situations themselves do not enable the child to express important abilities, characteristics, and skills. Accordingly, whenever possible, team members should maximize the ecological validity of the assessment by careful selection of tests and the use of informal as well as formal procedures (see Bailey & Wolery, 1989). By including naturalistic situations, for example, as part of the evaluation plan or by involving the family in the process whenever possible, the child's comfort level is increased, and different perspectives of the child's functioning can be obtained. The ecological validity of the assessments is enhanced as well by obtaining input from multiple sources (e.g., family, friends, teachers, child care workers, community professionals). Ultimately, it is the convergence and consistency of information from these multiple sources that will ensure that the interdisciplinary team assessment yields a meaningful outcome.

Recognizing Uncertainty

Variability in test performance and the existence of potentially conflicting information is likely even in the most ecologically valid assessments. Moreover, a simple snapshot of a child's performance must always be considered suspect, but confidence in the team's conclusions can be enhanced by obtaining other information, especially in relation to the stability of a child's developmental patterns. Issues of surveillance and timely reevaluations must be considered in this context, yet recognizing, accepting, and communicating the appropriate level of uncertainty remains an important principle.

Coordination and Nonredundant Testing

The gathering of prior information and scheduling and conducting the assessments require a high level of coordination. The stress on children and families is extraordinary, and the interdisciplinary assessment team must maximize smooth functioning among all facets of the process. Similarly, team members should ensure that testing is as nonredundant as possible, as many disciplines utilize similar assessment strategies and instruments. Moreover, the era of managed care has made it even more critical to select disciplines and tests that yield results in the most efficient and cost-effective manner possible.

Dynamic Nature of the Assessment

On the surface, the organization and scheduling of the process suggest a fixed series of events for the interdisciplinary team assessment. However, there are always surprises. It is not uncommon for new information to emerge during interviews with parents or providers or for major discrepancies to appear regarding the child's development in relation to past information. During the assessment itself, these developments must be communicated to team members and families as rapidly as possible so adjustments can be made prior to synthesizing information and developing recommendations.

Respect for Contributions of Other Disciplines

Extensive literature is available on interdisciplinary team functioning and the type of interpersonal relationships that should characterize an effective team.

For example, issues of communicative style, protocol, the ability to listen, leadership, and establishing common ground philosophies have been examined in considerable detail (Garner, 1994a, 1994b; Spencer & Coye, 1988; Stoneman & Malone, 1995). All of these concepts notwithstanding, perhaps the most fundamental requirement for establishing a true interdisciplinary team is an essential respect for each discipline's contribution to the overall process and, equally important, for the perspective each provides with respect to the biosocial and ecological-developmental approaches that constitute sound early intervention plans. Ideally, the training for each individual discipline included an understanding of contributions by other disciplines. If not, team members must work hard to learn from others, both within and outside the team's activities.

Cultural Competence

As the diversity of the population increases, considerable demands are placed on interdisciplinary team members to understand and relate to children and families whose cultural backgrounds differ radically from their own. The importance of becoming "culturally competent" is essential for the accuracy of any assessment and equally important in establishing an effective collaboration with the family (Lynch & Hanson, 1993). Clearly, for recommendations to meet the needs of families and to be realistic, differences in ethnic and religious backgrounds as well as family roles and expectations must be considered. Of course, these sensitivities should be part of any assessment centered around the family, yet the emergence of cultural issues poses a new level of complexity for the entire service and support system. Perspectives on the meaning of a child's disability and even the benefits of mildly intensive individualized interventions can become issues that must be thoughtfully addressed in a cultural context (Harry, 1992).

Role of Family

The central role of the child's family in the interdisciplinary team assessment process is well established. A family's input with respect to their child's development is absolutely critical, and, for the most part, parents are the team's clients. Because parents are responsible for their child's development, it is through their actions that the team's recommendations will be realized. Failure of the team to build an appropriate relationship with the family, to understand their values, and to communicate effectively will diminish the contributions of the entire process.

Indeed, concepts with respect to forming parent–professional partnerships and ensuring that families are empowered to carry out their responsibilities must be reflected throughout the entire assessment (Dunst & Trivette, 1989; Pearl, 1993). This principle implies that the family's perspective be accorded considerable, if not absolute, weight. In practice, however, there are circumstances that make this principle difficult to implement in its most complete sense. Occasionally, the team may perceive that the child's best interests and those of the family diverge, and there are instances in which the values of the team may not be concordant with the family's values. Disagreement may occur over priorities or attitudes within the family (e.g., insufficient time for recommended child therapies, lack of belief in efficacy). Some of these conflicts can be traced to cultural differences, as discussed previously. Unfortunately, no easy solution is likely in these instances, but a vigorous negotiation process should be initiated in which the team states its case in a context of open communication (see Bailey, 1987).

Finally, this principle also implies that the family should be able to participate in every activity and team discussion if they so choose. However, there may be instances in which the team or a subgroup wish to deliberate with the caregivers absent, such as when there are strong indications of parental abuse or neglect. Moreover, given the complex, dynamic nature of the interdisciplinary process, and the numerous hypotheses that are generated as part of any clinical activity, team members often feel most comfortable "thinking out loud" without familial scrutiny. Does this violate the essence of the parent–professional partnership? Although no simple answer to this question emerges, it seems that a useful operating strategy, and the one most consistent with this particular principle, is to include the family at all points in the process unless a clear reason not to do so is articulated and agreed upon by all team members. Each team should establish its own operating framework and try to apply it on a case-by-case basis. This case-by-case approach may be unsatisfactory to some, but it places the burden for excluding parents, even for a brief time, on having a well-developed framework and a corresponding set of arguments. If exclusion becomes more than a rare occurrence or considerable dissension exists among team members, the team should reevaluate its framework and operating principles. Of note, this entire family-focused process may prove to be a useful exercise in clarifying individual disciplines or the collective values of the team with respect to the roles of families.

Role of Community Providers

In order for the team's recommendations to be useful, it is essential not only that parents take responsibility, but also that community providers be involved as much as possible. For children already enrolled in an early intervention program, active participation of educators and other early intervention specialists is critical. It is less likely that the interdisciplinary team's recommendations, even general ones, will be translated into practice without extensive involvement of practitioners from the child's home community. Seeking input from key providers who are familiar with the child is certainly one vital part of this process, but conducting follow-up communications with providers—particularly the child's service coordinator identified as part of the IFSP or IEP process—is perhaps even more critical. If the circumstance permits, having the child's community service coordinator or other key provider participate as an observer and resource is ideal.

Inclusion and Support

The interdisciplinary process often leads to an initial dissection of the child into specific developmental domains before reconstructing the "whole child" within the larger family and community context. Nevertheless, this reconstruction process can easily fall short, as team members emphasize identified issues and link them to an often fractionated service system. To minimize this problem, teams should adopt the principle that their recommendations be designed to include the child and family in typical home and community activities. By having interdisciplinary teams address issues related to maximizing inclusion, particularly in relation to the child's social world, recommendations are more likely to address the child as an individual functioning within a larger ecological context. Increasing the inclusion of children and families has, of course, been a major theme since the mid-1970s in the field of developmental disabilities and is reflected in well-articulated ethical, legal, and value systems (Guralnick, in press).

Similarly, thinking about how best to organize and develop supports within the larger community for the child and family places the "whole" child at the center of the team's efforts. As thoughtfully articulated by Stoneman and Malone (1995) in the context of the interdisciplinary team assessment, the assessment itself and the recommendations that follow should consider strategies that involve the entire community of family, friends, providers, and others who can provide needed supports.

PURPOSE AND ORGANIZATION OF THIS VOLUME

The purpose of this volume is to provide an accessible reference for those considering developing interdisciplinary assessment teams, for new members of existing teams, and for students or trainees preparing for professional practice in the field of developmental disabilities focusing on young children. Although the intent and composition of interdisciplinary teams vary considerably, it is the expectation that the approach presented in this book can be readily applied to a variety of circumstances and needs. The goals, processes, and principles described in this volume may well be of fundamental relevance to interdisciplinary assessment teams in their many forms.

In Section II of this book, the perspectives of nine disciplines are presented. Although other disciplines are sometimes part of interdisciplinary teams, emphasis has been placed on the contributions of the following nine specialties: 1) audiology, 2) speech-language pathology, 3) neurodevelopmental pediatrics, 4) nursing, 5) nutrition, 6) occupational therapy, 7) physical therapy, 8) psychology, and 9) social work. Each of the nine chapters addresses the discipline's information-gathering strategies, commonly used assessment instruments, typical problems encountered, decision-making procedures, and approaches to interpreting assessments and making recommendations, as well as other issues relevant to the discipline.

Following these disciplinary presentations, Section III contains a series of case studies. It is through these cases that attempts are made to convey the nature of the five-step process outlined previously, how the principles described influence the team, the difficulties encountered, and the solutions proposed. Where appropriate, separate commentaries are provided in which points of interest are discussed.

Finally, Section IV provides an important international perspective on these issues. Interdisciplinary assessment teams have been established all over the world, and their conceptual frameworks and ways of operating are adapted to both current and historical conditions. Descriptions from Russia, Italy, and Sweden illustrate these points.

REFERENCES

American Psychiatric Association. (1994). *Diagnostic and statistical manual of mental disorders* (4th ed.). Washington, DC: Author.

Bailey, D.B. (1987). Collaborative goal-setting with families: Resolving differences in values and priorities for services. *Topics in Early Childhood Special Education, 7*(2), 59–71.

Bailey, D.B., Jr., & Wolery, M. (Eds.). (1989). *Assessing infants and preschoolers with handicaps.* New York: The McGraw-Hill Companies.

Baumeister, A.A., & Woodley-Zanthos, P. (1996). Prevention: Biological factors. In J.W. Jacobson & J.A. Mulick (Eds.), *Manual of diagnosis and professional practice in mental retardation* (pp. 229–242). Washington, DC: American Psychological Association.

Belsky, J. (1984). The determinants of parenting: A process model. *Child Development, 55,* 83–96.

Bowe, F.G. (1995). Population estimates: Birth-to-5 children with disabilities. *Journal of Special Education, 20,* 461–471.

Bronfenbrenner, U. (1979). *The ecology of human development.* Cambridge, MA: Harvard University Press.

Dunst, C., & Trivette, C. (1989). An enablement and empowerment perspective of case management. *Topics in Early Childhood Special Education, 8*(4), 87–102.

Garner, H.G. (1994a). Critical issues in teamwork. In H.G. Garner & F.P. Orelove (Eds.), *Teamwork in human services* (pp. 1–18). Woburn, MA: Butterworth-Heinemann.

Garner, H.G. (1994b). Multidisciplinary versus interdisciplinary teamwork. In H.G. Garner & F.P. Orelove (Eds.), *Teamwork in human services* (pp. 19–36). Woburn, MA: Butterworth-Heinemann.

Guralnick, M.J. (1997). Second-generation research in the field of early intervention. In M.J. Guralnick (Ed.), *The effectiveness of early intervention* (pp. 3–20). Baltimore: Paul H. Brookes Publishing Co.

Guralnick, M.J. (1998). The effectiveness of early intervention for vulnerable children: A developmental perspective. *American Journal on Mental Retardation, 102,* 319–345.

Guralnick, M.J. (in press). A framework for change in early childhood inclusion. In M.J. Guralnick (Ed.), *Early childhood inclusion: Focus on change.* Baltimore: Paul H. Brookes Publishing Co.

Hanson, M.J., & Carta, J.J. (1995). Addressing the challenges of families with multiple risks. *Exceptional Children, 62,* 201–212.

Harry, B. (1992). Values clarification for early interventionists. *Topics in Early Childhood Special Education, 12*(3), 333–350.

Holm, V.A., & McCartin, R.E. (1978). Interdisciplinary child development team: Team issues and training in interdisciplinariness. In E. Allen, V.A. Holm, & R.L.

Schiefelbusch (Eds.), *Early intervention—A team approach* (pp. 97–122). Baltimore: University Park Press.

Lipkin, P.H. (1996). Epidemiology of the developmental disabilities. In A.J. Capute & P. J. Accardo (Eds.), *Developmental disabilities in infancy and childhood: Vol. 1. Neurodevelopmental diagnosis and treatment* (2nd ed., pp. 137–156). Baltimore: Paul H. Brookes Publishing Co.

Lynch, E.W., & Hanson, M.J. (1993). Changing demographics: Implications for training in early intervention. *Infants and Young Children, 6,* 50–55.

Pearl, L.F. (1993). Providing family-centered early intervention. In W. Brown, S.K. Thurman, & L.F. Pearl (Eds.), *Family-centered early intervention with infants and toddlers* (pp. 211–243). Baltimore: Paul H. Brookes Publishing Co.

Rokusek, C. (1995). An introduction to the concept of interdisciplinary practice. In B.A. Thyer & N.P. Kropf (Eds.), *Developmental disabilities: A handbook for interdisciplinary practice* (pp. 1–12). Cambridge, MA: Brookline Books.

Sameroff, A.J. (1993). Models of development and developmental risk. In C.H. Zeanah, Jr. (Ed.), *Handbook of infant mental health* (pp. 3–13). New York: The Guilford Press.

Spencer, P.E., & Coye, R.W. (1988). Project BRIDGE: A team approach to decision-making for early services. *Infants and Young Children, 1,* 82–92.

Stoneman, Z., & Malone, D.M. (1995). The changing nature of interdisciplinary practice. In B.A. Thyer & N.P. Kropf (Eds.), *Developmental disabilities: A handbook for interdisciplinary practice* (pp. 234–247). Cambridge, MA: Brookline Books.

THE PERSPECTIVE OF INDIVIDUAL DISCIPLINES

Chapter 2

Interdisciplinary Team Assessment for Young Children with Possible Hearing Loss

Richard C. Folsom

The primary objective of early detection of hearing impairment in infants and young children is to initiate intervention that will reduce the impact of hearing loss on their development of language, academic achievement, and psychosocial development. Because hearing impairment is difficult to detect, extraordinary efforts must be made to assess hearing during infancy and early childhood, before irreversible impairments accumulate.

Hearing impairment occurs with sufficient frequency to warrant these assessment efforts. For example, 2 infants in 1,000 will be born with a severe-to-profound hearing impairment (Mason & Herrmann, 1998; Mehl & Thomson, 1998; National Institutes of Health [NIH], 1993). This degree of impairment will interfere with speech reception and, thus, will significantly affect oral language development and educational performance. The incidence of infants with mild or moderate degrees of hearing loss is estimated at 5–6 of every

1,000 births (Finitzo, Albright, & O'Neal, 1998). Furthermore, for children requiring intensive medical care during the neonatal period, 1 child in every
25–30 will have a hearing impairment (NIH, 1993; Swigonski, Shallop, Bull,
& Lemons, 1987; Thompson & Folsom, 1981). Finally, the most common disease of childhood, ear infection (otitis media), is associated with hearing loss.
Nearly 80% of children will experience some period of hearing loss related to
ear infection from birth through 3 years of age (Teele, Klein, & Rosner, 1980).

   Assessment of hearing early in life is a process that combines early identification and continued hearing assessment. The specific assessment tool available for this process largely depends on the developmental age of the child. That
is, for infants younger than 6 months of age, accurate assessment depends on
the use of a physiological measure to indicate response to sound (American
Speech-Language-Hearing Association [ASHA], 1992). For children older than
6 months of age, behavioral methods can be used to obtain reliable and valid
information about hearing (Moore, Thompson, & Folsom, 1992; Moore, Wilson, & Thompson, 1977; Widen, 1990). Regardless of the specific approach,
however, hearing assessment in young children is most commonly found within
the interdisciplinary team approach to child assessment. The relationships between hearing and oral language development, hearing and cognitive development, and hearing and psychosocial development define the need for early assessment within the interdisciplinary assessment team.

DIMENSIONS TO BE ASSESSED

The purpose of the audiological assessment is to determine the presence or absence of hearing impairment and, in the presence of hearing loss, to determine
both the extent and functional capacity of residual hearing. Traditional dimensions include frequency and intensity (corresponding to the perceptions of
pitch and loudness, respectively) as well as speech reception and speech understanding. Assessment of middle-ear function (acoustic immittance) is part of
the standard battery.

   In conventional pediatric hearing assessment, pure tones are used to assess sensitivity at specific frequencies (e.g., 250; 500; 1,000; 2,000; 4,000; 8,000
hertz [Hz]). Sensitivity is measured in decibels relative to the normal-hearing
population and is designated as *decibels of hearing level (dB HL)*. Responses at the
softest levels are called *thresholds* and are plotted on a grid displaying frequency
and decibels called an *audiogram*. Sounds are presented in two modes: 1) air
conduction testing, which refers to the presentation of sound through earphones or a loudspeaker and measures the complete auditory pathway and
2) bone conduction testing, which refers to presenting sounds through a vibrat-
ing device placed against the bones of the skull and measures the response of
the cochlea by circumventing the external and middle ear. Comparison of air
conduction and bone conduction measures leads to a determination of whether
a hearing loss is termed conductive or sensorineural. A child with conductive

hearing loss will hear bone-conducted sound normally because it bypasses the conductive apparatus (external and middle ear), and it is thus determined that a problem exists with the conductive mechanism. A child having a sensori-neural impairment hears the same by both air and bone conduction, so it is concluded that the site of damage is in the cochlea or neural pathway.

Hearing loss based on hearing threshold measurements can be classified descriptively as follows (Clark, 1981):

- 0 to 15 dB HL—normal hearing
- 16 to 25 dB HL—slight or borderline hearing loss
- 26 to 40 dB HL—mild hearing loss
- 41 to 55 dB HL—moderate hearing loss
- 56 to 70 dB HL—moderately severe hearing loss
- 71 to 90 dB HL—severe hearing loss
- greater than 90 dB HL—profound hearing loss

Classification of hearing loss based primarily on hearing threshold, none-theless, can be misleading when this criterion is used in isolation. For example, Knauf provided a word of caution:

> Although classifications based on hearing level are valuable in estimating the impact of a certain hearing level on an average child and in the early counseling of parents, there are many exceptions. Some unusual children with profound losses of 90 dB perform better in language and academic skills compared to other children with average intelligence and moderately severe losses of 70 dB. Similar individual variations will be found along the entire continuum of hearing levels. (1978, p. 550)

Conversational speech corresponds to approximately 50–60 dB HL. Thus, a child with an average hearing loss of 50–60 dB HL or greater will hear little speech without the use of a hearing aid. For many children, the common disease of otitis media with fluid will create a mild hearing loss that can reduce or eliminate the perception of some speech sounds.

The functional effect of hearing impairment is assessed through the use of speech stimuli. The *speech recognition threshold* (SRT) measures the lowest level at which speech can be understood and provides a reliability check for the pure tone thresholds. *Word recognition testing* (sometimes referred to as speech discrimination testing) measures the understanding of speech presented at comfortable listening levels. A complete understanding of the functional impact of a child's hearing loss, however, is not revealed solely by audiometric data but also through the observation of a child's use of amplification and his or her strides during rehabilitation audiology and subsequent school performance.

EXPECTED OUTCOMES OF ASSESSMENT

The expected outcome of a pediatric hearing assessment is the acquisition of sufficient data regarding hearing capacity to allow for the development of a management plan, if needed. Hearing in all infants and young children can be assessed. Whether an assessment yields "sufficient" data is, of course, driven by many factors. Age, behavior, cognitive level, medical status, and other factors combine to determine the adequacy of the assessment outcome.

Although the determination of the presence and extent of hearing impairment is an audiological diagnosis, the development of a management plan requires team input. Once hearing impairment has been identified, close ties between speech-language pathology, education, social work, medicine, psychology, and, sometimes, physical and occupational therapy are necessary for the development of the management plan. This plan is the initial step in establishing a partnership between parents and professionals that addresses family concerns about such issues as medical intervention, the influence of hearing loss on communication, the fitting of hearing aids, and referral to an intervention program. For example, intervention for hearing loss resulting from middle-ear disorders is usually carried out by the family physician, sometimes involving a referral to an otolaryngologist or otologist. Intervention for sensorineural hearing loss involves the combined efforts of audiology, medicine, education, and speech-language pathology. All plans should include the family as part of the team.

MAJOR CHALLENGES TO ACCURATE ASSESSMENT

Pediatric hearing assessment consists of acquiring relatively precise audiological information from an innately imprecise, highly variable young child or infant. Data regarding a child's hearing status rely heavily on that child's behavioral performance during structured tests of hearing rather than on informal observation. If adequate behavioral performance is not possible, information about the functional status of the peripheral auditory system can be obtained through physiological measures. From these measures, inferences can be made regarding hearing. There are few, if any, natural environments wherein the necessary dimensions of hearing can be assessed. The environment for a hearing evaluation is thus artificial and highly structured and uses, in large part, unfamiliar sounds. It is very difficult under these circumstances to obtain a sufficient number of consistent responses that will lead to an unambiguous conclusion about functional hearing. It is not sufficient to know whether a child has been reported to respond to speech because children can be remarkably responsive to a variety of sounds in the presence of significant hearing impairment. For example, children with unilateral hearing loss or hearing that is normal for some frequencies and impaired at others may be at risk for educational difficulties or speech-language delay, and yet they may show little or no obvious hearing impairment under superficial observation.

ASSESSMENT AND PROCESS

The purpose of a hearing assessment is to determine if a hearing loss exists and, if so, the extent and configuration of that loss. The tests that are selected for assessment will lead the audiologist and the family to decisions regarding audiological management and habilitation strategies. With infants and young children, the question of whether the loss impairs communication ability is usually addressed in terms of the likelihood that hearing loss will delay communication development.

Information Gathering

There are two primary approaches to assessing hearing in infants and young children: behavioral assessment, in which the child is an active participant, and physiological assessment, in which the child is a passive participant. These approaches can be complementary in that information about hearing obtained each way can be used to create a management plan. Hearing loss estimates obtained by each method should be in general agreement; indeed, physiological measures have long been used as a "cross-check" against which behavioral findings are compared (Jerger & Hayes, 1976). It is only through the use of a behavioral approach to assessment, however, that the concept of hearing can be addressed. A behavioral hearing assessment provides not only information about the sensitivity and functional state of the auditory system, but also evidence that a child is capable of using hearing to learn a task related to an auditory cue. Physiological assessment of hearing provides valuable data about the physiological integrity of the peripheral hearing mechanism, without the additional information of how sound may be put to use.

Deciding which approach to use for a child with developmental delay or disability is not always straightforward. As subsequent sections show, certain developmental landmarks are required for reliable behavioral assessment. In the absence of these landmarks, physiological tests can acquire sufficient hearing level data to proceed with intervention. Participation in the preassessment conference as part of the interdisciplinary team will help the pediatric audiologist determine the likelihood of a particular approach's success or failure. Nevertheless, the audiologist will usually decide on an assessment strategy and then, when necessary, modify that plan during the course of the evaluation. In young children with developmental delay, the earliest data often are physiological in nature because of the developmental skills required for reliable performance on behavioral tests of hearing. After the child reaches the appropriate developmental age, however, information about hearing from behavioral tests is available to plan the intervention.

Instruments Available

Two hearing test categories are available for reliable hearing evaluation in pediatric audiology: behavioral and physiological. Each approach has its own strengths and limitations, and the specific instruments for both are described next. Behavioral measures (those utilizing conditioned responses or play tasks) are the only true tests of hearing and are viewed as the gold standard for hearing. Physiological tests are measures of auditory function, not hearing, but can lead to valuable inferences about hearing status in infants and children.

Behavioral Testing

Behavioral hearing assessment requires special test techniques when assessing infants, toddlers, and preschoolers. Determining the appropriate technique is based, in large part, on chronological or developmental age. The techniques are behavioral observation audiometry (BOA), visual reinforcement audiometry (VRA), and conditioned play audiometry (CPA).

Behavioral Observation Audiometry

BOA is a procedure that is applied to very young infants (younger than 6 months of age) or children with developmental delays who cannot be conditioned to provide responses reliably through the use of reinforcement (Northern & Downs, 1991; Wilson & Thompson, 1984). In this procedure, the examiner observes any changes in behavior produced by the infant that are time-locked to the presentation of an auditory stimulus, such as noisemakers presented near the child or signals presented through the audiometer. Responses are unconditioned and can consist of virtually any behavior within the infant's repertoire. For example, responses may take the form of the following reflexive behaviors: a startle, an eye blink, eye widening, or a head turn toward the sound source. As the responses of the infant are not brought under stimulus control, there are inherent limitations in the use of BOA as a measure of hearing sensitivity (Wilson & Thompson, 1984). The probability of obtaining a response is dependent on the nature (novelty) of the auditory signal rather than its intensity at any point in time. Furthermore, response habituation is rapid during BOA testing and variability is high (Thompson & Weber, 1974). BOA can provide some information about hearing but, used alone, it is not a sufficiently precise infant hearing test to identify anything other than a bilateral, severe-to-profound hearing loss. As discussed previously in this chapter, this is one behavioral technique that is often combined with a physiological measure of hearing in an attempt to "piece together" an accurate estimate of hearing sensitivity.

Visual Reinforcement Audiometry

VRA is a powerful, operant conditioning test procedure that capitalizes on an infant's naturally occurring head turn toward interesting sounds by introducing visual reinforcement following the head-turn response (Wilson & Thompson, 1984). Interest in the auditory environment, resulting in auditory localization, is pervasive in typically developing infants after approximately 4 months of age. By 5–6 months of age, infants are cognitively able to learn that under some circumstances (e.g., when cued by sound) a head turn will result in reinforcement (Moore et al., 1977; Widen, 1990). Reinforcement in this behavioral approach consists of an animated, lighted toy situated at a 45°–90° angle to the side of the infant. Figure 2.1 shows the room arrangement most widely used in performing VRA. A head turn in the direction of the toy is an easily observed, unambiguous action on the part of the infant. Once an infant learns that the sound signals that the reinforcer is available for viewing, the intensity

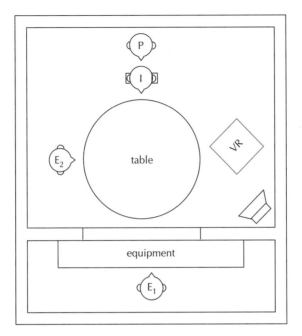

Figure 2.1.   Schematic diagram of test and patient room for carrying out visual reinforcement audiometry (VRA). (Key: E_1 = Experimenter 1; E_2 = Experimenter 2; P = Parent; I = Infant; VR = Visual reinforcer.) (From Greenberg, D.B., Wilson, W.R., Moore, J.M., & Thompson, G. [1978]. Visual reinforcement audiometry [VRA] with young Down's syndrome children. *Journal of Speech and Hearing Disorders, 43*[4], 448–458; ©American Speech-Language-Hearing Association. Reprinted by permission.)

level of the sound is reduced until the infant no longer responds and then raised until the infant responds again. In this manner, an infant's threshold for that sound can be determined. Figures 2.2a, 2.2b, and 2.2c show a schematic sequence of waiting at mid-line, head-turn response, and visual reinforcement. When applied under these conditions, visual reinforcement postpones habituation to the stimulus and allows for up to 30 or 40 responses, a sufficient number to obtain an audiogram on a child (Primus & Thompson, 1985). This is the procedure of choice for the behavioral assessment of hearing for infants between 5 and 24 months of age (Thompson, Thompson, & Vethivelu, 1989; Widen, 1990). The technique is equally as powerful in the assessment of infants and children with developmental delay, as long as a mental age equivalent of 8–10 months has been achieved (Greenberg, Wilson, Moore, & Thompson, 1978; Thompson, Wilson, & Moore, 1979).

Conditioned Play Audiometry
CPA is similar to the method of testing hearing that is familiar to most adults: A sound is presented and the individual raises a hand or pushes a button to signal that the sound was heard. CPA involves teaching a child a motor response that is time-locked to the presentation of the sound. In this procedure, the

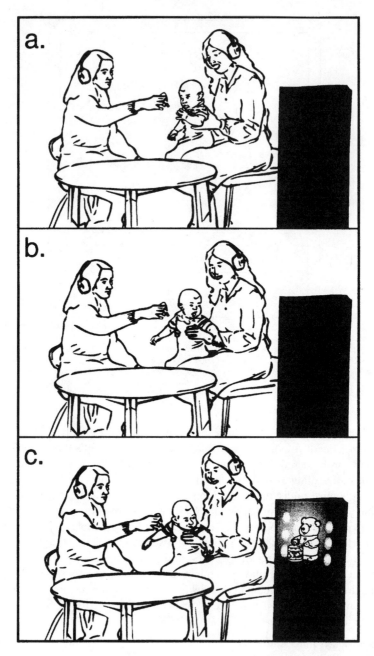

Figure 2.2.   Sequence of infant activity in visual reinforcement audiometry (VRA): a) Infant is directed with a toy to a "ready" position at mid-line. b) Infant turns head to left toward visual reinforcer following presentation of auditory stimulus. c) Visual reinforcer is activated following correct response on part of infant.

examiner selects a response that is consistent with the motor development of the child and one that presumably will be fun for the child to perform. For example, a child may be taught to drop blocks in a container, place rings on a spindle, or place a piece into a puzzle. Figure 2.3 shows a schematic sequence of anticipation of the sound and response. The aspect of this approach, which is most like an adult-oriented approach to hearing testing, is teaching the child the concept of waiting, listening, and then responding as soon as the auditory signal is presented. This concept of waiting requires some facility with language, self-restraint, experience with turn taking, and receptiveness to social reinforcement. Three-year-old children (and precocious 2-year-olds) can be tested satisfactorily with CPA (Thompson et al., 1989).

Table 2.1 displays a brief synopsis of behavioral tests of hearing. Test acronyms, appropriate age ranges, brief procedures, and expected outcomes and test limitations are summarized for each of the behavioral measures.

Physiological Testing
There are three main techniques used to conduct a physiological hearing assessment: acoustic immittance testing, auditory evoked potentials, and otoacoustic emissions (OAEs). These methods are discussed in detail next.

Acoustic Immittance Testing
An essential part of the pediatric audiology test battery is acoustic immittance testing (ASHA, 1990; Nozza, Bluestone, Karadatzke, & Bachman, 1994). This category of physiological assessment is made up of tympanometry and acoustic reflex testing. Tympanometry indirectly measures the function of the tympanic

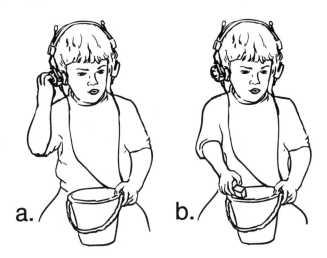

Figure 2.3. Sequence of child activity in conditioned play audiometry (CPA): a) Child is directed to hold block to ear in a listening posture. b) Child responds by dropping block in bucket following presentation of the acoustic stimulus.

Table 2.1.   Summary of behavioral tests of hearing

Test	Age/ developmental level	Procedure	Expected outcome and test limitations
Behavioral observation audiometry (BOA)	Birth–6 months or with pervasive developmental delay	Observation of unconditioned infant behavior following presentation of sound	Gross estimate of hearing or categorization of hearing responsiveness (i.e., evidence of hearing or no response) Not a reliable test of hearing sensitivity
Visual reinforcement audiometry (VRA)	5 months– approximately 24 months of age Applicable across a wide range of developmental delay	Conditioning of infant to turn toward a visual reinforcer following presentation of sound	Reliable minimum response levels (thresholds) can be obtained on individual ears Habituation to reinforcers is a limiting factor above 18 months of age Not appropriate for infants or toddlers with severe visual impairments
Conditioned play audiometry (CPA)	Approximately 24–48 months	Child engages in play task (e.g., ring on peg) in response to sound	Reliable thresholds to pure tones in individual ears Child must have sufficient motor skill for chosen task and must have concept of waiting for or anticipating a sound presentation

membrane and middle-ear structures by determining the relationship between presented and reflected sound energy in the ear canal under conditions of varying amounts of air pressure against the tympanic membrane. Acoustic reflex measurement involves the detection of the stapedius muscle contraction, following intense acoustic stimulation, by measuring its stiffening effect on the plane of the eardrum. This is determined by measuring changes in the energy reflected off the tympanic membrane following stapedial contraction.

These acoustic procedures are valuable in pediatric audiology as means to identify the presence of middle-ear dysfunction and, in some applications of the acoustic reflex, sensorineural hearing loss. Tympanometry is a relatively rapid, reliable tool that, when used in conjunction with hearing sensitivity data, will direct the audiologist in determining whether a hearing loss may be associated with a disorder in the conductive mechanism (Silverman & Silman,

1995). For example, when testing a child having otitis media with fluid, the most common conductive disorder in young children, the results of tympanometry are crucial to audiological management and decisions regarding referral for medical follow-up. Acoustic immittance procedures are not tests of hearing, and thus a determination of conductive hearing loss must be made through the combined used of pure tone, air, and bone conduction thresholds. Yet in cases of children having developmental delays, in which the audiologist is often fitting together multiple, abbreviated pieces of behavioral and physiological information regarding functional hearing status, the use of tympanometry is extremely valuable. Test sessions are often short or incomplete and the tympanometry results may be the only information available regarding the relationship between air conduction sensitivity and middle-ear status.

Auditory Evoked Potentials

In any pediatric population, there will be a subset of children for whom a physiological approach is necessary to augment the behavioral evaluation. These children may present with immaturity, developmental delay, noncompliant behavior, or physical limitations that make behavioral hearing assessment unreliable. Since the late 1970s, developments in the recording of auditory evoked potentials (particularly the short-latency, auditory brainstem response [ABR]) have made possible the accurate and reliable inference of hearing levels in infants and young children.

The ABR is recorded from the scalp in a manner similar to a clinical electroencephalogram (EEG). Three electrodes are attached (at the top of the head and behind each ear), and short, abrupt stimuli (clicks or tone-bursts) are presented through an earphone. A computer is required to extract the ABR from background EEG activity. The resultant waveform is shown in Figure 2.4, dominated by a positive-going peak labeled "V." This is one of three prominent peaks; the other two are labeled "I" and "III." Wave V is the largest and most robust at very low stimulus levels and can be recorded down to near the threshold of hearing. Its presence at low levels corresponds to normal function in the cochlea and lower brainstem.

In children for whom the behavioral hearing assessment does not provide a complete picture of a child's hearing capability, in particular those with developmental delays, the ABR has become a very powerful tool. It is particularly well suited for the purpose of hearing loss estimation for the following reasons: 1) the click-evoked ABR accurately approximates behavioral pure tone sensitivity in the mid to high frequencies (Gorga, Beauchaine, Reiland, Worthington, & Javel, 1984); 2) it does not habituate, that is, it is stable over time and is therefore suitable for acquiring the multiple waveforms necessary for hearing level estimation (Kuk & Abbas, 1989); and 3) it is unaltered by sleep or sedation and is thus useful for testing infants and children who are unable to cooperate during behavioral hearing testing but who are fully cooperative when sleeping. In addition, responses from infants and children have been

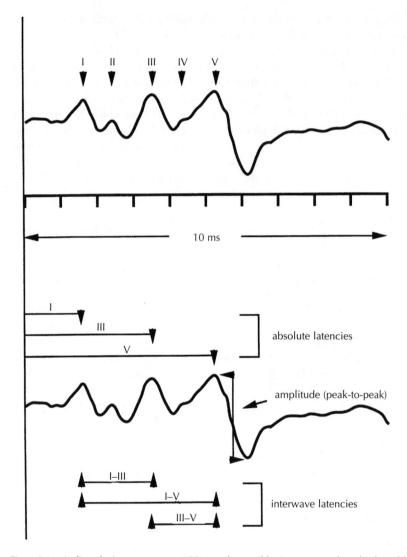

Figure 2.4.   Auditory brainstem response (ABR) waveform and basic measures of amplitude and latency. (Key: ms = millisecond.)

extensively described, providing a broad literature base for the clinical application of this tool in pediatric audiology (see Hall, 1992, for review).

Estimation of hearing sensitivity using an electrophysiology approach is most often necessary during early infancy, when behavioral responses to sound are unreliable, or with older children who are delayed or uncooperative and, therefore, not candidates for a behavioral approach in hearing assessment. Little is required of the child in this type of assessment. For many young children, testing during sleep is necessary because it is often beyond their ability to recline and relax so that movement artifacts do not interfere with the recording of the small electrical potentials that make up the ABR. Infants can often be tested during natural sleep by capitalizing on the timing of regular feedings and nap time. As sedation and accompanying sleep do not influence the ABR, a mild sedative can be used for older children who cannot be coaxed into natural sleep.

For the determination of hearing sensitivity, normative values are necessary in order to differentiate typical response patterns from those that are atypical. Because the ABR is influenced by a number of different stimulus and recording parameters, each clinic establishes its own set of normative data against which clinical decisions can be made.

When using the ABR to make inferences regarding hearing levels, each child is administered a series of stimuli at different intensities—just as stimuli might be presented to a child undergoing a behavioral hearing test. However, in this test situation, the child is not an active participant in the testing but, rather, a passive one (e.g., sleeping or awake but quiet). At each intensity, wave V is identified and measured. Figure 2.5 shows a series of ABR waveforms as a function of intensity. From this figure, it can be seen that, as stimulus intensity (dB nHL) decreases, the ABR wave V moves out in time and becomes progressively smaller (lower in amplitude) until it disappears into the noise floor.

The ABR is also used to determine whether the neural pathway is functioning normally. As previously described, the visual detection threshold is the level at which the ABR (usually wave V) can be differentiated from background noise and, by definition, is associated with the lowest stimulus intensity that just generates this response. For assessment of auditory pathway function, latency measurements are made on the waveform. Latency is the most widely used ABR measurement value. There are two basic latency values that can be obtained from the ABR waveform: absolute latencies and relative or interwave latencies (see lower part of Figure 2.4). Absolute latencies are defined as the elapsed time from stimulus onset to the wave peak. Interwave latencies are defined as the difference between the absolute latencies of two wave peaks (e.g., waves I and V). Because this implies that it is the time required to travel from one generator site to the next, it is often referred to as *central transmission time* or *neural conduction time*. Using absolute and interwave latencies, the ABR can be interpreted to reflect the integrity or maturation of the neural pathway.

Otoacoustic Emissions

OAEs are sounds generated by outer hair cells in the inner ear that can be recorded by sensitive microphones in the external ear canal (Kemp, 1978). They can be recorded noninvasively by placing a sensitive microphone in the external ear canal and are often used as clinical tools for monitoring cochlear status (e.g., Norton & Widen, 1990). OAEs are not in and of themselves neces-

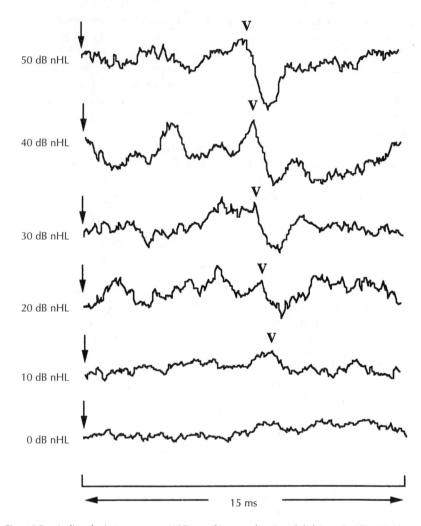

Figure 2.5.   Auditory brainstem response (ABR) waveforms as a function of click intensity (dB nHL). The position of wave V is indicated by "V." Note the change in the position of wave V in time domain (latency) and size (amplitude) across the range of intensities. (Key: ms = millisecond.)

sary for hearing nor are they a mechanism of hearing, but they reflect the status of structures that are necessary for hearing.

Emissions used in audiological assessment are those that occur in response to external auditory stimuli and are present in virtually all adults and children with normal hearing. These are termed *evoked OAEs*. Transient signals, such as the abrupt click used to evoke the ABR, are effective in generating transient-evoked OAEs (TEOAEs). Emissions can also result from the distortion in the cochlea created by the interaction between two pure tones presented at the same time. This method of generating emissions is called distortion-product OAEs (DPOAEs). Both types of evoked emissions are effective in revealing cochlear function across a wide range of frequencies.

Emissions can be recorded quickly, without active participation of the infant or child. As with the ABR, emissions are best recorded from quiet individuals. Sleeping provides the best recording circumstance in that movement artifacts and noise are at a minimum during sleep. Emissions represent a response of the cochlea for frequencies that are present in the stimulus. For example, high-frequency stimuli generate high-frequency emissions and low-frequency stimuli generate low-frequency emissions. Both the transient-evoked and distortion-product emissions can be used to assess cochlear status in infants and children as well as to screen for hearing loss in newborns. Evoked emissions are robust and easily recorded at all ages.

OAEs are present in virtually all adults and children whose hearing is known to be 20 dB HL or better (lower) and absent where hearing levels are approximately 35–40 dB HL or poorer (higher). OAEs therefore have the powerful capacity to indicate normal cochlear function when it exists. For pediatric audiology, in particular for children with developmental delays, this is especially helpful when used in conjunction with other hearing assessment tools such as behavioral hearing tests and tympanometry. For instance, in children with neurological involvement, an absent ABR can be the result of either severe cochlear impairment or lack of neural synchrony at the level of the brainstem (Starr, Picton, Sininger, Hood, & Berlin, 1996). A finding of normal evoked OAEs and normal tympanometry would indicate normal peripheral (middle ear and cochlea) functioning, thus isolating the disorder to the brainstem auditory pathway.

Table 2.2 displays a brief synopsis of physiological measures of auditory function. As with the behavioral tests, test acronyms, age ranges, procedures, and expected outcomes and limitations are summarized for each of the physiological measures.

REACHING AN INFORMED CLINICAL DECISION

In pediatric audiology, decision making is a dynamic operation with small decisions being made at multiple points throughout the assessment process. This discipline is helped significantly by the team evaluation, as the team preassessment conference can provide the pediatric audiologist with an initial strategy. Nonetheless, the evaluation of an infant or child with developmental delay is always evolving, and the evaluation procedures are subject to change at any time. The decision trees shown in Figure 2.6 illustrate the changeable nature of behavioral and physiological assessments of hearing. These trees are designed to provide the reader with insights into the logical flow of the decision-making process made by the pediatric audiologist at various steps during the assess-

Table 2.2. Summary of physiological measures of auditory function

Test	Age	Procedure	Expected outcome and test limitations
Auditory Brainstem Response (ABR)	No age limitations: test can be applied in the newborn period and at anytime during childhood Response undergoes change, most notably in latency, during first 18 months of life	Recording disks are attached to the scalp and abrupt stimuli are presented Brain activity is computer-averaged; the resultant waveform is scored for presence or absence and, most commonly, latency	Measures neural synchrony along the lower portion of the auditory pathway; can be interpreted as an estimate of hearing sensitivity A test of the function of the lower auditory pathway Requirement for neural synchrony makes it sensitive to disorders or maturation of the neural pathway Requirement for abrupt onset stimuli limits frequency specificity
Otoacoustic Emissions (OAE) Transient- (TEOAE) or Distortion-Product (DPOAE)	No age limitations; test can be applied in the newborn period and at any time during childhood	TEOAEs: Abrupt stimuli are presented through a probe in the ear canal; resultant emissions are computer-averaged and displayed in the frequency domain (i.e., a spectrum) DPOAEs: Two tones (primaries) are presented simultaneously and a third tone, a distortion product, is generated by the ear. This distortion product is recorded as an emission in response to multiple primary frequencies	OAEs measure outer hair cell function in the cochlea. When present and robust, OAEs can be interpreted as reflecting a normal functioning cochlea OAEs can be recorded rapidly and provide valuable information for both hearing screening and diagnosis of hearing loss Presence of OAEs represents the typical function of structures that are necessary for hearing Susceptible to excessive acoustic noise as well as external canal debris and middle-ear dysfunction

ment. An initial key decision, for example, would be whether a behavioral or physiological assessment approach (or, commonly, both) is appropriate and, upon making that decision, which specific assessment tool to apply. Each conclusion subsequently produces other points at which decisions must be made. It is not intended for decision trees to be viewed as independent, but as complementary. In pediatric audiology, both behavioral and physiological assessments are commonly conducted for an infant or child during the same session. The decision trees are presented separately to highlight the numerous steps within each approach, not to list them as two separate assessment avenues.

Examples of Decision Making Through Case Studies

The approach of choice is a hearing assessment based on behavioral response to sound. There are times, however, when the behavioral approach will not suffice. For infants younger than 6 months of age, children with severe developmental delays, or those with vision or motor impairments, physiological assessment is required. The next two case studies illustrate how referrals are triaged to develop an initial assessment strategy. An experienced pediatric audiologist will piece together information from the case history, parent interview, and informal observation of the child to decide on an assessment approach.

Matt

Matt was a typically developing 9-month-old. He was born in a hospital at term and spent 48 hours in a general newborn nursery. He was not screened at birth for hearing loss. Matt presented with no risk factors for hearing impairment (ASHA, 1994). His parents were concerned, however, about his inconsistent responses to sound since he was 7 months of age. They noticed that when Matt and his cousin were together, the two children responded differently to sound. His cousin, who was 1 month older, was highly attentive to voices and environmental sounds. Matt was inattentive and sometimes required touch to get his attention. He did not use his voice when playing and did not favor toys that made noise.

Matt's pediatrician was not concerned at this time and ascribed Matt's differences with his cousin as age related and as two children reacting to sounds differently. She cited Matt's history of several upper respiratory infections and the fact that he responded to voice when his back was turned. She doubted that an accurate test could be carried out at this age. A friend suggested that the parents seek out a pediatric audiologist.

Assessment

The purpose of Matt's visit to the audiology clinic was to address parental concerns regarding whether any auditory problem existed, to evaluate his hearing sensitivity, and, if a loss was present, to develop a management plan. The initial clinical decision was the formulation of an overall strategy to assess Matt's hearing. Based on an interview with Matt's parents and an informal observation of him in the waiting room, the clinicians planned a behavioral approach

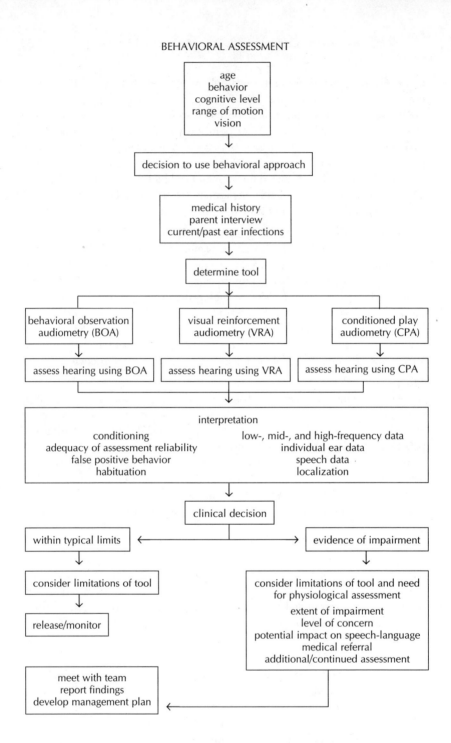

BEHAVIORAL ASSESSMENT

age
behavior
cognitive level
range of motion
vision

decision to use behavioral approach

medical history
parent interview
current/past ear infections

determine tool

behavioral observation audiometry (BOA)

visual reinforcement audiometry (VRA)

conditioned play audiometry (CPA)

assess hearing using BOA

assess hearing using VRA

assess hearing using CPA

interpretation

conditioning
adequacy of assessment reliability
false positive behavior
habituation

low-, mid-, and high-frequency data
individual ear data
speech data
localization

clinical decision

within typical limits

evidence of impairment

consider limitations of tool

consider limitations of tool and need for physiological assessment

extent of impairment
level of concern
potential impact on speech-language
medical referral
additional/continued assessment

release/monitor

meet with team
report findings
develop management plan

Figure 2.6.   Clinical decision trees for behavioral and physiological assessments of hearing.

Figure 2.6.   (*continued*)

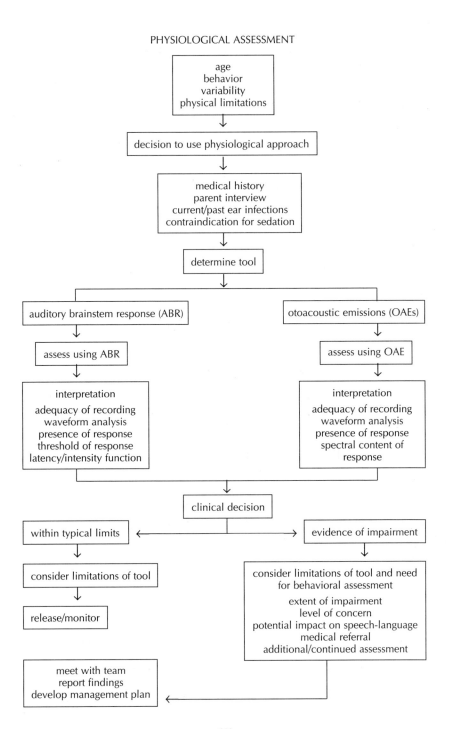

PHYSIOLOGICAL ASSESSMENT

age
behavior
variability
physical limitations

↓

decision to use physiological approach

↓

medical history
parent interview
current/past ear infections
contraindication for sedation

↓

determine tool

↓

auditory brainstem response (ABR)   otoacoustic emissions (OAEs)

↓   ↓

assess using ABR   assess using OAE

↓   ↓

interpretation   interpretation
adequacy of recording   adequacy of recording
waveform analysis   waveform analysis
presence of response   presence of response
threshold of response   spectral content of
latency/intensity function   response

↓

clinical decision

within typical limits   ←→   evidence of impairment

↓   ↓

consider limitations of tool   consider limitations of tool and need
                                       for behavioral assessment

↓   extent of impairment
                                       level of concern
release/monitor   potential impact on speech-language
                                       medical referral
                                       additional/continued assessment

meet with team
report findings
develop management plan   ←

to assessment. Matt's age, appropriate developmental landmarks, and good vision made VRA the logical choice. (Behavioral assessment is the approach of choice, when possible, because it is the most direct measure of hearing.)

Using insert earphones, Matt conditioned easily to the VRA protocol. Consistent, head-turn responses were observed for the frequencies 500 through 8,000 Hz. Matt's minimum response levels (MRLs) showed a mild hearing loss at 500 Hz, sloping to a severe loss at 4,000 and 8,000 Hz in each ear. (The term *minimum response level* is used in lieu of the common audiological term *threshold* when describing the responses of infants and toddlers.) Using speech, Matt responded to his name to both left and right ears at levels consistent with his pure tone responses. When testing by air conduction was finished, a bone conduction oscillator was placed behind Matt's ear on his mastoid and bone conduction MRLs were determined. These results were found to be equal to the air conduction scores. Tympanometry showed normal middle-ear function in each ear. TEOAEs showed reproducible emissions at below 750 Hz but no emissions above this frequency. These findings combined to indicate that the loss observed by air conduction was sensorineural in nature (i.e., it originated in the cochlea or VIIIth nerve).

Recommendations

Matt's parents were counseled regarding the extent of his hearing loss. They were told that his hearing loss ranged from mild in the low frequencies (with which he could easily detect their voices) to severe in the high frequencies (with which he would most certainly miss important aspects of speech). Because Matt heard the same through air and bone conduction presentations of sound, his hearing impairment was described to them as sensorineural and permanent in nature. The range of options for initial management and intervention were also presented so that the family could make an informed choice. A referral for genetic counseling was made to help the family answer questions about the etiology of the loss. A medical workup with an otolaryngologist was scheduled to rule out any medical contraindication to proceeding with hearing aids. Matt was fitted with binaural hearing aids and his parents enrolled him in a total-communication early intervention program for infants and children with hearing loss and their families.

Amy

Amy was a 5-week-old infant who was born prematurely (at 32 weeks of gestation) with a birth weight of 1,400 grams. Her Apgar scores were 4 (at 1 minute) and 6 (at 5 minutes), and she had received a 5-day course of antibiotics beginning at 12 days of life. Otherwise, she had a relatively mild period in the neonatal intensive care unit (NICU). Amy's hearing was screened in the NICU using TEOAEs. Results of this TEOAE screening showed no response in either ear. She was subsequently rescreened with the ABR prior to discharge from the hospital. This screening showed clear responses in both left and right ears at 70 dB nHL, but no response in either ear at 30 dB nHL. The lack of response at 30 dB nHL constituted a failure of the screen, and a follow-up diagnostic test was scheduled at roughly 4–6 weeks after discharge from the hospital. This appointment was scheduled as part of Amy's discharge summary and recommendations.

Assessment

The initial assessment decision in this case was to rescreen Amy's hearing prior to discharge from the hospital following an initial failure using TEOAEs. This approach (combining the two screening tools following failure of one) has been shown to reduce false positive findings and, thus, limit parental concern and program expense.

A second assessment decision point occurs at the time of diagnostic follow-up. Although a behavioral approach is the method of choice in infant hearing assessment, the acquisition of reliable behavior responses is dependent on developmental age. Specifically, for children younger than 6 months of age, clinical data using a behavioral approach are highly variable and poor indicators of hearing sensitivity. Thus, a physiological approach was indicated for Amy, who returned for her diagnostic follow-up assessment at 6 weeks corrected age.

Otoscopy showed that her ear canals were clear and her tympanic membranes were visualized. For physiological assessment of the auditory pathway and the estimation of hearing levels, both the ABR and OAE were used. Results of a click-evoked ABR showed clear responses in the left ear at above 50 dB nHL and for the right ear responses at above 60 dB nHL. Tone-burst evoked ABRs using abrupt, tone-burst stimuli at 500 Hz showed clear responses at 20 dB in each ear. An ABR to a click presented by bone conduction showed responses at above 50 dB nHL when the bone oscillator was placed on the left mastoid. Click-evoked OAEs showed clear responses only for frequencies below 1,500 Hz.

Recommendations

Clinical interpretation of the physiological assessment was that Amy had a bilateral, sensorineural hearing loss that ranged from normal in the lows (500 Hz) to moderately severe in the highs (above 2,000 Hz). Amy's parents were counseled regarding the estimated extent of her hearing loss, its potential impact on speech-language development, and the limitations of estimating hearing sensitivity with the ABR and TEOAE. Plans were established for Amy to return, at 5–6 months of corrected age, for a repeat, four-frequency, tone-burst ABR as well as a behavioral assessment. The repeat ABR (consistent with the initial findings) helped establish that, so far, Amy's loss was stable (i.e., not progressive). The range of options for initial management and intervention were presented so that Amy's family could make an informed choice. A referral for genetic counseling was made to help the family answer questions about the etiology of the loss. A medical workup with an otolaryngologist was scheduled to rule out any medical contraindication to proceeding with hearing aids. Following the repeat ABR, Amy's parents chose to proceed with hearing aids and enrollment in an early intervention program for infants and children with hearing loss as well as their families.

ISSUES RELEVANT TO PEDIATRIC AUDIOLOGY

The intent of this chapter is to familiarize the reader with how pediatric audiologists utilize available tools to assess the hearing status of infants and young children. It is not the case, of course, that the reader can follow the brief explanations presented here and carry out hearing assessment that leads to meaningful management of a child with hearing loss. Assessment of hearing status is more than collecting behavioral or physiological information and making comparisons to normative scales. On the surface, it appears that information or data gathered from an assessment lead directly to a management decision. In reality, assessment involves clinical judgment that the pediatric audiologist develops by combining knowledge and experience with clinical insight. Pediatric audiology has made gains in the development of technical procedures and instrumentation for hearing and auditory system assessment since the late 1970s. But without clinical insight and a family-centered approach, the acquired data do little to guide initial management strategies and long-term interventions for children with hearing loss and their families. It is through communication over time among families, teachers, speech-language pathologists, and pediatric audiologists that a complete understanding of the functional, long-term impact of a child's hearing loss, on both language development and school performance, can be assessed.

REFERENCES

American Speech-Language-Hearing Association. (1990). Guidelines for screening for hearing impairment and middle-ear disorders. *Asha, 32* (Suppl. 2), 17–24.

American Speech-Language-Hearing Association. (1992). Guidelines for audiological assessment of children from birth through 36 months of age. *Asha, 34* (Suppl. 5), 37–43.

American Speech-Language-Hearing Association. (1994). Joint Committee on Infant Hearing 1994 position statement. *Asha, 36,* 38–41.

Clark, J.G. (1981). Uses and abuses of hearing loss classification. *Asha, 23,* 493–500.

Finitzo, T., Albright, K., & O'Neal, J. (1998). The newborn with hearing loss: Detection in the nursery. *Pediatrics, 102,* 1452–1460.

Gorga, M.P., Beauchaine, K.A., Reiland, J.K., Worthington, D.W., & Javel, E. (1984). Effects of stimulus duration on ABR thresholds and on behavioral thresholds. *Journal of the Acoustical Society of America, 76,* 616–619.

Greenberg, D.B., Wilson, W.R., Moore, J.M., & Thompson, G. (1978). Visual reinforcement audiometry (VRA) with young Down's syndrome children. *Journal of Speech and Hearing Disorders, 43*(4), 448–458.

Hall, J.W. (1992). *Handbook of auditory evoked responses.* Needham Heights, MA: Allyn & Bacon.

Jerger, J.F., & Hayes, D. (1976). The cross check principle in pediatric audiology. *Archives of Otolaryngology, 102,* 614–620.

Kemp, D.T. (1978). Stimulated acoustic emissions from the cochlea. *Journal of the Acoustical Society of America, 64,* 1386–1391.

Knauf, V.H. (1978). Language and speech training. In J. Katz (Ed.), *Handbook of clinical audiology* (pp. 549–564). Philadelphia: Lippincott, Williams & Wilkins.

Kuk, F.K., & Abbas, P.J. (1989). Effects of attention on the auditory evoked potentials recorded from the vertex (ABR) and the promontory (CAP) of human listeners. *British Journal of Audiology, 27,* 665–673.

Mason, J.A., & Herrmann, K.R. (1998). Universal hearing screening by automated auditory brainstem response measurement. *Pediatrics, 101,* 221–228.

Mehl, A.L., & Thomson, V. (1998). Newborn hearing screening: The great omission. *Pediatrics, 101,* 4–9.

Moore, J.M., Thompson, G., & Folsom, R.C. (1992). Auditory responsiveness of premature infants utilizing visual reinforcement audiometry (VRA). *Ear and Hearing, 13,* 187–194.

Moore, J.M., Wilson, W.R., & Thompson, G. (1977). Visual reinforcement of head-turn responses in infants under 12 months of age. *Journal of Speech and Hearing Disorders, 42,* 328–334.

National Institutes of Health. (1993). Early identification of hearing impairment in infants and young children. *NIH Consensus Statement, 11,* 1–24.

Northern, J.L., & Downs, M.P. (1991). *Hearing in children.* Philadelphia: Lippincott, Williams & Wilkins.

Norton, S.J., & Widen, J.E. (1990). Evoked otoacoustic emissions in normal-hearing infants and children: Emerging data and issues. *Ear and Hearing, 11,* 121–127.

Nozza, R.J., Bluestone, C.D., Karadatzke, D., & Bachman, R. (1994). Identification of middle ear effusion by aural acoustic admittance and otoscopy. *Ear and Hearing, 15,* 310–323.

Primus, M., & Thompson, G. (1985). Response strength of young children in operant audiometry. *Journal of Speech and Hearing Research, 28,* 539–547.

Silverman, C.A., & Silman, S. (1995). Acoustic-immittance characteristics of children with middle-ear effusion: longitudinal investigation. *Journal of the American Academy of Audiology, 6,* 339–345.

Starr, A., Picton, T.W., Sininger, Y., Hood, L.J., & Berlin, C.I. (1996). Auditory neuropathy. *Brain, 119,* 741–753.

Swigonski, N., Shallop, J., Bull, M.J., & Lemons, J.A. (1987). Hearing screening of high risk newborns. *Ear and Hearing, 8,* 26–30.

Teele, D.W., Klein, J.O., & Rosner, B.A. (1980). Epidemiology of otitis media in children. *Annals of Otology, Rhinology, and Laryngology, 89* (Suppl.), 5–6.

Thompson, G., & Folsom, R.C. (1981). Hearing assessment of at-risk infants. *Clinical Pediatrics, 20,* 257–261.

Thompson, G., & Weber, B.A. (1974). Responses of infants and young children to behavior observation audiometry (BOA). *Journal of Speech and Hearing Disorders, 39,* 140–147.

Thompson, G., Wilson, W.R., & Moore, J.M. (1979). Application of visual reinforcement audiometry (VRA) to low-functioning children. *Journal of Speech and Hearing Disorders, 44,* 80–90.

Thompson, M.D., Thompson, G., & Vethivelu, S. (1989). A comparison of audiometric test thresholds for 2-year-old children. *Journal of Speech and Hearing Disorders, 54,* 174–179.

Widen, J.E. (1990). Behavioral screening of high-risk infants using visual reinforcement audiometry. *Seminars in Hearing, 11,* 342–356.

Wilson, W.R., & Thompson, G. (1984). Behavioral audiometry. In J. Jerger (Ed.), *Pediatric audiology.* San Diego, CA: College-Hill Press.

Chapter 3

Assessing Language and Communicative Development

The Role of the Speech-Language Pathologist

Truman E. Coggins and Geralyn Timler

The explosion of interest in and information about infants and young children has produced dramatic advances in clinical assessment. One of the most important changes has been the way in which experienced clinicians gather evidence from children with established developmental disabilities or presumed developmental delays. Most health care professionals would agree that an interdisciplinary approach is the only viable means of assessing the dynamic, interactive, and interdependent nature of developing systems (Gibbs & Teti, 1990; see Chapter 1).

The speech-language pathologist is an integral part of the interdisciplinary assessment team, as one of the most frequently mentioned areas of concern in young children with suspected developmental difficulties is speech-language impairments (Rossetti, 1986). In 1991, the U.S. Department of Education estimated that nearly half of all children receiving special education services had language-learning disabilities. Moreover, studies have reported that upward of one third of all children referred to mental health centers have undiagnosed speech and language problems (see Cohen, Davine, Horodesky, Lipsett, & Issacson, 1993). Given the centrality of language for educational success and socioemotional well-being, the speech-language assessment is vital for identifying children with disabilities and designing relevant interventions.

The purpose of this chapter is to explicate clinical decision making. The following discussion reveals how experienced speech-language pathologists assemble and review observations, gather useful and reliable information, and reach informed decisions regarding language and communication. It is hoped that the chapter illuminates some of the mental steps speech-language pathologists take as they are formulating "diverse and difficult decisions" (Kassirer, Kuipers, & Gorrey, 1982, p. 251). Decision trees and case histories are used in this chapter to illustrate how speech-language pathologists make judgments and reach conclusions. Although informed decisions cannot be reduced to "an algorithm and a few pages of text" (Yoder & Kent, 1988, p. v), experienced clinicians can specify the facts, knowledge, and attitudes that set the stage for learning how to think about clinical problems.

ASSESSMENT AND PROCESS

There are three fundamental reasons why speech-language pathologists assess children. First, identifying a child's level of communicative functioning is essential (Crais, 1995; Crystal, 1982). Clinicians seek to document a child's performance across critical developmental domains in an effort to estimate the existence and degree of impairment relative to a normative peer group. Members of the interdisciplinary assessment team rely on this type of data in reaching a diagnosis and documenting a child's eligibility for special services.

A second important reason for conducting a speech-language assessment is to facilitate treatment planning. Experienced clinicians often configure their assessment tasks to identify which treatment strategies might best meet the needs of a particular client. The resulting information can assist teachers and support personnel in moving children from where they are to where they need to be (Crystal, 1982). According to Olswang and Bain, "The decision regarding how to treat a language-impaired child grows out of the clinician's knowledge regarding assessment of children's current levels of performance and corresponding readiness for the acquisition of new behaviors, and the clinician's beliefs about the best way to bring about change" (1996, p. 415). The degree to which an assessment contributes to beneficial or functional treatment outcomes underscores the utility of the assessment findings (Hayes, Nelson, & Jarrett, 1987).

A third reason speech-language pathologists conduct clinical assessments is to evaluate intervention. Speech-language pathologists regularly assess children who have already been identified as having communicative impairments.

The purpose of a reassessment is to document the process of change rather than to determine the extent of a child's delay or disorder. Empirical evidence is necessary to demonstrate that behaviors generalize beyond a particular treatment environment as well as to document the durability of change. Assessing the effects, effectiveness, and efficiency of a child's treatment (Olswang & Bain, 1996) provides the type of useful information experienced clinicians require to reach informed decisions regarding what to treat, how to treat, and when to treat.

Procedures for Assessment

Clinicians have come to rely on three basic approaches for identifying impaired language and communication. Clearly, the most widely used methods for examining either the status of children or their unique needs are standardized tests. This approach establishes the presence of an impairment by referencing a child's deviation from average group performance. To complement the information obtained from standardized tests, clinicians routinely use nonstandardized measures to determine more precisely what children can and cannot do with their language. The final assessment technique relies on families providing information (through reports or questionnaires) about the language behavior of their children. Table 3.1 summarizes a set of commonly used assessment tools.

Standardized Assessment

Standardized assessment allows clinicians to compare the skills, abilities, and achievements of an individual child with those of a comparable (i.e., normative) referent group. Historically, standardized (i.e., norm-based) measures have been the instrument of choice for determining if an impairment exists and to establish its degree of severity. The long-standing popularity of norm-based standardized measures attests to their success in allowing clinicians to make meaningful comparisons of performance among children.

There are several reasons why standardized assessments have so many proponents. On a practical note, standardized tests typically have clear administration and scoring criteria that result in easily obtained tangible evidence. In addition, standardized tests provide numeric data that are purported to be valid and reliable. Thus, clinicians can readily compare the scores of one particular child to those of a large sample of children taking the same test. This comparative ability is important in that standard scores are usually required to qualify a child for early intervention services in an area such as speech-language. Moreover, it is possible to use standard scores to examine general changes in performance over time.

Nonstandardized Assessment

Nonstandardized assessment procedures are carefully designed to meet the needs and unique characteristics of an individual child. These elicitation tech-

Table 3.1.   Selected assessment instruments for speech-language pathology

Assessment	Type of assessment	Age range	Language processes assessed
Communication and Symbolic Behavior Scales (CSBS; Wetherby & Prizant, 1993)	Parent report Nonstandardized Naturalistic observation	9–24 months	Expressive language Receptive language Play skills
Infant-Toddler Language Scale (Rossetti, 1990)	Parent report Nonstandardized Naturalistic observation	Birth–36 months	Expressive language Receptive language Play skills
MacArthur Communicative Development Inventories (CDI; Fensen et al., 1993)	Parent report	8–30 months	Expressive language Receptive language Play skills
Peabody Picture Vocabulary Test–Revised (Dunn & Dunn, 1981)	Standardized	2 years, 6 months–Adult	Receptive language
Expressive One-Word Picture Vocabulary Test (Gardner, 1990)	Standardized	2 years–11 years, 11 months	Expressive language
Preschool Language Scale–3 (PLS-3; Zimmerman, Steiner, & Pond, 1992)	Standardized	2 weeks–6 years, 11 months	Expressive language Receptive language

niques allow clinicians the freedom to examine specific communicative behaviors in detail by systematically varying content and context. Although the procedures have neither standard stimuli nor generate standardized scores, there is consensus among speech-language pathologists that a nonstandardized approach can provide valid indices of linguistic performance (James, 1993; Miller, 1981; Olswang & Bain, 1996; Paul, 1995). Furthermore, because nonstandardized methods are flexible and child-centered, they "can be adapted to fit the needs and characteristics of the child being evaluated" (James, 1993, p. 204). This is a distinct advantage when faced with the limited attention span of a young child with developmental disabilities, the motor limitations of a toddler with reduced muscle tone, or the restricted social interaction of a child having an autism spectrum disorder.

The probing that is possible using nonstandardized procedures allows for fine-grain descriptions of language performance. Typically, these detailed descriptions are used to form baseline levels of functioning (Miller, 1981), to describe patterns of regularities in performance (Lund & Duchan, 1993), or to establish entry-level measurements across a range of pertinent domains (Bricker,

Bailey, & Slentz, 1990). Nonstandardized approaches rely on the examiner to structure and organize the situational context based on the behavior of interest and the individual needs of the child. They also allow the clinician to assess a particular behavior multiple times in a variety of relevant contexts to examine more precisely the nature of the presenting problem.

Naturalistic observation and structured elicitation tasks constitute two nonstandardized procedures that are often implemented to assess early linguistic and communicative abilities. Since the 1960s, naturalistic observation has been the predominant clinical methodology for assessing language and communication production in young children (e.g., Aram & Nation, 1982; Bloom & Lahey, 1978; Crystal, Fletcher, & Garman, 1976; Ingram, 1989; Miller, 1981). Much of what is known about language use in both children with typical skills and those with atypical development has been gained by observation in natural, or seminaturalistic, situations.

Elicitation tasks allow clinicians to separate contextual and linguistic variables that may influence a child's ability to understand or use language (Miller, Chapman, Branston, & Reichle, 1980). Indeed, this nonstandardized procedure is the method most frequently used to assess language comprehension. Elicitation procedures have been utilized successfully with infants and toddlers to evaluate their understanding of social-action games (Platt & Coggins, 1990), relational meanings (e.g., MacDonald & Nikols, 1974; Olswang & Carpenter, 1982), and social-communicative intentions (Carpenter, Mastergeorge, & Coggins, 1983; Coggins, Olswang, & Guthrie, 1987; Snyder, 1978; Wetherby & Prizant, 1993; Wetherby & Rodriguez, 1992).

Caregiver Report

Most families keep records of their children's language and communicative milestones. These observational records have proven valuable sources of information about the day-to-day progress of children during the first few years of life (Dale, 1996; Ingram, 1989). Fensen et al. (1993) argued that caregiver report has at least five inherent advantages over standardized and nonstandardized approaches to assessment: 1) Data are more representative because families observe their children in a much wider range of contexts; 2) performance factors are less likely to influence outcome; 3) it is a more cost-effective means of evaluating language and communication; 4) because caregiver report data can be gathered and analyzed before an evaluation, the information can assist clinicians in tailoring an assessment battery; and 5) as caregiver reports are based on everyday situations, they are valuable in monitoring the onset of new behaviors.

Despite these advantages, many clinicians have tended to shy away from using reports by caregivers as an assessment tool. Their reluctance in using this methodology revolved around issues of test–retest reliability. Until 1993, virtually all such report measures of early language development relied on recall memory. Caregivers were asked to think back on words, actions, and behaviors that their young children said, used, or did sometime in the past. Trying to provide an accurate report of past events from memory is a challenging task even for experienced clinicians, let alone caregivers without specialized training in language acquisition. Thus, it is not particularly surprising that findings from caregiver report measures using recall methodology have been viewed with suspicion.

In 1993, Fensen and his colleagues offered clinicians and researchers a new instrument to assess early communicative behaviors. Arguably, the MacArthur Communicative Development Inventories (CDI) provide professionals with the most effective and efficient means of sampling parents' knowledge of their children's communicative abilities. Rather than depending on a caregiver's "retrospective memory" (Miller & Paul, 1995, p. 14), the CDI is predicated on recognition memory. When a recognition format is used, current or emergent behaviors are the focus rather than past events, and parents select words their children say or know from a comprehensive list instead of all the words they recall from memory. These methodological changes have resulted in an instrument with strong internal consistency and high test–retest reliability (see Fensen et al., 1993). The CDI assesses early words—both receptive and expressive vocabularies—as well as gestures in infants (8–16 months of age) and expressive vocabulary and early sentences in toddlers (17–30 months old).

Process of Assessment

This chapter presents a primarily descriptive-developmental orientation toward early assessment (Bernstein, 1993; Miller, 1981; Paul, 1995). Such an approach assumes that children developing language typically provide the best way to identify the ability of a child with a language impairment to comprehend and produce language. McCormick and Schiefelbusch have aptly captured the essence of this approach.

> There is every reason to think that children with deficient language: (a) need language learning experiences as rich as those provided to normal language users, (b) will attend to, understand and talk about many of the same objects, events and relations as typical learners, and (c) want and need to experience the same control over their environment as their more competent peers at the same stage of development. (1984, p. 36)

Descriptive-developmental assessment focuses on a child's capacity to understand and produce linguistic elements. To comprehend and produce language, children must possess knowledge about formalizing, actualizing, and using language. The formulation of language centers on the meaning of words and word relationships (i.e., the semantic component). The actual form of language is determined by a set of abstract rules for combining words into sentences (i.e., the syntactic component). Finally, children must learn how to use their language to communicate effectively in different social contexts (i.e., the pragmatic component).

Assessing Comprehension

Assessing what children understand about language has always been a knotty assignment. Unlike spoken language that can be recorded on audiotape or videotape for later analysis, comprehension is far less tangible, as it is a private event that takes place in the listener's mind (Miller & Paul, 1995). The major task in assessing comprehension is appreciating the strong influence of context. This is challenging because context is a multidimensional construct encompassing 1) the physical context (including the layout of the room), 2) the social context (the history people have with one another), 3) the event context (why people have gathered together), 4) the affective context (emotional state and goals of the participants), and 5) the prior linguistic context (Lund & Duchan, 1993). Although these contextual variables are operative in the immediate situation, they also reveal the listener's past experiences which, according to Milosky, create "world knowledge and how selective aspects of world knowledge are activated in a given situation" (1992, p. 21).

Children first comprehend a few words in specific and predictable contexts. For example, some of the initial evidence that children understand parental speech is reported during social-action games: The mother of a 9-month-old claps her hands together and says, "Pat-a-cake, Pat-a-cake, baker's man," and her child begins to clap. Or the father of a 12-month-old holds his son up to the window and says, "Wave bye-bye," and the child waves. In these cases, the children's apparent understanding of the game and the verbal request is intimately tied to the context and the parents' sensitivity to their children's repertoire of actions (Chapman, 1981).

Parents typically scaffold important contextual variables until their children begin to master the linguistic form and content of a particular game as evidenced by their use of conventional behaviors associated with that game. By supporting their verbal messages with enough redundancy and context to ensure the child's understanding, parents may actually facilitate early language comprehension (Coggins & Olswang, 1987). Platt and Coggins (1990) found a positive relationship between the amount of structure parents provided during social-action games and their children's levels of performance. This finding stresses the importance of assessing a young child's performance with varying degrees of contextual support in order to obtain an indication of not only what a child can do but also what a child may be capable of doing.

Given the context-dependent nature of emerging language, the most relevant clinical question is how young children use context and their prior knowledge to comprehend messages. Chapman's insightful (1978) writings demonstrate that children actually comprehend little of what they hear during the first years of life. Instead, they use strategies that are based on prior experience to understand adult language. A comprehension strategy is a shortcut for arriving at the meaning of an utterance without "full marshaling of the information in a sentence" (Chapman, 1978, p. 309). Interestingly, children continue to rely on strategies well into the school grades. Preschool-age children, for example, know relatively little about the syntactic structure of sentences and depend heavily on their past experiences (i.e., knowledge of the world) to determine the meaning of the sentences they hear. Table 3.2 summarizes a set of strategies that infants, toddlers, and preschoolers may use to give the appearance of understanding entire sentences. Clinicians must be aware that children have "multiple avenues to meaning" (Chapman, 1978, p. 321) that do not require them to depend on adults' language.

Comprehension strategies may explain why certain children comprehend more in some situations than in others. For example, asking a child "What do you want to drink?" at a fast-food restaurant where a Coke machine is fully visible may be very different than asking the same question in the child's living room with no available objects to facilitate a response. In addition, some adults are quite skilled in using supportive gestures and materials to aid comprehension. They may create an interactive moment just before verbally requesting a child's participation, prosodically mark utterances to make them more discernible, or wait until the child has disengaged from a distracting activity before presenting an utterance to comprehend. In short, an assessment will provide a more accurate and complete picture of a child's comprehension skills if the clinician carefully samples a range of contexts that the child typically encounters during his or her daily routine.

Assessing Production

The reason children select a particular communicative gesture, word, or utterance is a function of their experiences and the multifaceted aspects of the context as they perceive it. Therefore, it is not surprising to find that the diversity,

Table 3.2.   Summary of comprehension strategies observed during the first 2 years of life

Age (months)	Comprehension ability	Comprehension strategy
9–12	Understands a few words in a predictable context	1. Look at objects adults look at 2. Act on objects noticed 3. Imitate ongoing actions
12–18	Understands a few words outside familiar events; still depends on immediate context	1. Attend to objects mentioned 2. Give evidence of notice 3. Act in usual manner
18–24	Understands single words outside predictable context; knows a few two-word combinations	1. Locate objects mentioned 2. Put objects in containers (or on surfaces) 3. Act on objects in way mentioned

From Chapman, R. (1978). Comprehension strategies in children. In J.F. Kavanaugh & W. Strange (Eds.), *Speech and language in the laboratory, school and clinic* (pp. 308–327). Cambridge, MA: The MIT Press; and Paul, R. (1995). *Language disorders from infancy through adolescence: Assessment and intervention.* St Louis, MO: Mosby; adapted by permission.

frequency, and even mode of a child's communication may vary depending on how an eliciting context is configured and perceived. This point is shown in the following example.

An interdisciplinary team assessed Byron, a 37-month-old boy who was suspected of having an expressive language delay. The child reportedly had an average sentence length of approximately 1.50 words. By the time most children celebrate their third birthday, they consistently put together three or more words into an average sentence. According to the team's psychologist, there were no concerns regarding Byron's cognitive skills. Furthermore, it was determined that this young child's understanding of language was well within the typical range.

As part of the speech-language assessment, Byron and his mother were observed playing together. Indeed, the child's average sentence length was near 1.50 words. However, there was concern that the context may have exerted a negative influence on Byron's expressive language. His mother's interactive style was quite directive. She asked an overabundance of *what* and *where* questions that required abbreviated responses. Furthermore, her utterances were almost exclusively concerned with toys and games with which her child had little, if any, experience. Finally, there were few genuine communicative opportunities in this unfamiliar situation for Byron to initiate social interactions.

The team asked Byron's mother if she would be willing to help with a simple experiment, to see if changing her verbal interactions and toys in the room could increase the length of Byron's utterances. She agreed, so three suggestions were offered. The first one was to be patient and to try to refrain from overpowering her son with requests or actions. She was asked to allow Byron space and time to perform and not to be afraid of "pauses." Second, it was suggested that Byron's mother follow her son's lead, using comments, questions, and responses that maintained Byron's topic of conversation. Finally, a familiar set of toys, with which Byron and his mother had played at home, was introduced. With these modest situational changes, Byron's average sentence length climbed from 1.50 to 2.50 words. According to Miller (1981), an average sentence length of 2.50 places this child within the expected range for his chronological age.

Contextual variables must be skillfully manipulated to reconcile variability in young children's communicative productions. Based on a review of selected experimental research, Coggins (1991) identified six contextual variables that have the potential to influence performance substantially. Five of these variables center on important nonlinguistic aspects of the environment; the sixth involves the adult's verbalizations. These six influential variables are summarized in Table 3.3.

Determining what a child is capable of expressing is a fundamental goal of assessment. To reach this objective, the clinician must establish the conditions under which communicative productions can be used in their most so-

Table 3.3. Six contextual variables and levels of support that may influence performance

Contextual variable	Level of support	
Nonlinguistic	**Minimal**	**Maximal**
Purpose of an activity or interaction	Naturalistic	Contrived
Experience with communicative partner	Unfamiliar	Familiar
Nature of stimulus materials	Novel	Familiar/thematic
Familiarity of activities	New/original	Event/routines
Responsivity of the listener	Immediate	Delayed
Linguistic		
Availability of cues or prompts	General statement	Elicited imitation

Adapted with permission from Coggins, T. Bringing context back into assessment. *Topics in Language Disorders,* 11, 43–54; ©1991, Aspen Publishers.

phisticated, conventional form (Coggins & Olswang, 1987). By creating situations that vary the nonlinguistic and linguistic contexts along a continuum from minimal to maximal amounts of support (see Table 3.3), it is possible to gain insight into a child's modifiability or potential for change.

REACHING AN INFORMED CLINICAL DECISION

Assessing language and communication within the interdisciplinary process is both complicated and humbling. It is complicated because clinicians are typically asked to gather exemplary information about interactive and dynamic systems in an unfamiliar environment; it is humbling because many assessment measures do not consider important knowledge regarding early linguistic development or make allowances for the activity level, attention span, and motor limitations frequently encountered in children who are developing atypically (Coggins, 1998). These limitations challenge the speech-language pathologist's ability to identify a child's current level of comprehension and production accurately. The task of assessing language, therefore, demands a fundamentally curious and creative person, with astute observational skills, who "feels compelled to keep up with developments in psycholinguistics, speech pathology and related fields" (Siegel & Broen, 1976, p. 75). These professional and personal qualities are the kind of attributes that interdisciplinary assessment demands.

How might a speech-language pathologist go about gathering relevant evidence? Figures 3.1 and 3.2 present decision trees that an experienced clinician might follow in trying to reach an informed decision. Figure 3.1 hypothesizes a sequence of mental steps for assessing comprehension, while Figure 3.2 addresses the assessment of communicative production.

There are four important referral concerns that obligate clinicians to assess comprehension (see Figure 3.1). These areas of concern include lack of compliance (or inconsistent compliance), questionable hearing, slow rate of development, and poor affective/social responses. When caregivers express one

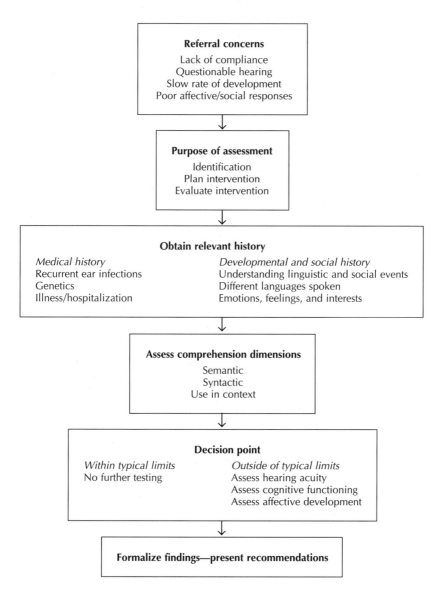

Figure 3.1.   A sequence of steps for assessing comprehension.

or more of these concerns, subsequent clinical assessment almost always documents an impairment in comprehension.

Families are invaluable sources of historical information. As noted in Figure 3.1, they can provide systematic accounts of salient medical episodes, developmental milestones, or problematic social events in the lives of their

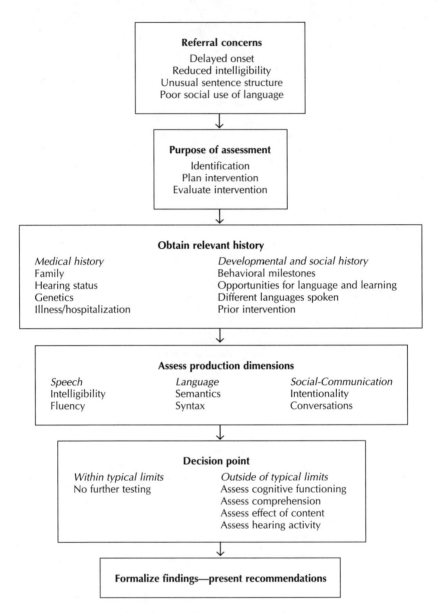

Figure 3.2.   A sequence of steps for assessing communicative production.

children. Knowing what parents think about their children's understanding of language helps clinicians to formulate the purpose of an assessment, decide on relevant procedures, and determine what linguistic components should be emphasized.

Speech-language pathologists take many of these same steps when deciding that language production should be assessed (see Figure 3.2). They review relevant records with an eye toward delayed onset of first words or sentences, unusual sounding words or sentences that the child is reported to express, and limited social uses of language. Families, teachers, or health care professionals are far more likely to refer a child for suspected delays in expressive language than receptive language. This is not to suggest that expressive language delays are more prevalent or more debilitating. Rather, sounds, words, and sentences a child produces are much easier to observe and document than trying to decipher the private world of comprehension.

Figure 3.2 summarizes the relevant medical and developmental and social histories that must be considered in any effort to understand why a child is having difficulties in expressing ideas, feelings, or desires.

Examples of Decision Making Through Case Studies

Case histories of two hypothetical young children are presented to illustrate the decision trees captioned in Figures 3.1 and 3.2. These data are frequently used in deciding what areas of language production (e.g., speech-language, social-communication) will receive special attention as an assessment plan is developed. Although Danny and Todd present different histories, their medical, developmental, and social histories put them at considerable risk for impaired language development. The case studies reveal how an accomplished speech-language pathologist, knowledgeable about presenting concerns and relevant histories, uses evidence to decide what linguistic features to assess and methodologies to employ.

Danny

Danny's mother was worried. Her son was 17 months old and had yet to say his first word. Many of his peers at the community child care center had been talking for some time; several were even starting to say short sentences. In addition, Danny's mother felt he was a "very active" child compared to his peers. He would not sit still to listen to stories and preferred running and climbing to quiet play with his toys. She had been told Danny was "not testable" because of his age and fleeting attention span. Moreover, several of her friends said that their children were also slow to talk but "grew out of it." Nevertheless, Danny's mother decided to have him evaluated by an interdisciplinary team. She was anxious to know if Danny would catch up on his own. Ultimately, she wanted to know why Danny was not talking and what she could do to promote his learning.

Assessment

Danny's assessment began with a parent interview. Danny's mother informed the team that her son had been a healthy child with no significant illnesses. Danny had had two ear infections but his mother was not concerned about hearing. Still, Danny was scheduled to see the interdisciplinary team audiologist as a precautionary measure. Danny's mother was also asked questions that highlighted prominent developmental and social milestones. In response to questions about family history, she reported that no one on either side of the family had had trouble learning to talk.

The interview questions were then focused on language and communication. Danny's mother completed the CDI, which provided a rich source of evidence regarding her son's early words, actions, and communicative gestures. She reported that Danny seemed to understand almost everything she said, including the names of family members, many everyday objects' names, and simple directions. Although Danny did not produce words, he was reported to use a variety of gestures to signal his wants and needs. As the interview progressed, it became clear that Danny had a variety of ways to make his intentions known to adults. For example, Danny employed gestures to initiate social-communication routines such as Pat-a-cake and Peekaboo. He also requested toys by pulling on his mother's shirt, waiting for her to look at him, and then pointing to the desired object. Questions about Danny's play skills were also asked to infer his overall level of cognitive abilities. Danny's mother reported he liked to play with a variety of objects and usually used them appropriately.

Evidence collected during the parent interview underscored the extent of Danny's delays. Whereas Danny had yet to say his first word, typically developing 17-month-olds would be producing somewhere between 25 and 50 different words. Interestingly, Danny's comprehension, at least in predictable situations and familiar settings, seemed age appropriate, and his social use of language and play behaviors appeared broadly within the expected range. Nevertheless, further evidence of Danny's social use of language, nonverbal problem solving, and comprehension in nonroutine situations was required. At this point in the assessment process, an expressive language delay was hypothesized.

Given Danny's age, limited attention span, and absence of expressive language, standardized measures did not comprise the primary assessment methodology. Instead, a nonstandardized approach was selected that tailored the content and context of the assessment to meet Danny's special needs. Naturalistic observation and structured elicitation probes determined what Danny understood about his language and the world around him. The goals used for Danny's assessment are summarized in Table 3.4.

A child-centered approach was used to assess Danny. This type of assessment milieu was most likely to capture Danny's interest and provide a representative sample of his behavior (Coggins, 1998). Danny and his mother were observed while playing with thematically related materials. Observing Danny in this context allowed the speech-language pathologist to gather evidence simultaneously about his expressive language, social interaction, cognition, and speech production skills.

To complement naturalistic observations, several "clinician-directed" activities were also used. These structured elicitation probes provided discrete

Table 3.4.   Assessment goals for Danny

1. Record and document speech-language production
   a. Analyze speech sound repertoire of consonant and vowel segments produced during the evaluation or reported by his mother
   b. Analyze frequency and variety of communicative functions and forms across both vocalizations and gestures
2. Document Danny's use of context and prior knowledge to comprehend messages
   a. Observe responses to directions and questions during low-structured tasks
   b. Record responses during high-structured tasks
3. Document cognitive skills that correlate with language acquisition
   a. Observe play skills for appropriateness and diversity
   b. Observe nonverbal, problem-solving strategies
4. Collect evidence to assist with intervention planning
   a. Determine propensity for imitating adult word models and communicative gestures
   b. Determine the effect of contextual variables on expressive language

opportunities to measure language comprehension and production abilities that might not be observed during low-structured play. The actions, behaviors, and responses obtained from Danny aided in understanding why he was not talking and what his mother could do to promote learning.

Danny exhibited a diverse set of appropriate play schemes. When his mother offered him a toy dollhouse and characters, Danny placed Big Bird in a high chair, gave him a drink from a cup, and pretended to scoop food off a plate with a spoon and feed Big Bird. These were expected play behaviors for children his age. Danny also demonstrated at least one multiple play episode and one extended multiple play episode (typically observed in children having reached 18 months of age) in his Big Bird routine.

Danny had little difficulty in gaining and maintaining the attention of his mother or the clinician. He was an assertive and responsive toddler who readily established eye contact and social interactions. Furthermore, he responded appropriately to most of the requests his mother made during their interaction. Danny also exhibited a range of communicative functions including commenting, requesting information, protesting, and showing off (e.g., smiling and looking at his mother after he threw the ball up high). When opportunities arose, Danny was presented with a selected set of "communicative temptations" (Wetherby & Rodriguez, 1992). For example, the clinician introduced an attractive windup toy that required adult assistance to operate. Danny vocalized, gestured, and combined vocalizations with gestures to request the windup toy. Finally, Danny's sound productions were analyzed for their frequency and diversity as well as for their intentionality.

From a speech-language perspective, Danny's play skills appeared age appropriate. Danny's expressive speech-language skills were characterized by both a limited variety of consonant and vowel production as well as limited word production. However, his demonstration of a variety of communication

gestures and social routines provided ample evidence of emerging and successful intentional prelinguistic communication skills typically observed by the
time most children celebrate their first birthday.

The preceding information was valuable, but it did not provide a complete picture of Danny's linguistic skills. Further knowledge about Danny's language comprehension skills during structured, clinician-directed activities was
required. Therefore, a series of structured probes were used to assess Danny's
comprehension of language. Although Danny was an "active" toddler, he was
curious about the stimulus materials, which provided ample opportunities to
present both familiar and unfamiliar requests.

The objective of structured comprehension tasks was to document the degree to which Danny depended on the nonlinguistic context (i.e., strategies) to
aid his understanding of adult directions and requests. When asked to perform
an illogical action, for example, "Kiss the ball," Danny just picked up the ball
and threw it to the clinician (i.e., the typical action one would perform with
a ball). His action suggested that he did not yet understand the semantic–
syntactic relation between words outside of familiar or predictable contexts. As
Danny was 17 months old, his performance on these tasks was developmentally appropriate.

Controlled contexts are also well suited for cognitive assessment. Means-
end (i.e., the ability to use a novel means to obtain a desired end) is one particularly salient cognitive structure that has shown a strong correlation with the
production of first words (Thal, 1991). Danny was able to use a stick to get an
object out of reach, and when a toy was placed in a matchbox type of box,
Danny was able to slide the box open to get the toy. This type of means-end
problem solving is typically observed in children by 15–19 months of age.

As Danny's favorite activities were identified, repetitive communication
games and routines were established to determine his readiness for reproduc-
ing gestures, sounds, and words. For example, Danny laughed when a ball was
thrown up to hit the ceiling. The clinician raised her hands while saying "up"
several times, pausing to allow Danny time to imitate the action and/or the
word. His mother copied the clinician's model and lifted Danny's arms. After
three turns, Danny lifted his own arms up and said "um" while looking expec-
tantly at the clinician. Danny's performance during the elicitation tasks provided further evidence about his developmental skills. Successful completion
of nonverbal problem-solving tasks supported the initial impression of age-
appropriate cognitive development. Danny's language comprehension also fell
in the normal range for his age. He appeared ready for imitation of gestures
and attempted a vocal imitation of the clinician model. His readiness suggested
one possible strategy for eliciting language production skills.

Danny's profile was consistent with an expressive language delay. His pro-
ductive abilities were characterized by limited word and consonant production
suggesting a concomitant delay in speech production skills. These production
delays were documented across several assessment methodologies. In contrast,

Danny's language comprehension and social communication skills appeared to be developing appropriately.

The speech-language pathologists shared their evidence and impressions with the team. The psychologist concurred that Danny's nonverbal cognitive skills were age appropriate. The developmental pediatrician reported that Danny was healthy. The audiologist noted that Danny passed his hearing screening. Accordingly, the team concurred that Danny exhibited an expressive language delay. His intact language comprehension, play, cognitive, and gestural communicative skills, as well as his supportive family environment, suggested his expressive delays might be resolved without direct speech-language intervention (Olswang, Rodriguez, & Timler, 1998; Paul, 1995).

Recommendations

These impressions were shared with Danny's mother. She was clearly relieved but still wanted to know how to promote Danny's communication skills. Collectively, the team decided that although Danny did not need direct intervention, he was an appropriate candidate for an indirect approach to treatment. This method emphasized the role of Danny's caregivers as the primary agents for change in Danny's language skills. The following suggestions were given:

1. A parent–child home intervention program, which provided written suggestions and models of language activities to facilitate expressive language production, was discussed with Danny's mother.
2. Danny was scheduled for a follow-up visit in 3 months to monitor his progress in expressive speech and to provide a more intensive center-based intervention program if necessary.

Todd

Todd was 4 years and 8 months old at the time of his first interdisciplinary assessment. He attended a developmental preschool. When he was 3 years and 8 months old, Todd was identified as a "focus of concern" by an assessment team from the local school district and enrolled in a preschool program for children at risk for developmental disabilities. For the previous year, Todd had attended the district's developmental preschool four mornings each week. Todd's parents brought him to the interdisciplinary center to answer three important questions: 1) What gains had Todd made over the 12 months? 2) What was the reason for his delayed development? 3) How could he be helped to reach his potential?

Todd's parents reported no familial history of developmental disabilities or learning problems. Indeed, Todd had a 6-year-old brother whose development was typical. In contrast, there had always been concerns regarding Todd. He was slow to walk and talk. He had had numerous ear infections and three sets of pressure equalization tubes. He also wore glasses to correct nearsightedness.

A review of the school district's initial diagnostic report revealed that Todd's comprehension and production of language ranged between the 12- to

15-month-old levels of functioning (whereas chronological age was 3 years and 8 months). He did not initiate many play schemes with his toys, follow multiple stage directions, or point to pictures in storybooks. Still, he demonstrated intermittent eye contact when his teachers requested his attention, was able to take a few turns in familiar communication games (e.g., Pat-a-cake), and enjoyed being bounced up and down on an adult's lap.

The teachers and therapists from Todd's school completed several preassessment questionnaires documenting his progress. Prior to Todd's interdisciplinary assessment, the information was thoughtfully reviewed by the clinic team. The school's occupational therapist reported that Todd was hypotonic and continued to receive both occupational and physical therapy. Todd's speech-language pathologist estimated Todd's expressive language skills to be near the 2-year-old level. Both she and Todd's classroom teacher reported he was able to follow classroom routines.

Todd's parents also completed several questionnaires in preparation for the upcoming interdisciplinary assessment. Fortunately, Todd's parents had completed the CDI 12 months earlier as part of the school district's initial speech-language assessment. When he was 3 years and 8 months old, Todd was producing 29 words; at the time of the interdisciplinary assessment, he was producing 225 words. This dramatic increase documented the gains in expressive vocabulary that his parents, speech-language pathologist, and teachers had observed. Although Todd's parents were justifiably pleased with his expanded vocabulary, Todd rarely used his words to talk with his classmates.

There was genuine confusion as to what Todd actually understood about language. The school speech-language pathologist believed that Todd "understood almost everything." In fact, she estimated his receptive language abilities at or near age level. Yet Todd's parents reported that their son had considerable difficulty at home following directions and answering their questions with relevant information. Todd presented other puzzling behaviors. His parents said that he had trouble interacting socially with other children, and he would not play with an unfamiliar toy until seeing someone else first play with it. When he eventually "played" with the toy, his actions tended to be imitations of what he had observed. In short, he seemed to lack imagination and curiosity when faced with new people, objects, or events.

The clinical team carefully reviewed the findings and impressions from Todd's initial school district assessment. This information, coupled with the concerns expressed by Todd's parents and teachers, led to the theory that, despite his expressive language gains (particularly his vocabulary production), Todd may have had an autism spectrum disorder.

Assessment

The assessment plan was designed to document Todd's linguistic and social-communicative competence and relevant cognitive processes. Two different assessment approaches were used to gather pertinent information across these three important domains. First, a standardized test was selected to examine Todd's linguistic competence without contextual cues, supports, or prompts. The Preschool Language Scale–3 (PLS-3; Zimmerman, Steiner, & Pond, 1992) was administered to obtain norm-referenced scores regarding language comprehension and production. A nonstandardized assessment approach was also employed, allowing the clinicians to gather a more fine-grained description of Todd's language performance and play skills in "context-supported" environments. The goals for this assessment are summarized in Table 3.5.

One assessment result was that Todd obtained a standard score on the PLS-3 of 63 and language age score of 3 years. Todd's strengths included his knowledge of colors, single-word object names, action words, and counting. However, Todd did not demonstrate comprehension of sentence level directions (e.g., "Show me he is on the stairs"), even when the clinician modified the test directions.

To assess Todd's comprehension using nonstandardized testing methods, he was asked to perform several simple actions on a set of familiar objects (following Miller & Paul, 1995). During these activities, Todd consistently followed two-word requests (e.g., "kiss apple") but was inconsistent with three-word instructions (e.g., "push big car") typically mastered between 30 and 36 months of age. In addition, Todd responded to yes/no questions (e.g., "Is this a cow?") and wh- questions (e.g., "Where's the baby?") by repeating the last word of the questions. Invariably, Todd repeated the last few words of all comments. In fact, other than occasionally labeling an object or action, Todd did not use his language to get or give more information or to continue social interactions.

Todd was then presented with a variety of thematically related toys (e.g., a kitchen set). Todd examined the toys but did not pick them up. When offered a dish, he put it on the floor and did not use this opportunity to initiate a reciprocal social interaction. It was decided to model play behaviors in an attempt to

Table 3.5.   Assessment goals for Todd

1. Document language comprehension skills
   a. Standardized assessment: Preschool Language Scale–3 (PLS-3; Zimmerman, Steiner, & Pond, 1992)
   b. Nonstandardized assessment: semantic relations, question comprehension
2. Document speech-language production skills
   a. Obtain language sample during low-structured activities
   b. Observe speech intelligibility during naming and conversational activities
3. Document social-communicative skills
   a. Observe communicative attempts with different communicative partners, activities, and contexts
   b. Determine conversational skills
4. Document play skills
   a. Observe schemes for relating to objects during play
   b. Determine if symbolic play is present

observe Todd's interest in and ability to imitate play behaviors. When the clinician performed several steps in a sequence, Todd imitated each step. He did not, however, contribute any new actions or "invite" others into his play. His parents, who were watching from a one-way mirror, stated that both Todd's communicative and play behaviors during this playtime were typical of what they saw at home.

Overall, Todd's comprehension and production of language remained substantially delayed. He was not yet using his words to construct multiword utterances, and the results of standardized tests and nonstandardized measures showed little clinically meaningful difference between Todd's expressive language and his comprehension. In addition, Todd's ready imitation of others' play behaviors suggested that his performance was likely to be influenced by predictable or familiar environments where he could use the structure of routines to facilitate understanding rather than rely on linguistic (i.e., semantic–syntactic) comprehension. Furthermore, Todd's impaired social use of language went well beyond what would be expected in a young child with a general developmental delay.

In sum, Todd's profile was not suggestive of simply delayed performance. Rather, his language and communicative impairments were similar to children with an autism spectrum disorder. This evidence and tentative hypothesis were presented to team colleagues. Both the team psychologist and the developmental pediatrician concurred that Todd's developmental history and current language and learning profile were consistent with the diagnostic features for an autism spectrum disorder.

Recommendation

A diagnosis of expressive and receptive language disorder, in conjunction with an autism spectrum disorder, suggested a direct treatment framework as documented by 1990s research of young children with autism. The interdisciplinary team suggested specific teaching strategies deemed successful for children with autism (see Dawson & Osterling, 1997) and recommended continued enrollment in Todd's developmental preschool classroom. The team further recommended that Todd's speech-language therapy focus on social-communication skills, specifically turn-taking (in both nonlinguistic and linguistic contexts), commenting on ongoing activities, and answering and asking early developing questions. It was proposed that Todd be paired with a peer model to afford him the opportunity of imitating socially appropriate behavior.

CONCLUSION

This chapter examines how speech-language pathologists assess young children with impaired language and communication skills. The purposes and processes of assessment are summarized in an attempt to illustrate informed decision making. An attempt has been made to conceptualize how experienced clinicians gather essential linguistic and social-communicative behaviors in young children with or at risk for developmental problems. The evidence that speech-language pathologists provide to members of the interdisciplinary team plays a vital role in identifying children with disabilities and designing functional intervention programs.

The heart and soul of clinical assessment is informed decision making. Informed judgment is the just balance between two essential qualities: knowledge and insight. The emphasis in this chapter is on the knowledge speech-language pathologists use to analyze, organize, and interpret evidence and information. It can be argued that knowledgeable clinicians are the ones who stay abreast of pertinent research literature in child development. They read professional publications, reflect on results, and, when appropriate, revise their assessment models or measures based on experimental data.

Nevertheless, although knowledge is essential, it is not sufficient to render informed clinical judgments. Clinically competent speech-language pathologists often display what seems to be a natural tendency to render insightful judgments about the nature of their clients' communicative impairments. What may at first appear to be a natural clinical inclination may in reality be an astute ability to observe behavior; astute observers are as sensitive as they are perceptive. The penetrating observations that thoughtful speech-language pathologists make about their clients are not simply "lucky guesses." By intellectually identifying with their clients, experienced clinicians often reach deeper levels of understanding about the nature of the problem and how to address it than is possible to achieve from test scores, questionnaires, or performance profiles. Thus, clinical insight is the proper balance between natural aptitude and scientific knowledge, and it can be learned from working with experienced and thoughtful clinicians.

As a professional discipline, speech-language pathology has made impressive gains in understanding and treating children with impaired communicative systems. Much of the field's new knowledge has come from the skillful ways in which experienced clinicians have gathered information from young children with atypical communicative development. Since the early 1990s, speech-language pathologists have been adopting and developing new methodologies to provide families and professionals with more clinically useful information. One of this chapter's goals is to show the reader why and when experienced clinicians use these assessment strategies. Because these newer methods yield contextually sensitive and socially relevant information, the findings from the speech-language assessment have become an even more important part of an interdisciplinary team assessment.

REFERENCES

Aram, D., & Nation, J. (1982). *Child language disorders*. St. Louis, MO: Mosby.

Bernstein, D. (1993). The nature of language and its disorders. In D. Bernstein & E. Tiegerman (Eds.), *Language and communication disorders in children* (pp. 2–23). Indianapolis, IN: Macmillan Publishing USA.

Bloom, L., & Lahey, M. (1978). *Language development and language disorders.* New York: John Wiley & Sons.

Bricker, D., Bailey, E., & Slentz, K. (1990). Reliability, validity and utility of the evaluation and programming system: For infants and young children (EPS-I). *Journal of Early Intervention, 14,* 147–158.

Carpenter, R., Mastergeorge, A., & Coggins, T. (1983). The acquisition of communicative intentions in infants eight to fifteen months of age. *Language and Speech, 26,* 101–116.

Chapman, R. (1978). Comprehension strategies in children. In J.F. Kavanaugh & W. Strange (Eds.), *Speech and language in the laboratory, school and clinic* (pp. 308–327). Cambridge, MA: The MIT Press.

Chapman, R. (1981). Exploring children's communicative intents. In J. Miller (Ed.), *Assessing language production in children* (pp. 111–136). Baltimore: University Park Press.

Coggins, T. (1991). Bringing context back into assessment. *Topics in Language Disorders, 11,* 43–54.

Coggins, T.E. (1998). Clinical assessment of emerging language: How to gather evidence and make informed decisions. In S.F. Warren & J. Reichle (Series Eds.) & A.M. Wetherby, S.F. Warren, & J. Reichle (Vol. Eds.), *Communication and language intervention series: Vol. 7. Transitions in prelinguistic communication* (pp. 233–259). Baltimore: Paul H. Brookes Publishing Co.

Coggins, T., & Olswang, L. (1987). The pragmatics of generalization. *Seminars in Speech and Language, 8,* 283–302.

Coggins, T., Olswang, L., & Guthrie, J. (1987). Assessing communicative intents in young children: Low structured observation or elicitation tasks? *Journal of Speech and Hearing Disorders, 52,* 44–49.

Cohen, N., Davine, M., Horodesky, N., Lipsett, L., & Issacson, J. (1993). Unsuspected language impairment in psychiatrically disturbed children: Prevalence and language and behavioral characteristics. *Journal of the American Academy of Child and Adolescent Psychiatry, 32,* 595–603.

Crais, E. (1995). Expanding the repertoire and techniques for assessing the communication skills of infants and toddlers. *American Journal of Speech-Language Pathology, 4,* 47–58.

Crystal, D. (1982). *Profiling linguistic disability.* London: Edward Arnold.

Crystal, D., Fletcher, P., & Garman, M. (1976). *The grammatical analysis of language disability: A procedure for assessment and remediation.* London: Edward Arnold.

Dale, P.S. (1996). Parent report assessment of language and communication. In S.F. Warren & J. Reichle (Series Eds.) & K.N. Cole, P.S. Dale, & D.J. Thal (Vol. Eds.), *Communication and language intervention series: Vol. 6. Assessment of communication and language* (pp. 161–182). Baltimore: Paul H. Brookes Publishing Co.

Dawson, G., & Osterling, J. (1997). Early intervention in autism. In M.J. Guralnick (Ed.), *The effectiveness of early intervention* (pp. 307–326). Baltimore: Paul H. Brookes Publishing Co.

Dunn, L., & Dunn, L. (1981). *Peabody Picture Vocabulary Test* (3rd ed.). Circle Pines, MN: American Guidance Service.

Fensen, L., Dale, P., Reznick, J.S., Thal, D., Bates, E., Hartung, J., Pethick, S., & Reilly, J. (1993). *MacArthur Communicative Development Inventories (CDI): User's guide and technical manual.* San Diego, CA: Singular Publishing Group.

Gardner, M. (1990). *Expressive One-Word Picture Vocabulary Test* (Rev. ed.). Novato, CA: Academic Therapy Publications.

Gibbs, E.D., & Teti, D.M. (Eds.). (1990). *Interdisciplinary assessment of infants: A guide for early intervention professionals.* Baltimore: Paul H. Brookes Publishing Co.

Hayes, S., Nelson, R., & Jarrett, R. (1987). The treatment utility of assessment: A functional approach to evaluating assessment quality. *American Psychologist, 42,* 963–974.

Ingram, D. (1989). *First language acquisition: Method, description and explanation.* Cambridge, United Kingdom: Cambridge University Press.

James, S. (1993). Assessing children with language disorders. In D. Bernstein & E. Tiegerman (Eds.), *Language and communication disorders in children* (pp. 185–228). New York: Macmillan Publishing USA.

Kassirer, J., Kuipers, B., & Gorrey, G. (1982). Toward a theory of clinical expertise. *The American Journal of Medicine, 73,* 251–259.

Lund, N., & Duchan, J. (1993). *Assessing children's language in naturalistic contexts* (3rd ed.). Upper Saddle River, NJ: Prentice-Hall.

MacDonald, J., & Nikols, M. (1974). *Environmental language inventory manual.* Columbus: Ohio State University Press.

McCormick, L., & Schiefelbusch, R. (1984). *Early language intervention: An introduction* (2nd ed.). New York: The McGraw-Hill Companies.

Miller, J. (1981). *Assessing language production in children: Experimental procedures.* Austin, TX: PRO-ED.

Miller, J., Chapman, R., Branston, M., & Reichle, J. Language comprehension in sensorimotor stages V and VI. *Journal of Speech and Hearing Research, 23,* 284–311.

Miller, J.F., & Paul, R. (1995). *The clinical assessment of language comprehension.* Baltimore: Paul H. Brookes Publishing Co.

Milosky, L. (1992). Children listening: The role of world knowledge in language comprehension. In R. Chapman (Ed.), *Processes in language acquisition and disorders* (pp. 20–24). St. Louis, MO: Mosby.

Olswang, L., & Bain, B. (1996). Assessment information for predicting upcoming change in language production. *Journal of Speech and Hearing Research, 39,* 414–423.

Olswang, L., & Carpenter, R. (1982). The ontogenesis of agent: Linguistic expression. *Journal of Speech and Hearing Research, 25,* 306–314.

Olswang, L., Rodriguez, B., & Timler, G. (1998). Recommending intervention for toddlers with specific language learning difficulties: We may not have all the answers, but we know a lot. *American Journal of Speech-Language Pathology, 7,* 23–32.

Paul, R. (1995). *Language disorders from infancy through adolescence: Assessment and intervention.* St. Louis, MO: Mosby.

Platt, J., & Coggins, T. (1990). Comprehension of social-action games in prelinguistic children. *Journal of Speech and Hearing Disorders, 55,* 315–326.

Rossetti, L. (1986). *High-risk infants: Identification, assessment and intervention.* San Diego, CA: College-Hill Press.

Rossetti, L. (1990). *The Rossetti Infant-Toddler Language Scale.* East Moline, IL: LinguiSystems.

Siegel, G., & Broen, P. (1976). Language assessment. In L. Lloyd (Ed.), *Communication, assessment and intervention strategies* (pp. 73–122). Baltimore: University Park Press.

Snyder, L. (1978). Communicative and cognitive abilities in the sensorimotor period. *Merrill-Palmer Quarterly, 24,* 161–180.

Thal, D. (1991). Language and cognition in normal and late-talking toddlers. *Topics in Language Disorders, 11,* 33–42.

Wetherby, A., & Prizant, B. (1993). *Communication and Symbolic Behavior Scales (CSBS) Manual* (Normed ed.). Chicago: Applied Symbolix.

Wetherby, A., & Rodriguez, G. (1992). Measurement of communicative intentions in normally developing children during structured and unstructured contexts. *Journal of Speech and Hearing Research, 35,* 130–138.

Yoder, D., & Kent, R. (Eds.). (1988). *Decision making in speech-language pathology.* Burlington, Canada: Decker.

Zimmerman, I., Steiner, V., & Pond, R. (1992). *Preschool Language Scale-3 (PLS-3).* San Antonio, TX: The Psychological Corp.

Chapter 4

Neurodevelopmental Pediatrics in the Interdisciplinary Team Assessment Process

Emphasis on Etiology

Vanja A. Holm and Nuhad D. Dinno

This chapter provides a neurodevelopmental pediatric perspective on the interdisciplinary team assessment of young children evaluated for developmental delays or disabilities. The process of establishing a diagnosis and communicating that diagnosis to families constitutes a vital task for the interdisciplinary team in general and neurodevelopmental pediatrics in particular. However, attempting to identify a medical etiology of the developmental disability is a unique contribution of the neurodevelopmental pediatrician to the team. When a medical diagnosis provides a basis for the child's developmental disability, specific information can often be given to the family regarding genetic and developmental implications and can identify likely immediate and long-term medical needs.

In many situations, possibly the majority, the medical etiology remains unknown. Sometimes a categorical diagnosis may be the best that can be accomplished. Diagnoses such as developmental delay or communication disorder are usually formulated during the team conference and shared with the family. These terms contribute meaningful information to families, even if not accompanied by definite etiologic or causative knowledge. Other categorical diagnoses, such as cerebral palsy or autism spectrum disorder, convey more specific information and imply a variety of possible etiologies, but considerable uncertainty still remains. In these cases, the role of the neurodevelopmental pediatrician is to communicate relevant medical and developmental information effectively to the family. In all instances, the neurodevelopmental pediatrician must be familiar with medical community resources so the family can be directed to the best follow-up care for both etiologic and incidental conditions uncovered during the medical assessment. Families often feel a sense of relief when a diagnosis is made, providing a framework for understanding their child's development across the life span (Piper & Howlin, 1992). Indeed, it has been well documented that coming to terms with a diagnosis has important implications for the parent–child relationship (Pianta, Marvin, Britner, & Borowitz, 1996).

The dimensions to be assessed in the neurodevelopmental pediatric evaluation are determined by the standard medical evaluation of present and past medical histories, a review of organ systems, family and social histories, and physical and neurological examinations. Certain aspects take on special importance when one is examining a young child with developmental disabilities, as discussed in this chapter. A more detailed account of the medical examination for each of these areas can be found in textbook chapters on neurodevelopmental disorders (Montgomery & Jones, 1996; Palmer, 1996; Shapiro, 1996). This chapter presents an outline of the assessment process in the context of the interdisciplinary team assessment, emphasizing a search for information that will contribute to a diagnosis.

ASSESSMENT PROCESS

A thorough evaluation of both genetic and environmental factors, along with careful physical and neurodevelopmental examinations, is necessary to identify conditions that are contributing to or causing a developmental disability. Sometimes laboratory tests are needed for further clarification. Assuming that a developmental disability does exist, the following material outlines the process utilized to identify the etiology of the developmental disability.

Information Gathering and Medical History

Collection of past medical information from birth records as well as previous and present treating physicians, clinics, and hospitals is an important part of the assessment process in neurodevelopmental pediatrics. Past medical history and prior laboratory test results need to be reviewed before the physician's first visit with the child and the family. Specific information, such as growth data, might need to be collected from several sources. Poor physical growth is a common problem in children with developmental disabilities.

Further information is also obtained from the child's caregivers. It is help-ful to understand their concerns about the child and at what age difficulties first became evident. Additional history taking requires a careful review of health data for both parents and their families. From this information, a fam-ily tree (pedigree) will be constructed. This is followed by an evaluation of the pregnancy, labor, birth, and the neonatal and postnatal periods. A detailed history of the child's developmental and behavior profiles is also crucial to the evaluation process (Palmer, 1996).

When children are adopted or in foster care, the procedure, by necessity, is different. Sometimes caseworkers for such children have access to medical records on the child and biological parents. At other times family members might be contacted. Often, however, the neurodevelopmental pediatric evalu-ation has to be performed with less than adequate information and, accord-ingly, is less precise.

For ease of communication and a means of organizing potential etiologies, possible causes of developmental disabilities are discussed in terms of pregesta-tion as well as the prenatal, perinatal and neonatal, and postnatal periods. In actuality, these periods are often linked (e.g., a genetic [pregestational] cause often is associated with prematurity [perinatal] or seizures [neonatal]).

Pregestational Data

Parental age at the time of conception is important. Older maternal age is a factor in chromosomal abnormalities such as Down syndrome. Older paternal age is a factor in autosomal dominant spontaneous mutations as in achondro-plasia. Maternal health factors such as diabetes and poor nutrition also have implications for pregnancy outcome. The clinician needs to inquire about the presence of certain conditions in the family history, such as mental retardation, learning disorders, neurological and mental disorders, congenital malforma-tions, and consanguinity, to construct a family pedigree.

Single-Gene Disorders

Obtaining a pedigree is important in diagnosing single-gene disorders that can result in developmental disabilities, such as visual and hearing impairments. Autosomal dominant conditions can be inherited from generation to genera-tion, but frequently a child might be more severely affected than the transmit-ting parent because of variable gene penetrance. This is seen in neurocuta-neous disorders, such as neurofibromatosis and tuberous sclerosis (TS). For an autosomal recessive inherited condition, both parents of an affected child are nonsymptomatic carriers. Examples of such conditions are phenylketonuria (PKU), cystic fibrosis, and Tay-Sachs disease. Consanguinity of parents makes it more likely that a child will be affected by a condition caused by autosomal recessive inheritance because the parents might be asymptomatic carriers of the same gene. In addition, a pedigree is essential in making a diagnosis of X-linked recessive conditions, such as fragile X syndrome, hemophilia, or Lesch-Nyhan syndrome, by revealing that only males are affected. Although most genetic disorders are rare in the general population, collectively they make up a significant part of the population of individuals affected with developmental disabilities. Table 4.1 provides examples.

Chromosomal Abnormalities

Rearrangements of chromosomes constitute another important group of genetic causes of developmental disabilities (see Table 4.1). Many chromosomal abnormalities are not compatible with life and result in spontaneous abortions. However, most surviving chromosomal abnormalities cause mental retardation or, on occasion, learning disabilities. A chromosome study is usually indicated in the laboratory workup where the etiology of the disability is unclear.

Polysomy (extra chromosomes) is usually associated with congenital malformations in addition to mental retardation. Trisomy 21 (three copies of chromosome 21 instead of two) is the etiology of Down syndrome, which is the most common chromosomal cause of mental retardation. Trisomies of chromosomes 13 and 18 are other examples of polysomy occasionally compatible with life but causing limited survival. Small pieces of extra chromosomal material or deletions of a part of a chromosome can also contribute to mental retardation. Cri-du-chat ("cat cry") syndrome, for example, is caused by a deletion of the short arm of chromosome 5.

Table 4.1.   Examples of genetic etiologies of developmental disabilities

Single-gene disorders
  Autosomal dominant
    Neurofibromatosis
    Tuberous sclerosis
  Autosomal recessive
    Phenylketonuria
    Galactosemia
    Hurler syndrome
    Tay-Sachs disease
  X-linked recessive
    Fragile X syndrome
    Nonspecific X-linked mental retardation
    Lesch-Nyhan syndrome
    Lowe syndrome (oculocerebrorenal syndrome)
Chromosomal abnormalities
  Polysomy
    Trisomy 21
    Trisomy 18
    Trisomy 13
  Autosomal deletion abnormalities
    Cri-du-chat syndrome
  Sex chromosome abnormalities
    Turner syndrome
    Klinefelter syndrome

Multifactorial Conditions

Many developmental disabilities are considered to have multifactorial etiology because they are caused by interaction of genes and factors in the biological environment (e.g., neural tube defects, hydrocephalus). Neural tube defects occur more often in pregnancies when sisters or mothers have neural tube defects; however, low folic acid levels in the intrauterine environment have also been found to predispose the fetus to neural tube defects.

Prenatal Period

Close review of history and pregnancy records can be helpful. The first 12 weeks (the first trimester) of the pregnancy are crucial because the central nervous system is being formed. During this same period, events are also simultaneously taking place in other developing body organs, and the ingestion of teratogens such as alcohol, Accutane for acne, and Dilantin or other anticonvulsants can result in multiple anomalies (dysmorphogenesis) and developmental disabilities, such as fetal alcohol syndrome (FAS). Table 4.2 shows some examples of nongenetic etiologies of developmental disabilities.

Nerve cell division and maturation begin during the first trimester and extend into mid-pregnancy and well into the perinatal period. Certain events

Table 4.2. Examples of nongenetic etiologies of developmental disabilities

Prenatal

Infections (cytomegalovirus, human immunodeficiency virus [HIV], German measles)
Maternal health (diabetes mellitus, hyperphenylalaninemia)
Maternal medications (e.g., Dilantin, Accutane)
Placental abnormalities
Exposure to radiation
Toxemia
Maternal alcoholism
Trauma

Perinatal and neonatal

Prematurity
Low birth weight
Abnormal presentation
Obstetrical complications
Multiple gestation
Seizures
Intraventricular hemorrhages
Hypoxia due to respiratory compromise
Sepsis or meningitis

Postnatal

Infection (e.g., encephalitis, meningitis)
Exposure to toxins (e.g., lead)
Head injury
Hypoxia due to near drowning or smoke inhalation
Psychosocial factors

during this time, such as radiation, maternal viral infection (e.g., German measles), alcoholism, and maternal conditions of hyperphenylalaninemia or diabetes, can result in an abnormally small brain (microcephaly) in the fetus. Maternal infections that have mild or no symptoms in the mother can be devastating to the fetal brain. For example, a cytomegalovirus infection is usually nonsymptomatic in the mother but can cause microcephaly, hearing impairment, cerebral palsy, and mental retardation in the child.

The history of maternal nutrition and poor weight gain during the pregnancy are important and must be documented. Severe malnutrition in times of war has been shown to have deleterious effects on the developing fetus. Important factors in late pregnancy that might predispose the fetus to a compromised outcome include toxemia, preeclampsia, hemorrhage, and premature birth.

Perinatal and Neonatal Period
The perinatal and neonatal period starts with labor, beginning with the rupture of membranes, and includes the first 4 weeks of life. Fetal distress, abnormal presentation, intracranial hemorrhage, delayed respiration, cyanosis, infection, jaundice, hypoglycemia, and neonatal seizures should be noted in the history taking. Apgar scores obtained from birth records are a significant part of the history.

Postnatal Period
This period includes events that have taken place after the first 4 weeks of life until the child is presented at the clinic for assessment. Important issues to consider in this part of the history include factors affecting the central nervous system, such as meningitis, encephalitis, trauma, child abuse, a near drowning event, or inadequate parenting. Of note, many genetic disorders such as fragile X syndrome, Hurler syndrome, and Tay-Sachs disease are not evident at birth; children become symptomatic in infancy or later childhood.

Physical Examination
A thorough physical examination is the primary instrument used by the neurodevelopmental pediatrician. Important aspects regarding the examination of a child with a developmental disability, or a potential disability, are emphasized.

Accurate Growth Parameters
Stadiometers are used to record height, and regularly calibrated balance scales provide exact weight measurements. The largest head circumference is obtained by encircling the forehead and the occiput with a nonstretchable tape measure. All these data are carefully marked on appropriate growth charts that display the child's percentile ranking in height, in weight, and in head circumference compared with age-mates. Weight for height can also be plotted in children who appear underweight or overweight. The latter information will identify children who need further anthropometric measurements and should be seen by the nutritionist. The height of unusually short or tall children should be compared with the height of their birth parents. Charts are also available to determine if a child's growth is within expectations for the family.

Vision Assessment

The evaluation of visual acuity is important. Significant visual impairments are usually associated with obvious physical eye findings, except when caused by neurological abnormalities of the optic nerve or the brain (cortical blindness). The inability to fix and follow bright or shiny objects can be detected in the first few weeks of life, but acuity screening using child appropriate charts is not possible until a child has a developmental age of at least 3 years. However, a trained pediatric ophthalmologist might be able to assess visual acuity in children having substantial developmental delays. Children with developmental disabilities have higher incidences of marked nearsightedness than typically developing children. Strabismus, or "lazy eye," is also more common in this population. Children with strabismus have to suppress the vision in one eye in order not to see double. Although this does not directly interfere with vision and does not constitute a visual impairment, it can cause permanent loss of vision in the "lazy" eye unless prevented by appropriate treatment. Strabismus might also interfere with depth perception. If visual status is a concern, ophthalmological referral is always indicated.

Hearing Assessment

Audiological screening is needed in all children with developmental disabilities. A treatable condition such as hearing loss needs to be ruled out. Language delay is a common presentation for children with a range of disabilities. Traditional hearing screens as performed in schools and physicians' offices require cooperation and maturity. However, more thorough assessments require special equipment, and the audiologist can assess hearing in any child regardless of age or disability (see Chapter 2).

Assessment of Extremities

Length and proportion of the extremities must be compared with the rest of the body. The hand and foot length can be measured and compared with published standards. The relationship between palm and finger length is very useful for diagnosing certain syndromes. The presence of unusual creases on the palms can be noteworthy. The fingers can be incurved (often seen in the fifth finger), short, or broad. Webbing between either fingers or toes may be significant. Toes can be broad, overlapping, or widely spaced. Nail growth and shape should also be assessed (Montgomery & Jones, 1996).

Evaluation of Other Body Parts

A variety of major and minor congenital malformations are seen in syndromes and are important in the evaluation for an etiology of developmental disabilities. Congenital heart disease, renal malformations, chest deformities, variations in the formation of the external genitalia in boys, and unusual placements of the anus are examples of malformations usually seen as single birth defects without significant hereditary or developmental consequences. However, when they are present in a child with a developmental disability, these characteristics take on a different meaning and are considered a significant finding that may point toward a specific condition or syndrome.

Examination of the Skin

The skin and the brain originate from the same embryonal tissue during early gestation; thus, the examination of the skin takes on special significance in evaluating a child with developmental disabilities. A careful check for neurocutaneous lesions should be part of the examination. The distribution, configuration, and extent of birthmarks or areas of hypopigmentation or hyperpigmentation can be very helpful in determining specific conditions and associated complications.

Neurological Examination

A careful neurological examination must be performed on each child with suspected developmental disabilities. What is done depends on the child's age and functional developmental status. Muscle tone needs to be carefully assessed. Hypotonia (poor muscle tone) is a common nonspecific finding in young children with developmental disabilities (Shapiro, 1996). It can also be an early manifestation of more serious neurological or muscle conditions. Both gross and fine motor coordination are carefully evaluated. In babies and in children who function at very low levels, the persistence of primitive reflexes may be found. In an uncooperative child, much useful information is obtained by observing the child playing with toys, running in the corridor, or handling papers and crayons.

Appraisal of the Presence of Facial Dysmorphic Features

It is essential to compare the child's facial features with those of family members. If family members are not available, it is important to ask if the child resembles parents or siblings. Photographs are helpful. Measuring the outer canthal distance (the outer corners of the eyes), the inner canthal distance (the inner corners of the eyes), and the palpebral fissure (the eye opening) and comparing them to age standards can be helpful; it will determine if the eyes are wide set, if the palpebral fissure is short, and so forth. The eyes may be slanted upward or downward, and the presence of speckling in the eyes may point the clinician toward certain conditions. The size, shape, and placement of the outer ears can be measured and compared with age standards. The nose can be prominent, upturned, or broad. The shape of the mouth can be unusual. Downturned corners of the mouth and full or thin lips are seen in certain syndromes. The chin can be prominent or recessed. The cheekbones may be flattened or prominent. All of these factors are relevant because the presence of unusual facial characteristics is often the first clue in the process of identifying a syndrome (Montgomery & Jones, 1996).

Behavior Observations

Observations of the child's behavior in the examining room and in parent–child interaction are an integral part of the neurodevelopmental pediatric evaluation. Does the child have poor or fleeting eye contact? Is the child excessively active for his or her age? Is the child fearful and withdrawn? Does the child flit from activity to activity? Are toys played with in an age-appropriate manner? Is the child passive or aggressive? How does the parent respond to transgressions? Does the child listen to the parent and examiner? Is the child manipulative, looking for adults to respond to obvious misbehaviors? In an interdisciplinary team environment, behavior observations made by the neurodevelopmental pediatrician should be compared with other team members' observations. This material is significant in the assessment of a child's behavior for both diagnosis and management recommendations.

REACHING AN INFORMED CLINICAL DECISION

The family history as well as prenatal, perinatal, and postnatal information about the child play significant roles in forming a diagnosis. These elements and the developmental course, coupled with physical, neurological, and behavioral findings, provide the information needed to develop a tentative list of medical diagnostic possibilities.

Syndrome Identification

Syndrome identification is an important component in the medical assessment of a child with a possible developmental disability. As previously noted, dysmorphic features that are not familial traits are clues to syndrome diagnoses. Growth disturbances coupled with developmental delays might also point to a syndrome. The combination of certain facial features and minor variations on hands and feet will give the astute clinician a gestalt that might lead to a specific diagnosis such as Down syndrome. In other conditions—for example, FAS—medical history, developmental and behavior characteristics, and physical findings are all crucial components of the diagnosis.

Exciting developments in molecular genetics are adding additional tools to syndrome identification. As described in Chapter 16, Prader-Willi syndrome was diagnosed solely on history and physical findings until the early 1980s, when special chromosome studies demonstrated a deletion on chromosome 15 in some individuals. Since the mid-1990s, molecular genetic techniques can be used to confirm the diagnosis in almost all people with the syndrome. In 1997, Williams syndrome also became confirmable by laboratory diagnosis: A DNA probe on chromosome 7 will verify the diagnosis of this disorder in more than 95% of typical cases.

In other syndromes, such as Sotos, Cornelia de Lange, and Rubinstein-Taybi syndromes, a genetic etiology is likely but less well understood. However, with ongoing research, it is anticipated that many such syndromes considered of unknown origin (called spontaneous mutations) may have clear genetic explanations. In any case, encountering a child with a developmental disability and unusual physical features should direct the clinician to reference books such as *Smith's Recognizable Patterns of Human Malformation* (Jones, 1997). Special computer programs have also been developed to aid in syndrome identification.

Abnormal Neurological Findings

When clearly abnormal neurological findings or a categorical diagnosis of cerebral palsy are present, the medical history takes on special importance. Perinatal, neonatal, and postnatal events might be causally significant. For example, children with intrauterine growth retardation (IUGR) have low birth weight and are small for gestational age. Even though they otherwise appear physically normal, they are at risk for central nervous system abnormalities. The brain development in such infants is immature and vulnerable to insults that can be withstood by babies of normal birth weight.

Infants born prematurely but with appropriate weight for gestational age are susceptible to perinatal insult. There are many possible causes for brain damage in such infants. Especially ominous is large intraventricular or subdural hemorrhage. The neurodevelopmental pediatrician often has to conclude that, despite neurological findings and even a diagnosis of cerebral palsy, the specific causal event cannot be determined.

In the past, birth injury in full-term infants was often blamed on obstetrical complications and frequently thought to be a major cause of cerebral palsy. Although such events do occur, they account for only a small percentage of children with cerebral palsy. Unfortunately, most of these obstetrical adversities are not medically preventable. Sepsis and meningitis in the neonatal period are the cause for some of these problems, while others are due to respiratory compromise of pulmonary dysmaturity or hypoxia of unclear origin.

It has become evident that about half of the cerebral palsy cases are mainly due to causes preceding birth. Certain genetic and prenatal events may make it difficult for a baby to adjust to the necessary physiological changes that take place during the transformation from an intrauterine to an extrauterine existence. Problems in the perinatal and neonatal period might be symptoms of a preexisting condition rather than being causally related to the later developmental disability. In such situations, the neurodevelopmental pediatrician must weigh the historical and physical findings in an attempt to judge what might be the most likely cause of the disability.

In almost 10% of children with cerebral palsy, the etiology is postnatal. Head trauma, cerebral infection, or asphyxia from near drowning or smoke inhalation are frequent causes. Such cases are usually clear cut: The child was healthy before the incident and experienced a marked developmental setback afterward.

Laboratory Studies

Possible medical diagnoses serve as guides for the indication of specific laboratory studies. One or several studies might be appropriate. These include chromosomal analysis, DNA molecular analysis for fragile X syndrome, and urine or blood samples for an amino acid screen and abnormal metabolites. Electroencephalogram (EEG) and computed tomography (CT) scan as well as magnetic resonance imaging (MRI) or other radiological studies might also be indicated. Clinical judgment should dictate the extent of a laboratory workup based on the individual child. Laboratory tests may be quite specific in the etiological diagnosis of some developmental disabilities. For example, if the clinical findings suggest a diagnosis of Williams syndrome, only one specific laboratory DNA test for this condition needs to be ordered. In cases for which medical history does not provide clues to the etiology for children with significant disabilities, urine metabolic screening, chromosome study, and DNA molecular analysis for fragile X syndrome are recommended. The evaluation for fragile X syndrome is mandatory when there is a family history of developmental disabilities such as learning disability, mental retardation, or attention-deficit/hyperactivity disorder.

When laboratory tests are inconclusive, the neurodevelopmental pediatrician, using clinical experience and judgment, might be able to make a tentative medical diagnosis based solely on the history and physical findings. In situations in which a categorical diagnosis is considered, the final diagnostic decision will await consultation with other members of the interdisciplinary team.

Examples of Decision Making Through Case Studies

The following case studies illustrate the work of neurodevelopmental pediatricians in assessing conditions and recommending interventions. In the first example, involving Michael, history and physical examination were instrumental in identifying the medical etiology of a child's developmental disability. The second study, which discusses Don's case, illustrates a situation in which an etiological diagnosis cannot be made and the team arrives at a categorical diagnosis.

Michael

Michael was referred to the interdisciplinary team for assessment of developmental delays at age 5. During the pediatric evaluation his parents expressed their concerns about coordination difficulties and delayed speech-language development. They asked what had caused his developmental delays.

Pregnancy, delivery, and immediate postnatal period were unremarkable. Michael's parents reported mild delays in all developmental milestones. Michael started experiencing grand mal seizures at 18 months of age and was being treated by a neurologist. He had received early intervention services since he was $2^{1}/_{2}$ years old, attended a special education preschool, and received occupational and speech-language therapy.

Michael's parents were healthy college graduates; his 3-year-old sister was described as healthy and typically developing. A maternal uncle, who had graduated from college, was being monitored for a seizure disorder. The family history otherwise revealed no significant medical information.

The general physical examination was remarkable only for a red papular rash over the malar region (cheeks, nasolabial folds, and chin), which did not fade when pressure was applied. There were several depigmented spots that measured between 1 and 2 centimeters in diameter over the lower extremities, the back, and the abdominal wall. He also had a macular erythematous-like rash over the back that was approximately 2 × 5 inches in diameter and with irregular distribution. Neurodevelopmental examination revealed unsteady gait, poor running skills, and mild intention tremor.

Assessment

The presence of skin lesions, combined with a history of developmental delay and seizures, raised the possibility of a neurocutaneous disorder, specifically TS. With this diagnosis in mind, the skin was further examined in a dark room using an ultraviolet light known as a Woods Lamp. Depigmented spots were noted, many with a typical configuration (described as Ash Leaf spots) classically seen in TS.

Investigations included a CT scan of the head that revealed calcifications projecting into the ventricular cavities. An ultrasound study of the kidneys showed renal hamartomas (a tumor-like mass representing anomalous development of an organ's own tissue), which presented as bilateral polycystic kidney changes. An ophthalmologic consultation showed retinal changes characteristic of retinal phakomas that are astrocytic tumors seen in TS. These investigations confirmed the diagnosis of TS.

An Explanation of Tuberous Sclerosis

TS is an autosomal dominant, genetically heterogeneous disease. The prevalence is estimated to be 1 in 6,000. The rate of new mutation (i.e., the fresh occurrence in a fetus of a gene that causes genetic disorders) is around 60%. The clinical presentation is variable. TS is characterized by malformations and tumors of the brain, with localized motor impairments as common neurological manifestations. Infantile spasms or partial or generalized seizures are present in about two out of three patients. Mental retardation is seen in about 40%–50% of people with this condition, and hyperkinetic behaviors may be observed in many children. Increased intracranial pressure resulting from hydrocephalus, due to giant cell astrocytoma of the foramen of Monro, is seen in about 3% of cases. Children with TS may have autistic features (40%–45%) or full-fledged autism (25%) and 1%–4% of individuals with autism also have TS (Smalley, 1998). A wide variety of skin changes occur in TS. Adenoma sebaceum, a papular rash in the malar region of the face, periungual fibromas involving the nail beds, hypomelanotic macules in the form of depigmented lesions on the skin, and shagreen patches are classic examples. Eye findings are found in the form of retinal phakomas and peripapular retinal hamartomas; kidney changes, seen in about 60% of symptomatic patients, manifest as multiple renal angiomyolipomas with multiple renal tumors and renal cysts; and the heart is involved about 30%–60% of the time in the form of rhabdomyomas, a type of hamartomas, with some pulmonary changes possibly noted (Aicardi, 1993; Gomez, 1988). TS is genetically referred to as Tuberous Sclerosis Complex (TSC) and has been linked to one locus on chromosome 9 (TSC1) and another one on chromosome 16 (TSC2). There are no significant clinical differences in families with different loci.

Recommendations

The diagnosis of TS was presented to the parents as part of the team process. Because of the genetic implications, the need for genetic counseling was emphasized. The maternal uncle's history of seizures could be a mild manifestation of TS in the mother's family, which would make genetic counseling crucial. If either parent was found to have mild TS, then Michael's sister needed an assessment to determine if she had the condition. That information would be important for her when the time came to make reproductive decisions.

Don

Don was 4 years and 6 months old when he was last seen in the interdisciplinary clinic for reevaluation at the request of his parents. He had originally been referred by his pediatrician when the doctor became concerned about delayed developmental milestones at Don's 2-year checkup, and he had been seen for an earlier reevaluation at age 3 years and 2 months.

At his initial team evaluation at 25 months of age, Don was found to be functioning at a 14-month level in gross motor skills and a 15-month level in fine motor skills. His receptive language was at the 13-month level, and his expressive language was at the 10-month level. Don's developmental motor quotient was 56, and his mental quotient was less than 50. The family history was unremarkable, the pregnancy was negative for any events known to adversely affect fetal development, and the birth had been uncomplicated. Physical growth was typical with no significant dysmorphic features. Mild hypotonia was the only neurological abnormality noted except for the delayed development. Chromosomal studies, DNA molecular studies for fragile X syndrome, and a metabolic urine screen were normal. The parents were told that Don had global developmental delays of unknown etiology at the time of the initial team evaluation.

Don's mother was pregnant with a second child. The parents were told that, because of the possibility of an undiagnosable recessive disorder, their risk of having another child with delayed development was slightly higher than the risk in the general population. A great deal of time was spent with them discussing how the future implications of Don's developmental delay were uncertain because of his young age. He was referred to a developmental center in their hometown for intervention, and a reevaluation in 1 year was recommended.

At the reevaluation at 3 years and 3 months of age, Don continued to show global developmental delays. His parents were pleased with Don's progress and expressed their satisfaction with the developmental center. They reported that his 10-month-old sister seemed to be more active and alert than Don had been at the same age. The parents were told that Don had showed developmental progress at a steady rate compared with the first evaluation but that his developmental rate continued to be significantly slower than that of the average child.

Assessment and Recommendations

At the time of his reevaluation at age 4 years and 6 months, Don's developmental delays compared with age-mates had become very apparent to his parents, and they noted that Don's younger sister was catching up with him developmentally. They had many questions about Don's future. He continued to show significant global delays, with an IQ score of 55 on the fourth edition of the Stanford-Binet Intelligence Scale (Stanford-Binet-IV; Thorndike, Hagen, & Sattler, 1986). His expressive language was at the 20-month level, which was his most seriously delayed area. His gross motor skills were his strongest area of development (34-month level). The parents were told that mental retardation requiring limited support would be the term most appropriately used to describe Don's cognitive functioning in the future and that this diagnosis would secure educational and other services he might need over time. Recommendations were made for planning for the move from the developmental center to an inclusive public school program and to include speech-language and occupational therapy services.

As had been done on both previous parent conferences, Don's parents were told that the cause of their son's developmental delays remained undetermined. It was explained that the cause most likely was of prenatal onset due to an unknown prenatal process. They were again reassured that the cause was not due to anything they had done, or neglected to do, at any time either before or after his birth.

INTERPRETATION AND RECOMMENDATIONS

The degree of confidence with which the clinician can inform the family about their child's diagnosis of disability varies greatly. Once a specific medical etiological diagnosis is identified, as in the first case study, specific information can be shared with the family. The child's immediate and long-term needs can be discussed. Identifying a specific syndrome assists in establishing a prognosis, even though there is extensive variability in outcome within syndromes. The day-to-day care of a young child with a disability might not change, even if the underlying cause is known. However, the family's accurate understanding of the reason for their child's difficulties often seems to improve their ability to cope with a difficult situation.

When a vague categorical diagnosis is the only one that can be made, as in the second case study, the clinician's degree of confidence in the diagnosis is significantly lower. The younger the child, the more uncertain the prognosis, hence the diagnosis of developmental delay. As of 2000, the etiology of developmental disabilities remains totally unknown in an estimated 30%–40% of cases despite a careful history and assessment.

When no specific etiology is identified, as seen in the second case study, it is important to assess the family's perspective of the medical history and their understanding of the cause of the disability. For example, there are often occurrences surrounding the birth that were very traumatic to the parent even though, in retrospect, they do not explain the child's present disability. The parents may need to have this put into perspective. Whether she expresses these thoughts or not, a birth mother invariably questions if there was something she did or did not do during the months she was carrying the child that caused the disability. In the majority of cases the answer is a reassuring no, but this issue needs to be addressed at some point during the assessment, whether it is during the medical evaluation, at the parent conference, or at both times.

When dealing with families of children having other categorical diagnoses such as cerebral palsy and autism, the clinician's confidence in the diagnosis certainly is increased, and it will be more definite and detailed as the child grows older. In children with cerebral palsy, it is often unclear what specific event or events caused the damage to the brain, as discussed in previous sections, and families often need repeated and detailed discussions on the medical aspects of this diagnosis. In autism, a profound neurodevelopmental disability, a most puzzling aspect to professionals and families is the lack of noteworthy medical events and the absence of deviant physical findings. Only a very small percentage of children with autism have a recognizable medical etiology to their disability (e.g., TS, fragile X syndrome).

On rare occasions, the cause of a child's developmental disability needs to be determined quickly. If the mother is in the early stages of a new pregnancy at the time of the evaluation, it may be possible to diagnose a chromosomal anomaly, metabolic error, or neural tube defect in the developing fetus in time for her to make important reproductive decisions.

One of the more helpful areas available to families with children with developmental disabilities is the growing number of parent support organizations. These may be devoted to specific medical conditions or directed at categorical disability diagnoses. Families can receive information and have opportunities to communicate and share advice regarding the management of their children's problems. Since the end of the 20th century, even those living in remote areas can interact with others through support groups on the Internet. Many World Wide Web sites have been created that are devoted to specific developmental disabilities.

ISSUES PARTICULARLY RELEVANT TO THE DISCIPLINE

Determining an etiology for a developmental disability might not be possible on the initial evaluation. In the very young child, the medical picture changes with time. Hypotonia is a common, nonspecific symptom in infants. In some, it heralds cerebral palsy because spasticity (increased muscle tone) or athetosis (fluctuating muscle tone, sometimes called *dystonia*) might develop later. Moreover, facial features, characteristic for many syndromes associated with developmental disabilities, are frequently not recognizable at birth but develop over time. In an occasional case, the child's developmental course changes, with regression in functioning. This might indicate a degenerative process. Finally, the medical information relating to developmental disabilities is forever growing, and etiologies that cannot be determined today may be understandable tomorrow. Thus, the search for the etiology of developmental disabilities is a dynamic process often requiring repeated assessments.

The proper use of medical consultants is another important issue in neurodevelopmental pediatrics. The neurodevelopmental pediatrician is trained in the assessment and care of children with developmental disabilities, but if during the medical examination a child is suspected of having scoliosis, an orthopedic referral is needed, and the referral is initiated either through the neurodevelopmental pediatrician or the child's primary physician. Similarly, if hydrocephalus is suspected, a neurosurgical consultation is appropriate. Follow-up care and treatment of the occasional child found with psychosis is clearly the purview of child psychiatry. Similarly, psychopharmacological treatment of severe behavioral manifestations of developmental disabilities may also require consultation.

The relationship between a child's community physician and the consulting neurodevelopmental pediatrician is an important one. Oral and written communications are vital to assure follow-up care. Children with developmental disabilities typically have more medical difficulties, more complex health problems, and a family that needs support. An active general pediatrician or family practitioner should ideally be the child's primary health care provider.

Finally, young children with developmental disabilities and their families have complex needs that present challenges to many professions. Give-and-take during personal interactions on a well-functioning interdisciplinary team provides the neurodevelopmental pediatrician with a most satisfying and stimulating place to practice the newly recognized pediatric subspecialty of neurodevelopmental disability.

REFERENCES
Aicardi, J. (1993). Tuberous sclerosis. *Internal Pediatrics, 8*, 171–175.

Gomez, M.R. (1988). *Tuberous sclerosis* (2nd ed.). Philadelphia: Lippincott, Williams & Wilkins.

Jones, K.L. (1997). *Smith's recognizable patterns of human malformation* (5th ed.). Philadelphia: W.B. Saunders Company.

Montgomery, T.R., & Jones, K.L. (1996). The dysmorphology examination. In A.J. Capute & P.J. Accardo (Eds.), *Developmental disabilities in infancy and childhood: Vol. I. Neurodevelopmental diagnosis and treatment* (2nd ed., pp. 283–291). Baltimore: Paul H. Brookes Publishing Co.

Palmer, F.B. (1996). The developmental history. In A.J. Capute & P.J. Accardo (Eds.), *Developmental disabilities in infancy and childhood: Vol. I. Neurodevelopmental diagnosis and treatment* (2nd ed., pp. 271–282). Baltimore: Paul H. Brookes Publishing Co.

Pianta, R.C., Marvin, R.S., Britner, P.A., & Borowitz, K.C. (1996). Mothers' resolution of their children's diagnosis: Organized patterns of caregiving representations. *Infant Mental Health Journal, 17*(3), 239–256.

Piper, E., & Howlin, P. (1992). Assessing and diagnosing developmental disorders that are not evident at birth: Parental evaluation of intake procedures. *Child: Care, Health and Development, 18,* 35–55.

Shapiro, B.K. (1996). Neurodevelopmental assessment of infants and young children. In A.J. Capute & P.J. Accardo (Eds.), *Developmental disabilities in infancy and childhood: Vol. I. Neurodevelopmental diagnosis and treatment* (2nd ed., pp. 311–322). Baltimore: Paul H. Brookes Publishing Co.

Smalley, S.L. (1998). Autism and tuberous sclerosis. *Journal of Autism and Developmental Disorders, 28*(5), 407–414.

Thorndike, R.L., Hagen, E.P., & Sattler, J.M. (1986). *Stanford-Binet Intelligence Scale* (4th ed.). Itasca, IL: The Riverside Publishing Co.

Chapter 5

The Nursing Role within an Interdisciplinary Assessment Team

Diane Magyary and Patricia Brandt with Gail Kieckhefer

This chapter discusses the contributions of an advanced practice nurse to the interdisciplinary team assessment approach for young children with special health care or developmental needs and their families. An advanced practice nurse specializing in this field is prepared at the master's or doctoral level in nursing. In addition to participating in the assessment and the development of an interdisciplinary care plan with individual families, the advanced practice nurse provides coordination, advocacy, and leadership in population-based program planning and evaluation (University of Kentucky, 1994). Nurses with doctoral degrees also add the skills of designing and directing research projects that meet the emerging needs of young children and their families.

This chapter primarily emphasizes the advanced practice nurse's roles in the assessment and planning processes and in care coordination. To provide the broadest possible illustration, a clinical case example in which the nurse is the service coordinator is presented. Nursing practice, diagnostic decision making, the clinical utility of assessment, issues relevant for nursing, and recommendations for the future are discussed.

PURPOSE OF ASSESSMENT
The advanced practice nurse functions in health promoting, health supporting, and health restoring roles. Throughout the assessment process, nursing care emphasizes collaborative relationships with children, families, and their communities, in addition to other professionals on the team, to fulfill the following functions: 1) determine family strengths, concerns, and unmet needs pertinent to the assessment and plan of care; 2) identify how the child and family health and developmental patterns are expressed in the context of daily living and the community environment as well as how these health patterns can be promoted, supported, or restored; and 3) participate as a team member in the assessment and planning process to obtain information pertinent to the child's goals and needs; then jointly develop an intervention plan that is culturally sensitive, developmentally appropriate, comprehensive, coordinated, and individualized to the child and family.

DOMAINS OF NURSING PRACTICE
The scope of nursing practice involves diagnostic decision making and interventions that are aimed toward the responses of individuals, families, or communities during health and illness (American Nurses Association, 1994). The assessment, diagnostic, and planning processes are but three components of the nursing process that also includes intervention and outcome evaluation. Each element of this process is part of a constant feedback loop. The diagnostic statements that develop are not fixed but function as working hypotheses to be constantly evaluated in the context of new information derived.

The nursing diagnostic taxonomy commonly used to guide an assessment is based on Gordon's (1995) typology of 11 health pattern responses. The North American Nursing Diagnosis Association (NANDA, 1994) continually revises this nursing diagnosis taxonomy for assessment. By having standardized criteria to guide the assessment, nursing accountability and thoroughness during the data collection process are enhanced. Nursing diagnoses are based on cultural, developmental, social, psychological, genetic, and biophysiological factors.

In the *National Standards of Nursing Practice for the Care of Children and Adolescents with Special Health Care and Developmental Needs* (University of Kentucky, 1994), 10 health patterns are described—with minor modifications in wording from the original 11 patterns—as being useful for guiding the assessment of children with disabilities and their families. These standards were developed by a consensus committee composed of nursing leaders in the field of childhood disabilities, and they serve as guidelines for nurses in this specialty. The 10 health pattern responses are as follows: 1) health perceptions and health management practices that include individual and community resources; 2) nutritional needs and metabolic functioning; 3) factors that affect sleep–wake patterns, activity, exercise, self-help, and recreation and vocation—such as neuromuscular, cardiovascular, respiratory, and developmental functioning; 4) elimination patterns; 5) cognitive and perceptual functioning; 6) roles, relationships, and social supports; 7) coping and stress responses, including family strengths and resources; 8) self-perception/self-concept; 9) problems and concerns with sexuality or reproductive functioning; and 10) family and community values, beliefs, concerns, and priorities (University of Kentucky, 1994, pp. 11–12).

A nursing diagnostic statement is formed within the nursing scope of practice and with consideration of input from the other disciplines on the team. For example, the cognitive and perceptual health pattern does not include the diagnosis of mental retardation. However, the nursing diagnosis of knowledge deficit is within the domain of nursing. Inappropriate developmental expectations for their children may be based on parents' lack of understanding about developmental milestones and the parameters of typical development. A nursing diagnosis of knowledge deficit in parenting provides the basis and justification for an intervention directed at enhancing parenting knowledge and skills (NANDA, 1994).

The diagnosis is obtained through data collection procedures that are planned and analytical (Shoemaker, 1984). The determination of whether a health pattern is health promotional depends on a process of comparing the assessment data to baseline information and established developmental norms, as well as cultural, social, and other relevant information (Gordon, 1987). Furthermore, the interrelationship among health patterns needs to be evaluated to understand the overall functioning exhibited by the child, the child's interaction with the family, and community responses.

REACHING AN INFORMED CLINICAL DECISION

Historically, one of nursing's most important contributions to the interdisciplinary team has been the comprehensive scope of a nursing assessment. Comprehensiveness is defined with respect to both breadth and depth of assessment. The breadth of focus can be compared to a wide-angle lens adjusted to perceive all of the health patterns, and it is inclusive of individual, family, and community responses. The depth of focus narrows the lens to obtain a close-up perspective of health patterns relevant to a particular child's and family's presenting concerns. During the assessment process, the adjustment of the lens is dynamic because both a close-up and a wide-angle view may be needed at different or concurrent time points, and one health pattern may interrelate with another. The following sections examine how breadth and depth in assessment are employed during the two phases of assessment: the preassessment stage and the assessment itself.

Preassessment Phase: Breadth of Focus

Typically, the family, primary care provider, or other professionals in the community have expressed a particular concern about the child's health, development, or behavioral-emotional status. If an assessment solely focuses on the most prominent or initially identified factors, the identification of other relevant issues may not occur. Thus, a comprehensive yet efficient screen for other concerns may ensure that the depth of a singular focus does not preclude a quick screen of many foci. A broad-based screening process invites the family's systematic review with the nurse of the child's developmental and health patterns and the family health patterns relevant to the child. A comprehensive screening conveys to the family that the interdisciplinary team desires to understand the child in an holistic and individual way.

Screening generates data indicative of typical or questionable findings. Questionable findings are followed by a more in-depth assessment. Systematic screening of health patterns may occur in a variety of ways. For example, the nurse could use the health pattern criteria and apply NANDA's 1994 diagnostic guidelines. Each component would be reviewed with the family to determine if they had any other concerns or priorities in addition to the presenting concerns. This type of approach is guided by the *Prenatal and Child Health Screening and Assessment Manual* (Region X Nursing Network, 1989), developed to screen across the health pattern responses of children ages birth–36 months and their families.

The timing for screening health patterns varies with each agency or particular clinic as well as with who is involved in the assessment process. Screening questions could be incorporated into the initial intake. This would involve a deductive reasoning process during assessment as the approach moves from general to specific. The screening begins with a broad focus to cover all of the health patterns and then progresses to an in-depth assessment of health patterns deemed as the most pertinent to the particular child and family.

In contrast, the inductive reasoning process occurs when the screening moves from specific to general. In this method, data collection begins with an in-depth look at the presenting concern and then progresses to a wider screening of the other health patterns. Those patterns most likely to interface with the health responses relevant to the presenting concern would receive priority screening. For example, as the family and child discuss the presenting concern, information revealed in the conversation may prompt the nurse to consider other health factors that appear to influence the child and family. Regardless of whether an inductive or deductive approach is used, screening, assessment, and accurate diagnostic decision making require interplay between breadth and depth.

Assessment Phase: Depth of Focus

During assessment planning, the service coordinator balances the cost and the benefits of the number of professionals involved and examines the array of assessment approaches. The thoroughness of behavior sampling and the number of perspectives obtained needs to be determined by considering multiple factors such as the type and complexity of child and family concerns, team membership, time allotted for the assessment process, cultural considerations, and cost to the family and agency. Sometimes during the assessment, the emerging data may suggest the involvement of additional disciplines; thus, the process is dynamic and fluid. The service coordinator strives to be comprehensive yet efficient and focused on the family's priorities.

The service coordinator needs to keep each member of the interdisciplinary team informed of others' assessment approaches and domains to minimize redundancy and maximize corroboration when needed. The interdisciplinary assessment process is analogous to a puzzle: Each team member and the family work together to identify and assemble the different pieces to create an accurate and useful treatment plan.

The actual content of the assessment is guided by the nursing discipline's protocols of care as well as national guidelines that are applicable across disciplines. Nurses would likely use *Nursing Standards for Children with Special Health Care Needs: Guidelines for Practice* (Magyary, Brandt, Padget, Fleming, & Kieckhefer, 1990) in addition to clinical paths such as *A Clinical Path for Assessment: Children with Nutritional Problems* (Magyary, Brandt, & Rowley, 1995). Both of these clinical paths were developed and field-tested by faculty, students, and expert clinicians affiliated with the graduate training grant Nursing Graduate Program for Leadership: Children and Adolescents with Special Health Care Needs, Families and Communities, funded by the Maternal and Child Health Bureau. Standardized protocols such as *Nursing Systems Toward Effective Parenting–Preterm* provide additional assistance in assessing a child who has sleep, eating, and parent–child interactive difficulties (Johnson-Crowley & Sumner, 1987).

Diagnostic Decision-Making
Process in an Interdisciplinary Context

To arrive at reliable and valid nursing diagnoses that interrelate with information from other disciplines, multiple measures, methods, time points, sources, contexts, and environments need to be considered as well as the integration of physiological and psychosocial data (Yin, 1995). The assessment process involves using a variety of measures and, whenever appropriate, standardized instruments. The use of standardized instruments depends on knowing on what type of sample the tool was normed and having a thorough understanding of the instrument's development, purpose, procedural guidelines for data collection, interpretation, and recording techniques. Nonstandardized instruments and interviews also provide valuable information and opportunities to hear real-life experiences from the family's perspective. Some commonly used assessment instruments for infants and toddlers are described in Table 5.1.

Methods

Different methods of data collection—such as questionnaires, interviews, observations, standardized instruments, physical exams, laboratory tests, and

Table 5.1.   Commonly used assessment instruments/protocols for infants and toddlers

Instrument	Ages	Description
Nursing Child Assessment Training (NCAT): Nursing Child Assessment Feeding Scales (Barnard, 1994b)	Birth–1 year	Standardized observation guide Assesses characteristics in six key areas found important to the interaction/adaptation process between child and parent during a feeding episode: parent sensitivity to cues, parent response to infant distress, parental fostering of socioemotional growth, parental fostering of cognitive growth, clarity of the child's cues to parent, child's responsiveness to parent Observations completed in typical feeding environment
Nursing Child Assessment Satellite Training (NCAST): Nursing Child Assessment Teaching Scales (Barnard, 1994a)	Birth–3 years	Standardized observation guide Assesses characteristics in six key areas found important to the interaction/adaptation process between child and parent as the parent teaches the child a new activity: parent sensitivity to cues, parent response to infant distress, parental fostering of socioemotional growth, parental fostering of cognitive growth, clarity of the child's cues to parent, child's responsiveness to parent Suggests specific age-appropriate activities for the parent to teach
Nursing Child Assessment Training (NCAT): Nursing Child Assessment Sleep/ Activity Record (Barnard, 1979)	Birth–1 year	Seven-day diary record kept by parents to enable the identification of patterns of activity that are emerging in their child Activities useful to track: sleep, feedings, crying episodes, awake periods, diaper changes, specific parent–child interactions Knowledge of patterns can reassure parents, form the basis for interventions
A Clinical Path for Assessment: Children with Nutritional Problems (Magyary, Brandt, & Rowley, 1995)	Birth–3 years	Multistep clinical guide Help organize, deliver, and evaluate children with special health care needs in terms of their nutrition/metabolic health pattern and four additional areas often disrupted when feeding problems exist Outcomes are considered at initial, short-, and long-term assessments: support for optimal growth and wellness, parental/care providers' management of the feeding plan, ability to deal with stress associated with the feeding, positive influence of family roles and relationships on feeding, child's developmental skills that support the feeding

Table 5.1.   *(continued)*

Instrument	Ages	Description
Nursing Standards for Children with Special Health Care Needs: Guidelines for Practice (Magyary, Brandt, Padget, Fleming, & Kieckhefer, 1990)	Birth–3 years	Comprehensive guide to assess children with special health care needs; eleven functional health patterns: nutrition/metabolic, elimination, sleep/rest, activity/exercise, cognitive perceptual, health perception/management, self-concept/self-perception, roles/relationship, sexuality/reproductive, coping/stress tolerance, values/beliefs
		Includes listing of common etiologies for problems, important goals, useful screening and assessment tools for each pattern
Protocol Manual: Nursing Systems Toward Effective Parenting–Preterm (Johnson-Crowley, & Sumner, 1987)	Birth–1 year	Standardized format
		Comprehensive assessment of preterm infants and intervention with their families
		Format includes designated visits with specified assessment instruments and intervention strategies
		Specific handouts included
Prenatal and Child Health Screening and Assessment Manual: Pregnancy and Birth to 36 Months (Region X Nursing Network, 1989)	Birth–3 years	Standardized format
		Screens and assesses eleven functional health patterns during prenatal period and first 3 years of life
		Patterns include nutrition/metabolic, elimination, sleep/rest, activity/exercise, cognitive/perceptual, health perception/management, self-concept/self-perception, roles/relationship, sexuality/reproductive issues, coping/stress tolerance, values/beliefs

records—are important to include in the assessment process. Each method provides a slightly different view of the entire picture. The nurse searches for patterns that emerge when data corroborate across different methods.

Time Points
Different time points provide evidence of the stability or instability of patterns over time. Therefore, it is helpful to evaluate the family's perspective about the child's feeding patterns, for example, both on weekdays and weekends or in mornings and evenings.

Sources
Data collected from different sources—including other professionals, the child, the mother, the father, or siblings—provide for consideration of multiple perspectives. One can obtain information about the child's sleep patterns from both the mother and the father as well as how each responds to the interrup-

tions in the night. Anyone relevant to the pertinent health patterns needs to be involved. In addition to the immediate family members, information is required from other sources such as the child care provider or an extended family member consistently involved in the child's care. When the child has communication and language skills, it is helpful to plan the assessment so that the family and the child can be seen together and alone to provide information regarding differences and consistencies.

Contexts
Data collected across contexts about a particular health pattern provide feedback on how behavior is manifested in different situations. For instance, obtaining material about the father–child relationship in both feeding and structured play teaching scenarios helps determine what types of interactive situations lead to the emergence of both problematic and nonproblematic patterns. The identification of nonproblematic components assists in generating an intervention plan that capitalizes on child and family strengths.

Settings
The collection of data across various environments, such as clinic, home, and school, provides information on how behavior is expressed in different environments. The plan of services and supports can then be better developed, with approaches subsequently directed toward the environments in which difficulties are expressed.

The service coordinator needs to analyze the appropriateness, feasibility, benefits, and cost of home and school visits. Certainly, if data derived from the clinic observation and parent interview conflict or are incomplete, having information about a particular health pattern from another environment would clarify and enhance the profile of the data obtained. Ecologically valid information is found in the home, while the clinic affords an opportunity for the family to participate in the assessment free from the everyday stresses in their natural environment. A home visit should be considered if a caregiver states that his or her interaction with the child differs from that at home or in the child care center. If a home visit is not possible due to the particular agency's policies, obtaining information from a child care provider or a community health nurse may be a useful alternative.

Integration of Biophysical and Psychosocial Data
The integration of biophysical and psychosocial data provides a holistic perspective of the particular health response pattern. For example, a child's weight and height ratio, a food diary completed by a parent, and the nurse's and nutritionist's observations of a feeding interaction between parent and child will confirm or disconfirm data about this health pattern.

Through the assessment process, evidence is accumulated in support of inferences about a particular health pattern and its interrelationship with other health patterns. A nursing diagnosis is confirmed by constantly evaluating consistency and inconsistency within the data set as manifested across measurements, methods, time points, sources, environments, contexts, and biophysical and psychosocial data. The process of diagnostic decision making and clinical judgment involves a search for patterns and variations in those patterns. A diagnosis is not based on a few isolated pieces of data but, rather, on multiple pieces of data that corroborate with each other and converge on a particular factor. A valid and reliable clinical decision about the child's and family's health patterns is substantiated by looking for consistency across multiple pieces of data.

Nursing Diagnoses

Nursing diagnoses in an interdisciplinary context usually are made in conjunction with information collected and diagnoses generated by other disciplines. Taken together, data gathered by various disciplines describe the nature of an individual's health, development, functional status, and needs. The nature of the interdisciplinary team is an important consideration as the nurse begins the assessment process. When a professional from a closely related discipline is a member of the team, discussion with that person is critical to ensure the domain is assessed in the most efficient yet comprehensive manner, with duplication of efforts only in desired areas. For instance, if the nursing screening data indicated a potential concern in the nutrition or metabolic pattern, the selection of assessment strategies would differ depending on whether a nutritionist is part of the interdisciplinary team. If a nutritionist is on the team, the assessment plan may dictate that both the nurse and the nutritionist observe and evaluate a feeding, noting different and similar components. However, only the nutritionist would be responsible for eliciting a 24-hour diet recall from the family to determine the variety and quantity of food intake.

Utility of Assessment Yields Recommendations

The assessment process is not conducted with the sole purpose of rendering diagnostic statements. It also serves to provide direction for the implementation and evaluation of interventions. Recommendations determined by this linkage of assessment and intervention are referred to as *treatment utility of assessment* (Hayes, Nelson, & Jarrett, 1987).

The results of the assessment and implications for interventions are based on perspectives jointly shared by and discussed between the family and the interdisciplinary team, with the service coordinator serving as the group process facilitator (see Chapter 1). Parent conferences are too often structured to deliver a particular diagnosis and to make intervention plan recommendations, but this should be a collaborative process. The extent to which parents are actively encouraged to participate in the generation of ideas or tailoring them for relevance and feasibility varies dramatically from one team to another. In addition, a follow-up conference with the family may reveal a valuable perspective—the extent to which the family found the assessment process and final conferencing session useful. Perhaps a series of family sessions would provide opportunities for a family to understand the material more fully. In turn, they could then be more active participants in the development of an intervention plan that includes identifying and eliciting specific community resources.

The notion of intervention utility for assessment is vividly depicted in a 1995 article by Taffel, a family therapist and the director of the Family and Couples Treatment Services at the Institute for Contemporary Psychotherapy. Taffel poignantly described what it was like to have his child evaluated at an early childhood center by an interdisciplinary team of experts. He highlighted two points that provide ideas for changing health care practices.

Family's Daily Life and Routines

Taffel's first recommendation was that professionals need to be curious about the ordinary. Despite hours of testing, the details of the family's daily life and routines are often not explored. Details of what occurs in the home on a daily basis offer the professional clues on how to dialogue further with family members and build relevant interventions with them. Ideally, the assessment yields information for intervention approaches that are jointly developed with the family. The prompt "tell me about a typical day" is often used by nurses to elicit everyday details. This style of interviewing could be further developed and studied for its usefulness. Taffel suggested an expansion of this question into the following set of three queries:

1. "Tell me what your routine is like on weekdays. How about Saturday and Sunday?"
2. "Describe to me the important transitions—the morning chaos, after school, the evening grind, and bedtime."
3. Describe for me some typical interactions around the house concerning conflict, communication, and having fun." (1995, p. 27)

Child and Family Strengths

Taffel's (1995) second recommendation was to highlight the child's and family's positive aspects. During the assessment of Taffel's child, family strengths were not addressed with the same rigor as family problems. As many clinical phenomena exhibit variations, exceptions or unique outcomes are critical to understanding what is occurring. Assessment approaches that concentrate on positive patterns within a problematic situation are commonly referred to in literature as *solution-oriented approaches* (Berg, 1994; DeJong & Berg, 1996; White & Epston, 1990). Although these positive variations may be atypical, they can offer insight about potential solutions and amplifying potential strengths.

The exceptions to problems and strengths provide key ideas for developing an intervention that augments the child's and family's strong points. Since the early 1990s, assessment and intervention approaches that systematically identify and highlight strengths have gained popularity (Berg, 1994; DeJong & Berg, 1996; White & Epston, 1990). Further development and testing of solution-focused assessment and intervention approaches by nurses fit with the strong nursing tradition that emphasizes health promotion and individual, family, and community strengths.

Examples of Decision Making Through a Case Study

The following case study illustrates the clinical concepts related to screening, assessment, service plan development, and care coordination. The parents of Johnny, a 30-month-old Asian American child, and their primary care provider requested a team evaluation and expressed two concerns. The main issue was that Johnny's parents were having difficulty feeding him. In addition, the primary care provider had documented that Johnny had a developmental delay, but the degree of delay and its etiology were undetermined and needed further investigation. The parents thought that Johnny was a "bit slow but that, eventually, he would grow out if it."

The advanced practice nurse on the team was designated as the service coordinator. Upon reviewing the intake information and prior health record, the nurse decided to screen for other potential health patterns before determining the full complement of disciplines to be involved in the assessment. The presenting data indicated that a comprehensive well-child screening had not occurred since Johnny's visit at 18 months of age. Due to the feeding issues and age of the child, priority was placed on seeing the family within the month.

The screening was guided by the Child Health Standards Screen (Region X Nursing Network, 1989). This instrument is a standardized checklist of several questions that pertain to each of the 11 health response patterns (Gordon, 1995). The suspected problems are then recorded on the Standards Screen Summary Sheet (Region X Nursing Network, 1989). In the service coordinator role, the advanced practice nurse began the screening process using a collaborative approach with the family (see Brandt, 1993). The family's expectations for the complete process (assessment, diagnosis, and planning) and their goals were discussed and clarified. The nurse introduced the screening intake procedure to the parents by acknowledging the family's primary concern and explaining to them that she would like to assess Johnny comprehensively to ensure that no other problems would be overlooked. The nurse then asked the parents to share their expert opinion of Johnny by inviting them to answer interview questions.

The results of the screening process indicated that in addition to the initial issues of feeding and development, the following areas were found to be of concern to the parents and, thus, were included in the more in-depth assessment plan: 1) sleep pattern, 2) parent–child relationship pattern, 3) coping/stress tolerance pattern, and 4) health perception and management pattern. The child's sleep patterns were irregular and had begun to interrupt his parents' sleep. Subsequently, the parents found it more and more difficult to interact with Johnny or to have successful outcomes regarding his sleep and eating patterns. His parents had also experienced several major life changes within the year that added to their parenting challenges and difficulties in finding a relaxed time to feed Johnny. They were becoming increasingly frustrated because they were having little success improving his eating and, therefore, their sense of competence as parents was eroding. In addition, discipline was becoming an issue in their relationship with Johnny. His parents acknowledged during the screening process that they were beginning to have second thoughts about Johnny outgrowing his delays in development. They believed that they would benefit by obtaining a better understanding of Johnny's delay; thus, they concurred that the etiology and prognosis of Johnny's delay needed to be added to the priorities for assessment.

Assessment

The overall assessment plan was then developed by the advanced practice nurse as the care coordinator, with the family members and pertinent disciplines consulted. Table 5.2 shows the primary domains related to the major concerns and the disciplines involved.

The parent–child relationship and interactive patterns were assessed in a variety of ways. In this instance, an open-ended interview question was asked: "What has it been like for you to have this challenge of helping Johnny with his eating?" The parents noted that at every well-child visit they felt that they were not good parents because Johnny was losing weight, so they had decided to be more forceful during eating times to ensure Johnny would eat. The nurse observed the parent–child interactive pattern in a feeding situation using the Nursing Child Assessment Training (NCAT) Feeding Scales (Barnard, 1994b). The parents developed a feeding style that ignored Johnny's disengagement cues during feeding, and, subsequently, they tended to overstimulate him. Johnny, in turn, became irritable and often tried to withdraw from the feeding episode.

Table 5.2.   Primary domains related to and disciplines involved in assessing major concerns for Johnny

Etiology and severity of the developmental delay
  Speech-language pathology
  Pediatrics
  Psychology
  Occupational therapy

Nutritional patterns, parent–child feeding interactive patterns
  Nursing
  Nutrition
  Occupational therapy

Parent–child relationship patterns and interactive patterns in nonfeeding situations, child and family sleep patterns, coping/stress tolerance pattern, and health perception/management patterns
  Nursing

Although Johnny's parents' intentions were appropriate, the feeding strategies they selected were counterproductive, and the interactive issues were not resolved. Both parents corroborated that this interactive pattern had been ongoing over the past few months. In addition, Johnny's growth parameters had fallen below his own growth curve (the 25th percentile) to the 5th percentile.

The feeding interactive patterns were complicated in that Johnny exhibited difficulty in providing clear engagement and disengagement behavioral cues during the feeding episode. Johnny's atypical motor coordination during the feeding episode was confirmed by the occupational therapist's evaluation. Temporal data were collected over time from a parental log of the feeding schedule and associated feeding approaches during the week and weekends by using the NCAT Sleep/Activity Record (Barnard, 1979).

A parent–child interaction during a teaching situation also was observed using the Nursing Child Assessment Satellite Training (NCAST) Teaching Scales (Barnard, 1994a). The feeding and teaching observational scales provided a comparison of interactions in two different situations. Johnny's parents also completed the Parenting Stress Index Questionnaire (Loyd & Abidin, 1985) to provide information regarding the stress they each experienced during feeding and other interactions with Johnny. An understanding of the cultural implications of the family's challenges regarding feeding is also a criterion of the nursing diagnostic guidelines. Beginning knowledge of cultural influences on the family's practices can be obtained through an interview question such as, "In your culture, are there particular ways recommended for trying to help the child eat better?"

By asking Johnny's parents about daily experiences, both the parents and the nurse arrived at a better understanding of Johnny's sleep–wake patterns in the context of family activities. Subsequently, the intervention was planned by having the family identify which routines they believed could be modified and would likely then improve Johnny's sleep–wake cycles. The aim was to increase regularity involving Johnny's sleep as well as to improve his inherent capacity for sleep–wake organization.

Recommendations

Although Johnny and his parents had difficulty engaging in a reciprocal interactive pattern during the feeding episodes, the teaching interactions proved otherwise. The teaching interactive episode as measured by the NCAT Feeding Scales (Barnard, 1994b) revealed that Johnny and each parent were able to engage in playful social behavioral exchanges. Johnny was found to exhibit clearer social cues of engagement and disengagement, and his parents were able to identify these cues and to respond appropriately. Thus, the teaching interaction served to reinforce a sense of competence for each parent. It also provided the exceptions needed to begin building an intervention plan that would generalize and extend the positive aspects of teaching experiences to the feeding interactions.

With respect to Johnny's clinical care, *A Clinical Path for Assessment and Management: Children with Nutritional Problems* (Magyary et al., 1995) provided the blueprint to relate the intervention plan systematically to the assessment findings. The intervention plan included Johnny's being enrolled in an early intervention program coupled with the parents' desire to enroll in a parenting support group provided by the Asian American community. His parents and the nurse coordinator collaborated regarding how to implement the specifics of the intervention plan. The extent to which the nurse coordinator remains a service manager versus relinquishing the role to a professional at the early intervention program depends on the breadth of services required, the community-based professionals' scope of practice, and parent preferences.

Throughout this assessment process, the nurse searched for patterns in the data set that could be corroborated across different methods of data collection (interview, observation, questionnaire), different sources (mother, father, and professionals from other disciplines), and different interactive situations (feeding and structured play teaching). The physical growth data, coupled with the feeding interactive data, corroborated the pattern of an altered parent–child feeding interactive process that resulted in serious ramifications on the child's nutritional and caloric intake. However, the altered feeding interactive pattern did not generalize to the structured play teaching situation.

At this stage in the assessment process, whether a home visit or another clinic visit would be considered depends on the clinic resources, the severity of the problem, and the contextual factors that may influence the validity of the assessment data. Perhaps a home visit would be warranted in the initial stages of developing, activating, and evaluating an intervention plan.

ISSUES RELEVANT TO NURSING AND FUTURE RECOMMENDATIONS

An advanced practice nurse's functions also include service coordination, community assessment, program development, and the provision of culturally competent care. Issues associated with these roles and recommendations for using them in the context of an interdisciplinary assessment are discussed in this section.

Service Coordination

With the increased emphasis on service coordination as a key component of cost-effective and quality health care, the future holds creative opportunities for interdisciplinary child assessment teams to provide coordination and advocacy services within a health care arena that is becoming progressively dominated by managed care. The service coordinator role holds special promise for the interdisciplinary team's articulation with managed care. However, clear answers are needed with respect to the type, purpose, functions, and goals of service coordination provided by the interdisciplinary team. Thoughtful solutions to the following questions are needed: How can the process of assessment be streamlined and coordinated to eliminate unnecessary and redundant steps as well as to promote quality and the timely delivery of services? How can the collaborative process between the service coordinator and the family be enhanced to create informed decision making, family-directed care, service coordination, and advocacy functions? What strategies enable the service coordinator to facilitate communication and decision making among family members and a variety of professionals and agencies in an opportune and cost-effective manner?

Numerous terms have been used to describe service coordination over the years depending on the nature of the organization, the type of services, the population targeted, and the coordinator's field. The advance practice nurse providing service and resource coordination for families within a single agency is described as the *internal case manager* or, when across agencies, as the *external case manager* (Case Management Society of America [CMSA], 1995). Over the years, the common provisions of service coordination have consisted of timely identification of problems, promoting access to supports, and organization and monitoring of quality services. In addition, cost-effective approaches have played a central role in providing service coordination in which the primary goal is to meet the complex health needs of individuals of all ages within the context of their families and communities (CMSA, 1995, p. 8).

The extent of follow-through on the interdisciplinary assessment team's intervention plan may be compromised without a designated coordinator who works with the family to ensure that the various components of the recommended intervention plan, including access to community-based resources, are executed and evaluated. Whether by default or plan, the role-defined boundaries of an internal versus external service coordinator often merge to guarantee implementation and evaluation of the plan. With the increase in service coordination as a key component of cost-effective and quality care, interdisciplinary teams can ensure that the intervention plan developed is with family realities in mind and that revisions to the plan are made in the implementation phase when the family deems them necessary.

Since the 1990s, nurses have been increasingly designated as service coordinators in health care organizations, given their breadth of focus and integrated approach to health care (CMSA, 1995). The nursing profession has been instrumental in developing strategies and techniques that enhance service coordination, such as clinical paths (Zander, 1991). Clinical paths function as blueprints for guiding assessments and interventions over time and across service providers with respect to client-defined outcomes of supports and services.

A Clinical Path for Assessment and Management: Children with Nutritional Problems (Magyary et al., 1995) provides an ideal instrument to assist the advanced practice nurse in coordinating and ensuring continuity of the community-based interventions. The clinical path serves as a guideline whereby the essential components of care are organized as intervention outcome statements with respect to the health response patterns of nutrition, activities and development, roles and relationships, coping and stress tolerance, and health perception and management. The components of care are organized across an initial phase, the short-term follow-up phase, and the long-term follow-up phase. The nurse coordinator, in collaboration with the family and the interdisciplinary team, prioritizes the components of care and develops a community-based intervention plan. The nurse coordinator and the family jointly problem-solve regarding the identification of community resources that could potentially interface with the plan. As the intervention plan is put into action, the nurse coordinator and the family continually evaluate the child's prognosis and the extent to which the intervention plan proves to be realistic, meaningful, efficacious, and accessible in the community. Periodically, the nurse as service coordinator and the family consult with the other disciplines to discuss an intervention plan that needs modification.

Program Development and Evaluation

Nursing has long recognized that human beings' responses to health and illness situations are influenced by their culture and environment (American Nurses Association, 1995). Therefore, the nurse coordinator needs to understand the community context and culture that influence families' health response patterns. An involvement in the community outside of the child development center's walls is valuable for generating outreach programs as well as for fostering population-based services within the community. The interplay between gathering data on individual families and the collection of aggregate data on populations is dynamic. As the advanced practice nurse in a service coordinator role interacts with individual families at an interdisciplinary child development center, the systematic collection of data across families may generate child and family profiles that suggest a need to complete a broader-based community assessment to document program and social policy needs on behalf of families and communities.

The successful implementation of an individualized and family-centered intervention is often contingent on the availability and appropriateness of community-based services. As the interdisciplinary team and the family generate a community-based intervention plan, the accessibility of community resources needs to be analyzed. This analysis requires the nurse as service coordinator not only to be aware of community resources but also to advocate for community resources that sustain intervention plans. Nursing interventions are both direct and indirect (American Nurses Association, 1995). Direct interventions are conducted through interactions with families, whereas indirect interventions are performed on behalf of families through interactions with health care environments and communities. "The nurse, in collaboration with the family and other providers, pursues strategies to enhance access to and utilization of adequate health care, social and educational services" (University of Kentucky, 1994, p. 23).

Inherent in program development is program evaluation. The advanced practice nurse, in collaboration with colleagues at the child development center, participates in the clinical evaluation component of care. The quality, effectiveness, and cost benefits of clinical services are monitored and evaluated in relation to child, family, and community outcomes (University of Kentucky, 1994). The ongoing evaluation data are used to revise how services are provided within the interdisciplinary team as well as how those services interface with community programs. Family and community input into the overall design, for monitoring and appraising the process and outcome dimensions of program evaluation, have proven useful in generating meaningful data and interpreting the implications of the data for program revisions (Ogles, Lambert, & Masters, 1996; Sperry, Brill, Howard, & Grissom, 1996). Nurses who practice at an advanced level do so by systematically studying and evaluating their practice in collaboration with other disciplines, families, and communities; they then use the results to support practice changes.

The issue of program development and evaluation needs to be considered in the context of culture so that culturally sensitive and competent services and supports are provided. Professional providers increasingly experience more opportunities to interact with a diverse population of clients. Consideration of one's culture entails understanding the various group norms as well as individual differences within group norms and, thus, seeking clarification from the child and family regarding how they perceive their culture. Culture shapes health beliefs that are in turn linked to health practices. The family's values, beliefs, and customs have important implications for assessment and intervention. The tendency to stereotype families according to cultural groups may be minimized by professionals eliciting information about and being sensitive to the ways in which a particular family's health beliefs and practices are consistent or inconsistent with the group norms of their self-defined cultural group. Community partnerships with representatives from diverse communities will enhance culturally competent care provided at child development centers (Anderson & Fenichel, 1989).

CONCLUSION

Constant change in the delivery and accountability of health care prompts interdisciplinary collaboration in the discovery of new ways to provide quality services and supports to families and their children. Interdisciplinary teams provide opportunities for collaboration as one way to respond to the challenges outlined by the Pew Health Professions Commission (1995). The evolving health care system places value on the coordination of interdisciplinary services, with an emphasis on improving efficiency and effectiveness—including client satisfaction. Interdisciplinary collaboration needs further exploration for a better understanding of the best ways to interface each discipline's expertise on behalf of families. Health care systems are placing more significance on

consumers by increasing partnership building between families and professionals. Valuing how individual families prefer to collaborate requires embrac-
ing diversity in one's conceptualization of creating partnerships. Finally, expectations for professional accountability are becoming a norm given the growing
scrutiny of cost–benefit analysis. How best to provide comprehensive assessments that have clinical utility for both short- and long-term outcomes requires
additional study by the interdisciplinary teams involved in these assessments.
Responsive client-oriented and cost-balanced approaches are needed to meet
the challenges emerging in the arena of health care reform.

REFERENCES

American Nurses Association Nursing's Social Policy Statement Task Force. (1994).
    Nursing's social policy statement. Washington, DC: American Nurses Publishing.
Anderson, P.P., & Fenichel, E.S. (1989). *Servicing culturally diverse families of infants and tod-
    dlers with disabilities.* Arlington, VA: ZERO TO THREE: National Center for Infants,
    Toddlers, and Families.
Barnard, K. (1979). *Nursing child assessment training (NCAT): Nursing Child Assessment
    Sleep/Activity Record.* Seattle, WA: NCAT Publications.
Barnard, K. (1994a). *Nursing child assessment satellite training (NCAST): Nursing Child Assess-
    ment Teaching Scales.* Seattle, WA: NCAST Publications.
Barnard, K. (1994b). *Nursing child assessment training (NCAT): Nursing Child Assessment Feed-
    ing Scales.* Seattle, WA: NCAT Publications.
Berg, I.K. (1994). *Family based services: A solution-focused approach.* New York: W.W. Nor-
    ton & Company.
Brandt, P. (1993). Negotiation and problem-solving strategies: Building partnerships
    between families whose children have special health care needs and professionals.
    *Journal of Infants and Young Children: An Interdisciplinary Journal of Special Care Practices,
    5*(4), 1–6.
Case Management Society of America. (1995). *Standards of practice for case management.* Lit-
    tle Rock, AR: Author.
DeJong, P., & Berg, I. K. (1996). *Interviewing for solutions.* Milwaukee, WI: Brief Family
    Therapy Center.
Gordon, M. (1987). *Nursing diagnosis: Process and application* (2nd ed.). New York: The
    McGraw-Hill Companies.
Gordon, M. (1995). *Manual of nursing diagnosis 1995–1996* (p. 2). St. Louis, MO: Mosby.
Hayes, S.C., Nelson, R.O., & Jarrett, R.B. (1987). The treatment utility of assessment:
    A functional approach to evaluating assessment quality. *American Psychologist, 42*(11),
    963–974.
Johnson-Crowley, N., & Sumner. G.A. (Eds.). (1987). *Protocol manual: Nursing systems to-
    ward effective parenting–preterm.* Seattle, WA: NCAST Publications.
Loyd, B.H., & Abidin, R.R. (1985). Revision of the Parenting Stress Index. *Journal of
    Pediatric Psychology, 10*(2), 169–177.
Magyary, D., Brandt, P., Padget, D., Fleming, J., & Kieckhefer, G. (1990). *Nursing stan-
    dards for children with special health care needs: Guidelines for practice.* Seattle: University of
    Washington Press.
Magyary, D., Brandt, P., & Rowley, M. (1995). *A clinical path for assessment: Children with
    nutritional problems.* Seattle: University of Washington Press.
North American Nursing Diagnosis Association. (1994). *NANDA nursing diagnoses: Defini-
    tions and classification 1995–1996.* Philadelphia: Author.

Ogles, B.M., Lambert, M.J., & Masters, K.S. (1996). *Assessing outcome in clinical practice.* Needham Heights, MA: Allyn & Bacon.

Pew Health Professions Commission. (1995). *Critical challenges: Revitalizing the health professions for the twenty-first century.* San Francisco: Center for Health Professions.

Region X Nursing Network. (1989). *Prenatal and child health screening and assessment manual: Pregnancy and birth to 36 months.* Seattle: University of Washington Press.

Shoemaker, J. (1984). Essential features of a nursing diagnoses. In M.J. Kim, G. McFarland, & A. McLane (Eds.), *Classification of nursing diagnoses: Proceedings of the Fifth National Conference.* St. Louis, MO: Mosby.

Sperry, L., Brill, P.L., Howard, K.I., & Grissom, G.R. (1996). *Treatment outcomes in psychotherapy and psychiatric interventions.* Levittown, PA: Brunner/Mazel Publishing.

Taffel, R. (1995, November/December). Honoring the everyday. *Networker,* 25–28, 56.

University of Kentucky, Consensus Committee, Leadership Development for Nurses in Early Intervention (Grant MCJ-215052 from the Maternal and Child Health Bureau). (1994). *National standards of nursing practice for the care of children and adolescents with special health care and developmental needs.* Lexington: University of Kentucky Press.

White, M., & Epston, D. (1990). *Narrative means to therapeutic ends.* New York: W.W. Norton & Company.

Yin, R.K. (1995). *Case study research: Design and methods: Vol. 5. Applied social research methods series.* Newbury Park, CA: Sage Publications.

Zander, K. (1991). Care maps. *The New Definition, 6,* 3.

Chapter 6

Nutrition Assessment for Young Children with Developmental Disabilities

Betty L. Lucas and Peggy L. Pipes

The quality and quantity of children's diets are the most constant environmental factors affecting growth and development. An adequate food intake provides the energy (calories) and necessary nutrients for increases in body size, resistance to infection, and the accumulation of nutrient reserves. Good nutrition is essential for health and quality of life. Food, feeding, and the satiation of hunger are also important factors in parent–infant bonding, parent–child interactions, and the child's ability to attend to his environment and to learn.

Feeding progresses from the newborn's total dependence on adults for breast milk or formula to the typically developing 6-year-old who can feed herself, use utensils, give clear signs for hunger and satiety, and obtain her own food. For adults, feeding their children is emotionally tied to adequate parenting. When this process does not go well or is not successful, feeding interactions and behaviors can become negative for all concerned.

105

Children with developmental disabilities are vulnerable to inadequacies in energy and nutrient intake. Many experience nutrition problems more frequently and with greater chronicity than do typically developing children. Rapidly growing children will soon deplete their reserves if adequate food is not consumed. Medications, such as anticonvulsants, may interfere with absorption or metabolism of nutrients or may depress the appetite. Medical conditions, including cardiac and pulmonary diseases, and excessive movement frequently increase energy needs. Other conditions, such as hypotonia (low muscle tone) or spastic cerebral palsy, limit activity and decrease energy requirements. Metabolic diseases (e.g., phenylketonuria), malabsorption, and other disorders require dietary modification. Children with poor self-feeding skills, oral-motor feeding problems, or limited food acceptances are at risk for inadequate energy and nutrient intake. Table 6.1 lists nutrition risk factors for young children with developmental disabilities.

THE NUTRITIONIST'S INTERDISCIPLINARY TEAM ROLE

Nutrition is a science derived from physiology, biochemistry, biology, food science, and other basic sciences. The application of nutrition science in a clinical setting utilizes many behavioral sciences as well, particularly in obtaining intake information through dietary interview. As many other disciplines employ a number of the same basic sciences in their clinical practice, there is sometimes overlap in the information collected. The tool that belongs solely to the nutritionist is assessment of foods as sources of nutrients. This enables nutritionists to quantify and assess the adequacy of an individual child's food intake in terms of energy and nutrient intake, to compare the intake data to appropriate guidelines, and to make recommendations for the addition or deletion of specific foods or supplemental nutrients. With this information, nutri-

Table 6.1.   Nutrition risk factors for children with developmental disabilities

Low birth weight, prematurity

Increased energy needs (due to cardiac or pulmonary conditions, excessive movement, etc.)

Decreased energy needs (due to short stature, decreased mobility, metabolic differences)

Delayed progress in feeding development

Chronic medication use

Atypical or dysfunctional oral-motor patterns

Dependent feeder

Allergies, food intolerances

Poor or excessive appetite

Frequent infections or hospitalizations

Pica (i.e., eating nonfood items)

Inappropriate parent–child interactions

Specific dietary needs or restrictions

tionists can also design diet changes for medical conditions and develop appropriate nutrition education programs.

Goals of Nutrition Assessment

The expected outcomes of the nutrition assessment are to collect all information necessary to document the adequacy and extent of the child's nutritional status and to develop a nutrition care plan that is realistic within the family context. In order to accomplish these outcomes, the following assessment components should be addressed.

Family Involvement

Determine the family's primary concerns regarding nutrition, diet, and feeding, as well as their understanding of any problems. Building initial communication with caregivers is important for soliciting their priorities and their history of nutrition or feeding concerns and for collecting complete dietary information.

Nutrition Intake

Define the adequacy of the child's energy and nutrient intake from food. Then compare the energy and nutrient intake from food and supplements to the child's age, size, activity level, medical diagnosis, feeding skills and abilities, and use of medications.

Growth

Ascertain the child's current growth parameters as well as patterns of growth over time. Current growth data should be compared to National Center for Health Statistics (NCHS) growth charts or diagnosis-specific growth charts, with consideration given to limitations in ambulation, body composition differences, prematurity, and diagnosis. Other body measurements may indirectly estimate body fat and protein stores. Sequential rates and patterns of physical growth are key to assessing children whose growth is outside of the standard parameters.

Effect of Food Intake

Establish the effect of food intake on the child's physical growth. Is the diet adequate to support continued growth in height and weight, to provide for catch-up growth, or to promote weight management for the overweight child?

Appropriateness of Diet

Determine the appropriateness of the diet composition relative to the child's developmental progress. The quality of the diet in terms of texture, consistency, and requirements for self-feeding must be compared to the child's developmental level and estimated age of feeding development.

Etiology

Discern the etiology of problems encountered in achieving an adequate energy and nutrient intake. Many factors can affect the child's ability to obtain an adequate diet: medical conditions, previous medical treatments that have negatively influenced feeding, limited or increased physical activity, caregiver abilities to provide food or feedings in an appropriate manner, oral-motor delays or impairments, and frequent illness or hospitalization. Even if some of the issues have been resolved, ongoing secondary impact on diet and feeding can persist.

Family and Community Resources

Identify family and community resources available to assist in the provision of food and nutrition education. Family resources include parents and other caregivers who feed the child; the availability of food in the home; and caregivers' nutrition knowledge, food preparation, and sanitation skills. Examples of community resources are the Special Supplemental Nutrition Program for Women, Infants, and Children (WIC); the Child Nutrition Program in child care, Head Start programs, and public schools; food stamps; and food banks.

The dimensions to assess in the nutrition evaluation depend on the child's age, health status, and presented problems. They may include 1) family concerns and questions regarding diet, growth, and feeding; 2) the child's medical, developmental, and growth history; 3) nutrients and energy provided by the child's diet; 4) anthropometric data such as length or height, weight, and skinfold measurements; 5) biochemical indicators of nutritional status; 6) clinical evaluation to identify any symptoms of malnutrition; 7) physical and psychosocial factors that may interfere with the ingestion of an adequate food intake; 8) the effect of medications on food intake and nutrient metabolism; 9) the family's use of community resources for food assistance and nutrition education; and 10) physical and medical factors that may modify a child's energy and nutrient needs.

It is important to recognize that nutritional deficiency develops over time in the following sequence (see Figure 6.1). First, an inadequate dietary intake or physical factors interfere with absorption or utilization of nutrients. Then tissue reserves of the nutrient become depleted. With depleted reserves, biochemical lesions can be measured (i.e., low blood levels). Clinical lesions are the final stage in the development of nutritional deficiency, which may be followed by death. In developed countries, few acute deficiency diseases are likely to be found. Instead, tissue depletion and subclinical lesions, underweight, and obesity are issues that most often need to be addressed.

Challenges

There are several challenges to accurate nutritional assessment of young children with developmental disabilities. Energy and nutrient requirements vary from one child to another depending on genetics, body composition, and activity level. In infants and young children with developmental disabilities, nutrient needs can also be influenced by a medical condition (e.g., congenital heart disease, bronchopulmonary dysplasia), the long-term use of medications, chronic infections, and reduced weight-bearing capabilities and mobility. Although the Dietary Reference Intakes (DRIs), which include the Recommended Dietary

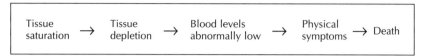

| Tissue saturation | → | Tissue depletion | → | Blood levels abnormally low | → | Physical symptoms | → | Death |

Figure 6.1.   Stages of development of nutritional deficiency. (From Beaton, G.H., & Benga, J.M. [Eds.]. [1973]. *Nutrition and preventive medicine* [World Health Organization Monograph No. 62]. Geneva, Switzerland: World Health Organization; adapted by permission.)

Allowances (RDA; Food and Nutrition Board, Institute of Medicine, National Academy of Sciences, 1997), provide guidelines for populations, decisions have to be made as to the appropriate intake specific to the infant or child being assessed. For instance, an appropriate energy intake is based on linear growth and weight gain in relation to the child's current energy intake, level of activity and mobility, and medical conditions that may alter the energy needs. Differences in children's physical size and weight at any age mandate that the DRIs be applied with caution. For example, some children with developmental disabilities are short in stature for their age or have slower growth rates. Their energy needs may be reduced compared to those of same-age peers, but the need for nutrients such as protein, vitamins, and minerals may be the same or greater than that of same-age peers. Meeting the unique nutritional needs of these children can be difficult.

A second challenge is the accuracy and reliability of the dietary information that is obtained, especially when the data source is frequently the memory of the child's caregivers. Each dietary collection tool has its limitations in terms of validity and reliability; using more than one tool helps increase the accuracy of the information. In addition, because feeding is such a visible sign of parenting, information provided by caregivers may be influenced by their feelings of adequacy in this area.

Another challenge is the constantly changing food supply. Not only are new foods added to the market daily while others are discontinued, but foods that have been available for years are often fortified with nutrients, making new nutrient sources available. The nutritionist is constantly challenged to remain aware of foods as sources of nutrients. A related issue is the use of vitamin and mineral supplements, other nutrition supplements and products, and the popularization of unproven dietary regimens. Families of children with developmental disabilities are particularly susceptible to the marketing appeal of supplements and products and to undocumented nutritional therapies found in the mass media and on the Internet.

NUTRITION ASSESSMENT PROCESS

The process of nutrition assessment includes screening to identify problems and concerns and referral to a qualified nutrition professional for a complete assessment. The results of the nutrition assessment are the basis for developing a nutrition care plan appropriate for the child and family.

Screening

For most young children with developmental disabilities, screening is typically performed by other health professionals such as primary care providers, nurses, or therapists. Early intervention providers, educators, and parents may also identify nutrition concerns. The consistency of screening and the elements included vary among environments and programs. The basics of screening should be comprised of growth, dietary intake, feeding problems, and family questions or concerns. If nutrition problems are identified by the screening, the child and family should be referred for a nutrition assessment to a nutritionist who specializes in children with special health care needs (American Dietetic Association, 1995). The process of nutrition screening and assessment is shown in Figure 6.2.

Assessment Components

A comprehensive assessment of nutritional status requires the collection of dietary intake, anthropometric, and biochemical data as well as a clinical evaluation. For young children, progress in feeding development and acquisition of skills is also a key factor in the assessment. A comprehensive nutrition evaluation can be costly, but it is unlikely that all the data will be necessary for an individual child's nutrition assessment in a community or outpatient setting. As nutritional inadequacy and growth alterations proceed progressively over time, information collected will serve to identify how and why the at-risk status has developed. In most circumstances, an assessment of dietary intake, current and past growth parameters, feeding skills, and clinical evaluation will be indicated.

Because the nutrition, growth, and feeding issues of young children affect overall growth and development, an interdisciplinary assessment is appropriate and useful (Wodarski, 1990). Depending on where services are delivered, other health care professionals (e.g., nurses, occupational therapists or speech-language pathologists, social workers, primary care providers) may obtain some components of the nutrition assessment. In situations in which the feeding, nutrition, and growth of infants and young children are complex and challenging, specially trained feeding teams can provide coordinated assessment and effective interventions. Representing a variety of disciplines—but including a nutritionist, a feeding therapist, and a behavioral specialist—these teams can reduce multiple family contacts, thereby avoiding the dissemination of conflicting or excessive advice and information to families.

Anthropometry

Assessment of children's growth is an important part of the nutrition evaluation. Height or length, weight, and head circumference accurately taken and recorded over time reflect nutritional status. Other measurements, such as mid-arm

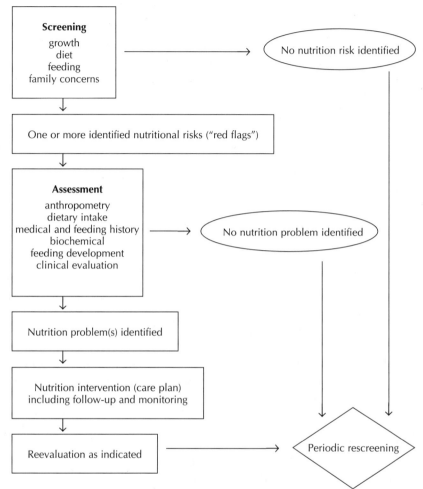

Figure 6.2.   Nutrition screening and assessment.

circumference and skinfold thickness, reflect present nutritional status. Individual children whose growth does not appear to be proceeding normally may require additional methods of assessment (e.g., bone age determination).

Height, Length, and Weight
Height (or length for children younger than 36 months old) and weight values, plotted on growth charts for age, give information as to how children rank in size in relation to other children of the same sex and age (Hamill, Drizd, Johnson, Reed, & Roche, 1977). Several measurements of height or length and weight at different ages plotted on the charts enable the practitioner to deter-

mine if the child's growth is progressing as might be expected. Most children stay in approximately the same percentiles over time. They grow in spurts, however, and changes in percentiles may be noted from one measurement to the next, with children usually returning to their predetermined growth channel over time. The growth parameters for infants born prematurely should be corrected for gestational age when plotted on NCHS growth charts.

The NCHS growth charts, based on a healthy U.S. population, do not always adequately describe all children. The growth of some children with developmental disabilities may be altered due to chromosomal abnormalities or other central nervous system insults. For instance, short stature is common in children with Down syndrome or fetal alcohol syndrome. Nevertheless, any impact on growth due to diet and nutrition should also be assessed.

Growth expectations also need to take into consideration any chronic disease, prenatal central nervous system insult, genetic condition, or disability. Interpretation can then be made regarding what is "normal" for an individual child. In addition, specialized growth charts exist for certain conditions, including Down syndrome, Turner syndrome, spina bifida, and Williams syndrome (Ekvall, 1993). Some of these growth charts include only one or two parameters, however, so the NCHS growth charts and other anthropometric data are also needed to assess physical growth (see Table 6.2).

Weight for length or height is used to determine the proportionality of the child's growth parameters. It assesses weight in relation to length or height for prepubertal children. For instance, the height and weight of a 3-year-old boy may be at or below the 5th percentile, yet his weight for height may be at the 25th percentile. Another way of interpreting weight and height is body mass index (BMI). It is used as a noninvasive clinical assessment of chronic energy deficiency or overweight in children older than 1 year of age (Cronk & Roche, 1982). BMI is expressed as a ratio of weight in kilograms to height in meters squared. The calculation of BMI adds a useful dimension in the assessment of body composition. When plotted over time on the BMI percentile curves (Hammer, Kraemer, Wilson, Ritter, & Dornbusch, 1991), relative changes of BMI can be visualized.

Some young children are difficult to measure and weigh due to the inability to stand, highly flexed limbs or contractures, or scoliosis. For those children, alternative growth parameters are indicated, such as sitting height, crown-rump length, arm span, and limb segment length. Techniques and equipment are standardized in obtaining the measurements, but comparison data is limited to healthy children (Ekvall, 1993; Trahms & Pipes, 1997). Nonetheless, these alternative measurements are useful in monitoring change and progress over time in an individual child. Table 6.3 describes some of these other measurements.

Indications that nutrition may have influenced the child's growth include 1) height or length for age or weight for age that is below the 10th percentile

Table 6.2. Specialized growth charts

Growth chart	Sample	Limitations	Used with NCHS	Reference
NCHS (current)	20,000 children, 1963–1974; NHES & NHANES I; 5th–95th percentiles	Data are longitudinal for infants, cross-sectional for children		Hamill et al., 1979
NCHS (new)	Previous data + NHANES III data; large sample; 3rd–97th percentiles			Centers for Disease Control and Prevention, in press
Down syndrome	Longitudinal, 400 males, 300 females, 1960–1986	Included children with congenital heart disease, reflects tendency to be overweight	Used with NCHS for weight/length, weight/height, BMI	Cronk et al., 1988
Turner syndrome			Used with NCHS for weight/age, weight/length, weight/height, BMI	Lyon, Preece, & Grant, 1985
Williams syndrome	61 females, 47 males	Retrospective and cross-sectional data, small number	Used with NCHS for weight/length, weight/height, BMI/age	Morris, Demsey, Leonard, Dilts, & Blackburn, 1988
Achondroplasia	189 males, 214 females for height	Small number	Compared to NCHS on chart; used with NCHS for BMI/age	Horton, Rotter, Rimoin, Scott, & Hall, 1978
Cerebral palsy	360 children	Longitudinal and cross-sectional data, small number	Compared to NCHS on chart	Krick, Murphy-Miller, Zeger, & Wright, 1996
Prader-Willi syndrome	56 males, 36 females	Longitudinal and cross-sectional data, small number	Compared to NCHS on chart; used with NCHS for BMI/age	Holm, 1995

Key: NCHS = National Center for Health Statistics, NHES = National Health Examination Survey, NHANES = National Health and Nutrition Examination Surveys, BMI = body mass index.

Table 6.3.   Alternative growth measurements

Measure	Sample	Limitations	Used with NCHS	Reference
Crown-rump	Approximately 75 females, 75 males	Longitudinal data	Used with NCHS weight/age	Hansman, 1970
Sitting height	NCHS population	Caucasian children and African American children	Used with NCHS weight/age	Hamill, Johnston, & Lemeshow, 1973; Johnson, Fulwood, Abraham, & Bryner, 1981
Incremental growth	Children who grew "close" to NCHS	Caucasian children	Used with NCHS weight/age, length or height/age	Roche & Himes, 1980
Mid-arm circumference	NCHS population	Use after 2 years of age	Used with NCHS weight/age, length or height/age	Johnson et al., 1981
Triceps skinfold thickness	NCHS population	Use after 2 years of age	Used with NCHS weight/age, length or height/age	Johnson et al., 1981
Subscapular skinfold thickness	NCHS population	Use after 2 years of age	Used with NCHS weight/age, length or height/age	Johnson et al., 1981
Parent-specific adjustment for length/stature		Note parent height on chart	Used with NCHS length or height/age	Himes, Roche, Thissen, & Moore, 1985
Knee height	13,821 ambulatory children; NHES I,II,III, 1960–1970	Use equation for race (85% Caucasian children)	Used with NCHS weight/age	Chumlea, Guo, & Steinbaugh, 1994

Key: NCHS = National Center for Health Statistics, NHES = National Health Examination Survey.

or above the 90th percentile, 2) weight for length or height that is below the 10th percentile or above the 90th percentile, and 3) dramatic increases or decreases in growth percentiles in any of the parameters over time.

Mid-arm Circumference and Skinfold Thickness

Mid-arm circumference, using the standardized technique and equipment, provides an index of body stores and protein mass. It is noninvasive and relatively easy to obtain. Although it can be used as an independent measure, it is most often used with skinfold thickness to calculate arm muscle circumference.

Because approximately half of the total body fat is deposited in subcutaneous adipose tissue, the fatness of an individual can be estimated by measuring the thickness of the skinfold at selected sites with special calipers that have been calibrated to provide a constant tension. In general, one truncal (subscapular) measurement and one limb (triceps) measurement are advised. If only one measurement is to be used, the triceps is preferred because it is the easiest site to measure and is representative of body fatness.

Percentiles for mid-arm circumference, arm muscle circumference, and triceps skinfold measurements have been compiled from a cross-sectional study of Caucasian individuals 1–75 years of age (Frisancho, 1981). These measurements are useful as an evaluation complement to growth charts and in any decision to modify energy or nutrient intake. Athletic, muscular children may appear overweight or obese if only height and weight are used as criteria for judgment. On the other hand, children with poor muscle tone or those who are not ambulatory (e.g., children with cerebral palsy) often plot at a lower percentile for weight for height even though they may have an adequate amount of fat stores.

Dietary Intake

A variety of means exist for collecting dietary intake information, each tool having limitations and different degrees of reliability. The choice of tool depends on the purpose of the interview, the time availability of the professional, and the cooperation of the family. Information sought will vary with the problem. Only one method is used in some instances, whereas a combination of tools is appropriate at other times. The tools most often used in the clinical setting are a 24-hour recall, dietary history, 3- and 7-day food records, and food frequency.

The interview is the most important aspect of these tools. The validity of the information obtained is dependent on the caregiver's understanding of the reasons for the interview and the information sought as well as the interviewer's skills at probing for and validating information. The dietary assessment data are only as valid as the parent's ability and willingness to share information with the interviewer. It is important that families feel comfortable with the interview and the individual conducting the assessment. The interviewer should set the stage and establish rapport with a warm greeting, a clear definition of the purpose of the interview, and the reasons for the "how much" and "how often" questions asked. For young children, obtaining dietary intake from caregivers works best when done in the context of the child's daily routine. Some parts of the routine—including naps, therapy, child care, preschool, and family meals—often trigger times the child is offered something to eat or drink.

Providing an adequate diet for children is an important aspect of parenting. Some caregivers may feel threatened when questioned about a child's food intake unless there is sufficient understanding on their part. In addition, the interviewer must have reasonable expectations for the respondent. Parents who have several children cannot be expected to give information as precisely for one child as do parents who devote time to an only child. A number of meals may be consumed at child care or at school, and parents may not know what children eat in these settings.

During the interview, the interviewer must be careful to avoid suggesting times, meals, specific food, or amounts consumed. For example, the question "When does your child first have something to eat or to drink?" is appropriate, whereas "When does your child first eat breakfast?" is inappropriate. Infant feeding practices, food habits, and the common foods consumed vary in different cultures, so the interviewer must be nonjudgmental in gathering information. Silence must be accepted comfortably, and parents should be permitted time to formulate answers and to ask questions of their own. In some situations, a language interpreter will be needed for the nutrition interview.

24-Hour Recall

Although the 24-hour recall is the most common method used for collecting dietary data in clinical settings, it cannot be substituted for more intensive methods when judgments regarding the adequacy of an individual child's food intake are to be made. The 24-hour recall method is more appropriately used to characterize the nutrient intake of populations, to screen children for nutritional risk, and to determine compliance with a dietary regimen during clinical follow-up.

Families are asked to relate, in portion sizes, all food consumed by the child for the past 24 hours. Underestimation of food intake is more likely than overestimation. Errors are reported to result from the inability of parents to remember exactly what was eaten, difficulties in estimating portion sizes, and lack of commitment (Todd, Hudes, & Calloway, 1983). There is no assurance that the recall of the day selected is typical of other days. The accuracy of portion sizes can be increased by the use of food models and by skillful probing.

Dietary History

One method used to review dietary intake in retrospect is the research history method developed by Burke and modified by Beal (Beal, 1967; Burke, 1947). During an interview, the nutritionist obtains an estimate of the frequency and amounts of food and nutrient supplements consumed in a specified period, usually 1–6 months. Parents are questioned about the child's food preferences and aversions. If early feeding problems or experiences are suspected to be factors in the nutrition concern, information is elicited on early feeding history. The interview is often cross-checked with a 24-hour recall, a 3-day food record, or a food frequency questionnaire.

Several researchers have cautioned against using this tool as the sole source of data. One study compared the research-type dietary history with 10–14 days of weighed food records and 24-hour recalls and found that dietary

histories gave distinctly higher values than 7-day food records and 24-hour recalls (Medlin, 1990).

3- and 7-Day Food Records

The 3- or 7-day food record of all food and beverages consumed is commonly
used to characterize current intakes of individual children. Families are asked
to maintain the child's usual eating routines, to measure portions of food offered and amounts not eaten, and to record the amounts consumed. Families
report that measuring food poses no problems, but they find the rigidity of
recording each time the child eats difficult. Sometimes they forget to record
foods that are added to other foods (e.g., catsup, butter, jelly). Therefore, it is
important to present careful instruction as to how to record food intake. Training with food models has been shown to be effective in improving the accuracy
of the portions recorded for 1 week. The effect, however, did not persist for all
the portions studied for a 4-week period (Bolland, Ward, & Bolland, 1988).
Debriefing, reviewing food records, and clarifying information on the records
can increase the accuracy of information because portion sizes, brand names,
and constituents of recipes can be defined (Garrahie, Humphrey, Witschi,
Stephenson, & Ellison, 1991).

Food Frequency

A food frequency tool lists foods and asks for portion sizes as well as the frequency of their consumption (i.e., per day, week, or month). The advantages
of this tool are that it is easy to administer and is a good screen for nutrient
sources that are low or missing or provided in excess. Yet it does not provide
information regarding the frequency and regularity of a child's feedings, the
portion sizes offered at a feeding, or feeding environments. In addition, food
frequency tools do not include a variety of ethnic food items. However, the
food frequency can be used in screening or in combination with food records
or a diet history.

Interpreting Dietary Intake Information

After the dietary intake information has been collected, the adequacy of the
child's energy and nutrient intake can be assessed. Decisions as to which
method of evaluation should be used and which nutrients will be calculated are
based on the precision and reliability of the information collected, the foods
that appear in the dietary records, the nutritionist's knowledge of foods as
sources of nutrients, and the problem presented for evaluation.

In some instances, intake data may be compared to food groups. When
parents are unable to give information that can be quantified, the analysis of
food groups or foods as sources of nutrients is appropriate. Nevertheless, if the
child is underweight or overweight or if food sources of a particular nutrient
appear on the record only occasionally, calculations of energy and nutrient intake are important. Foods that are present or absent in the dietary history may
sufficiently indicate the presence or absence of nutrient intake problems.

If precise and complete information has been collected, software or manual calculations of nutrients in the foods consumed by the child can be made. When calculations are complete the data is compared with a standard. Often children who consume less than two thirds or three fourths of the RDA of any nutrient are defined as being at nutritional risk. For a population of young children with developmental disabilities, additional considerations in determining nutrient adequacy include medications used, body size, and rate of growth, as well as ambulation and activity level.

Biochemical Evaluation

When dietary or medical information indicates a nutrient of concern, biochemical tests are often requested. They are helpful in defining nutritional status because they define marginal nutrient deficiency before overt clinical symptoms appear. Results must be interpreted according to the standardization and experience of each laboratory. It is important to recognize that, in most instances, blood levels generally reflect recent dietary intake, not long-term nutritional status. Thus, results should not be considered alone but as part of the clinical evaluation. The most common biochemical parameters considered in children are those used to define iron deficiency: hemoglobin and hematocrit. If there are questions about the adequacy of protein intake, serum prealbumin may be obtained. If anticonvulsants are prescribed, an assessment of vitamin D status is indicated. Most often serum calcium, phosphorus, and alkaline phosphatase are initially requested, but if they are at elevated levels, more specific biochemical tests may be indicated. Table 6.4 includes common biochemical parameters assessed in young children.

Table 6.4.   Common nutrition biochemical parameters in children

Laboratory test	Indicator	Normal values
Hemoglobin	Iron status	
	1 month	10.0–18.0 g/100 ml
	6 months	9.5–13.5 g/100 ml
	2 years	10.5–13.5 g/100 ml
Hematocrit	Iron status	
	1 month	31%–55%
	6 months	29%–41%
	2 years	33%–39%
Ferritin	Storage iron	Females 15–160 mg/1
		Males 25–160 mg/1
Percent transferrin saturation	Iron deficiency Hematopoiesis	204–360 mg/100 ml
Serum alkaline phosphatase	Elevated with vitamin D deficiency	(up to 7 years of age) 95–380 IU/l
Serum prealbumin	General protein status	Infant: 2.9–5.5 g/100 ml
		Child: 3.8–5.4 g/100 ml

Key: g = gram, ml = milliliter, mg = milligram.

Clinical Evaluation

During the physical exam, the child will be observed for symptoms of undernutrition or malnutrition. Selected clinical signs indicative of malnutrition are shown in Table 6.5. Many signs of malnutrition are nonspecific and may be caused by nonnutritional factors. Identification of the signs is subjective and interexaminer differences are often considerable. Clinical examination is most valuable when the deficiency of one or more nutrients has reached the stage of overt disease, but this is not common in the United States. Table 6.6 shows the clinical signs of malnutrition usually seen in children in relation to their overall nutrition. The presence of any sign should not be interpreted as a conclusive diagnosis of a nutrient deficiency, but it should be used for further dietary and biochemical studies.

Feeding Development and Skills

The development of feeding behavior depends on central nervous system maturation, which controls fine, gross, and oral-motor skills. This feeding development proceeds in an orderly and predictable manner for typically developing children. Assessing children's developmental levels of function and their readiness to progress in eating and self-feeding is necessary to define reasonable expectations for caregivers. Changes in food and feeding behavior should be effected when children are developmentally 6–7 months of age, when they demonstrate readiness to self-feed and to begin using a cup. Table 6.7 defines important developmental landmarks and suggests food appropriate for changes in feeding behavior.

Children with developmental disabilities are more likely to have feeding and eating difficulties than the general pediatric population. The etiology of these feeding problems can include 1) overall delayed development with related delays or immaturity in feeding progress; 2) neuromotor dysfunction with oral-motor impairments, positioning difficulties, and fine motor limitations;

Table 6.5.   Clinical signs of malnutrition

Affected area	Symptom	Nutrient of concern
Hair	Dull, dry, thin, easily plucked	Protein
Face	Pale	Iron
Skin	Hyperpigmented, dry, flaky, lack of fat underneath	Protein, Energy
Skeletal system	Bowed legs, knock knees, beading of the ribs	Vitamin D
Psychomotor	Listless, lethargic	Energy, Iron
Subcutaneous tissues	Lack of or excessive fat stores	Energy
Teeth	Decay Mottled enamel	Carbohydrate Fluoride

Table 6.6. Clinical signs of malnutrition seen in children

Diagnosis	Symptom	Nutrient of concern
Undernutrition	Low weight in relation to height, mental and physical lethargy, skinfold measurement below the 10th NCHS percentile	Energy, iron, protein
Failure to thrive	Lack of appropriate gain in weight and length over time (2–3 months), depending on age	Energy, protein, zinc
Obesity	Excess weight in relation to height, skinfold measurement above the 90th NCHS percentile	Energy
Iron deficiency	Pallor of the mucous membrane, lethargy	Iron
Vitamin D deficiency (secondary to anticonvulsant use)	Beading of the ribs, knock knees, muscular hypotonia	Vitamin D

Key: NCHS = National Center for Health Statistics.

3) medical or physical conditions such as a cleft lip or palate, gastroesophageal reflux, swallowing dysfunction, or the use of nasogastric or gastrostomy feeding tube; 4) behavior or emotional interactions that negatively affect eating (e.g., force-feeding, control issues between caregiver and child, neglect, a lack of response to the child's cues for hunger and satiety); and 5) any combination of these issues.

Screening for feeding problems can be conducted during the nutrition evaluation. The early feeding history identifies problems in formula and food acceptance, delays in texture progression and self-feeding skills, and medical procedures or conditions influencing early feeding. Obtaining the current dietary intake data for a child, using the framework of a typical day's routine, can identify feeding problems such as poor signals for hunger and satiety, lengthy mealtimes, the use of bribery or punishment, negative noneating behaviors during meals, gagging, spitting, choking, parental anxiety, and food intake dictated by the child. Observation of a characteristic feeding is ideal, either at home or at school, but not often possible for the professional. Tools are available for both screening and comprehensive evaluation of feeding and eating problems (Pipes & Glass, 1997).

REACHING AN INFORMED CLINICAL DECISION

The assessment of a child's nutritional status is based on a careful evaluation of the collected data. The results of the different assessment components are integrated to summarize the child's current situation and to give positive feedback or to make recommendations for intervention. The steps of clinical decision making for nutrition assessment are shown in Figure 6.3.

If the assessment indicates that adjustments need to be made in the kinds or portions of food offered to the child, or if a therapeutic diet is indicated,

Table 6.7. Developmental stages of readiness to progress in feeding behaviors

Developmental landmarks	Change indicated	Examples of appropriate foods
Tongue laterally transfers food in the mouth Voluntary and independent movements of the tongue and lips Sitting posture can be sustained Beginning of chewing movements (up and down movements of the jaw)	Introduction of soft, mashed table food	Tuna fish; mashed potatoes; well-cooked mashed vegetables; ground meats in gravy and sauces; soft diced fruit such as bananas, peaches, pears, liverwurst, flavored yogurt
Reaches for and grasps objects with scissor grasp Brings hand to mouth	Finger-feeding (large pieces of food)	Oven-dried toast, teething biscuits, cheese sticks (food should be soluble in the mouth to prevent choking)
Voluntary release (refined digital grasp)	Finger-feeding (small pieces of food)	Bits of cottage cheese, dry cereal, peas
Rotary chewing pattern	Introduction of more textured food from family menu	Well-cooked chopped meats and casseroles, cooked vegetables and canned fruit (not mashed), toast, potatoes, macaroni, spaghetti, peeled ripe fruit
Approximates lips to rim of cup	Introduction of cup	
Understands relationship of container and contained	Beginning self-feeding (messiness should be expected)	Food that when scooped will adhere to the spoon, such as applesauce, cooked cereal, mashed potatoes, cottage cheese
Increased rotary movement of the jaw Ulnar deviation of wrist develops	More skilled at cup and spoon feeding	Chopped fibrous meats such as roast and steak Raw vegetables and fruit (introduce gradually)
Walks alone	May seek food and get food independently	Food of high nutrient value should be available
Names food, expresses preferences; Prefers unmixed food Goes on food jags Appetite appears to decrease		Balanced food intake should be offered (child should be permitted to develop food preferences)

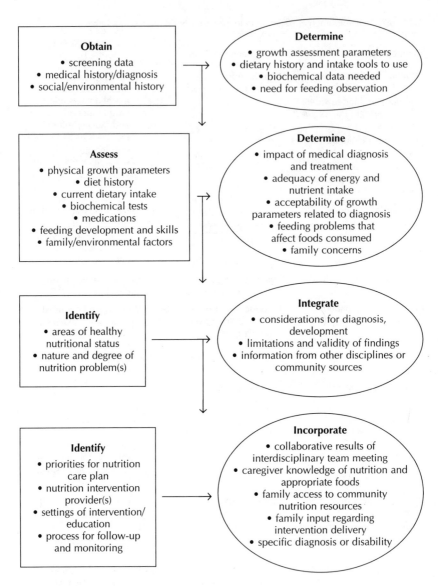

Figure 6.3.   Nutrition assessment decision making.

plans for modifying food intake should be made with the child and the family. The nutritionist can screen for and make referrals regarding delays in feeding skills or eating patterns as well as problem feeding behaviors and interactions. Oral-motor feeding issues are typically evaluated by occupational therapists or speech-language pathologists; behavior feeding problems might be assessed by specially trained psychologists, social workers, or nurses. Young children with feeding problems are best served by interdisciplinary developmental teams or specific feeding teams.

Example of Decision Making Through a Case Study

The following case study describes a nutrition assessment and the clinical decision-making process involved. Luis was an 18-month-old Hispanic boy referred by his developmental program to a tertiary interdisciplinary team for an overall developmental evaluation. He was born at 31 weeks' gestation and was hospitalized for 7 weeks. Luis was gavage fed for the first 2 weeks of life and received oxygen for 3 months. His program reported that Luis refused foods that were not smooth or puréed. On the nutrition screening form, Luis' parents indicated that they were concerned about Luis' underweight and poor appetite. Luis had recently been diagnosed with a seizure disorder and was on an anticonvulsant. He received therapy twice per week, once at home and once at child care. He lived with his parents and a 3-year-old sister in a rural county. Luis's father was a seasonal farm worker; his mother worked part-time at a convenience store. Spanish was their primary language, but they spoke and understood English.

Plans were made for assessing this child. First, the following needed to be obtained: Luis' growth history, current growth parameters, feeding history, and current intake. With parental permission, the clinician would also observe Luis being fed. Because toddlers in general are at risk for iron deficiency anemia, a hematocrit would be necessary. Finally, the family's priorities, as compared to program's priorities, would be clarified.

Assessment

During his evaluation, Luis's length, weight, and head circumference were taken and plotted on NCHS growth charts and corrected for the 9 weeks of prematurity. An interview with the mother included early feeding history, developmental feeding progress, and current diet intake. This was cross-checked with a food frequency. Luis's length was at the 25th percentile, his weight below the 10th percentile, and his weight for length at the 10th percentile. Luis's mother was surprised that he was on the growth chart; further discussion revealed that his growth had not been corrected for gestational age consistently by community health providers. Although Luis's arm circumference was below the 5th percentile, his triceps fatfold was in the 10th–25th percentile. Luis's diet consisted of milk (four to five 7-ounce bottles per day), rice cereal, banana, and jarred baby food. The child's mother stated that she had tried to give Luis lumpier food when he was between 6 and 10 months old, but he would cry, gag, and choke. Closer to the time of assessment, Luis would gag and also spit out food with lumps. The mother said that WIC had urged her to wean Luis from the bottle, but she was hesitant to do so because her son was underweight and would not eat many solids. In addition, relatives who provided child care felt it was easier to give Luis the bottle, especially as he was just learning to crawl and was developing slowly. Hematocrit results showed borderline anemia. Luis had been taking phenobarbital for 3 months; he took no vitamin supplements. A bottle feeding as well as solids fed by his mother was observed by the nutritionist and the occupational therapist.

The energy intake of 12 calories per centimeter of length was low, even with Luis's limited mobility. Approximately 60%–70% of his energy intake came from milk, and he received marginal or inadequate levels of iron, zinc, and vitamin B_6. Luis's growth parameters were typical of children with cerebral palsy, including a body composition more reduced in muscle mass than in fat stores. Nonetheless, his weight for length and triceps thickness suggested mild underweight. Health care providers had not been consistent in correcting Luis's age, so the family was unclear regarding the concept of corrected age. The parents and extended family had still considered Luis a "baby" and had been more concerned about weight gain than the feeding progress. The feeding observation revealed that Luis was approximately 10–12 months old in his oral-motor feeding abilities but had had little consistent practice with appropriate foods or utensils. In addition, there seemed to be a behavioral component in his response due to negative neonatal feeding experiences and being offered textures before he could handle them.

Luis's parents had done a good job of providing a healthy diet, despite his feeding challenges. His growth was within low normal limits for children with cerebral palsy, but somewhat higher stores of protein and fat (close to the 25th percentile) would have been more desirable. His intake at the time of assessment would not likely support that growth goal, especially with his activity level increasing. Dietary goals included increasing energy and iron intake, decreasing the volume of milk, and expanding the variety and amounts of solids. With ongoing anticonvulsant use, regular biochemical evaluation of bone mineralization would need to be done by the primary care provider or a neurologist.

Recommendations

A feeding evaluation suggested that Luis should have been able to accept and eat foods with textures and to begin some finger feeding. However, it was decided that this would probably be best introduced from a community therapist working with the family and the relatives who cared for Luis. It may have been hard for the family to see the behavioral component as something that needed to be addressed with a consistent approach.

Luis's parents were willing to make changes in his diet in order to increase energy and iron, such as reducing the amount of milk in each bottle. They agreed to give him an iron supplement. The parents opted to have the anemia follow-up and growth and nutrition monitoring done at the WIC clinic; they would share the nutrition recommendations with WIC. The community therapist was available by telephone during the parent conference, and she agreed to begin to work on increasing Luis's texture acceptance at each therapy visit.

The parents preferred this because they were not sure they could do this on their own—especially with Luis's tendency to cry and choke. The team occupational therapist provided specific suggestions for feeding progression, including the use of utensils and positioning. The psychologist provided behavioral resources for the family and a developmental program.

ISSUES PARTICULARLY RELEVANT TO NUTRITION

Each dietary intake tool will have different limitations. One may overestimate a child's actual intake; another may underestimate it. Combining diet history with current food records provides more data on which to make evaluations of energy and nutrient intake. However, due to barriers of language, culture, time, and motivation, some families may be able to provide only limited information. In some situations, other environments and caregivers can provide the needed diet and feeding information.

As a pediatric nutrition assessment includes physical growth status, accurate and appropriate anthropometric data are essential. Obtaining this information requires utilizing standardized equipment and technique. The usefulness of this growth data can be insufficient at times due to the variety of environments where measurements are made, inconsistent or unreliable equipment and techniques, lack of longitudinal data, and inadequate training of personnel.

Judgments about the quality of a child's food intake must be made recognizing the limitations of current methodology, the ranges of nutrients found in foods grown in different locations, and the bioavailability of nutrients. Also, because much of the information collected is dependent on careful observations and recall by parents, who may not be aware of food eaten away from home or of the amounts consumed at home, the reliability of information collected must be constantly evaluated. Making decisions about the validity of gathered material requires the expertise of the nutritionist who is a registered dietitian (RD) with a specialization in pediatrics.

A key element in preventing nutrition problems or providing nutrition services for young children with developmental disabilities is the availability of nutrition screening in health care or programmatic environments. Nutrition screening is not administered uniformly or consistently, with children too frequently receiving nutrition assessments only when in a crisis state. Therefore, educators, therapists, and other health professionals who have regular contact with these young children are ideal people to receive training and to administer nutrition screening.

Another relevant issue is families' access to nutrition services. Early identification and preventive nutrition services can alleviate malnutrition, growth retardation, frequent infections, dehydration, and other medical consequences. Yet health plans severely limit coverage and reimbursement for nutrition evaluations, especially when not accompanied by a specific medical diagnosis—the symptoms of which still may not be apparent in the young child. Cost-effective studies of nutrition services are difficult to conduct but important to document when health care resources are limited. A 1998 report included the cost considerations and nutrition and health outcomes for a case series of children with special health care needs who received either nutrition services or feeding team services (Lucas & Feucht, 1998).

RECOMMENDATIONS FOR THE FUTURE

The rapid increase in knowledge of cellular function, metabolic processes, and methods of determining body composition will enable greater precision in defining individual energy and nutrient requirements. In turn, the approach to nutrition assessment and intervention will become much more individualized as methodology is refined. Recommendations for dietary intervention will also have a stronger scientific basis as nutrient functions are more fully described. In addition, nutritionists in the 1990s witnessed the identification and characterization of genes associated with many nutrition-related conditions. Nutrients may influence the transcription and translation of specific gene markers. Nutritionists must be aware of developments in molecular biology and respond to changing needs for nutrition care in the future (Bowers & Allred, 1995).

Like any other child, a young child with developmental disabilities should be evaluated as an individual, with nutrition assessment incorporating all current scientific, metabolic, nutritional, and technological knowledge. At the same time, a family-centered, coordinated, and community-based approach must be maintained. With appropriate nutrition screening, assessment, and intervention, a well-nourished child will be able to resist infections, attend school regularly, participate fully in therapy and educational programs, and have better overall functioning in everyday life.

REFERENCES

American Dietetic Association. (1995). Position of the American Dietetic Association: Nutrition services for children with special health needs. *Journal of the American Dietetic Association, 95*, 809–812.

Beal, V.A. (1967). The nutrition history in longitudinal research. *Journal of the American Dietetic Association, 51*, 426–432.

Beaton, G.H., & Benga, J.M. (Eds.). (1973). *Nutrition and preventive medicine* (World Health Organization Monograph No. 62). Geneva, Switzerland: World Health Organization.

Bolland, J.E., Ward, J.Y., & Bolland, J.W. (1988). Improved accuracy of estimating food quantities up to 4 weeks after training. *Journal of the American Dietetic Association, 88*, 1250–1407.

Bowers, D.F., & Allred, J.B. (1995). Advances in molecular biology: Implications for the future of clinical nutrition practice. *Journal of the American Dietetic Association, 95*, 53–59.

Burke, B.S. (1947). The dietary history as a tool in research. *Journal of the American Dietetic Association, 12*, 1041–1046.

Centers for Disease Control and Prevention, National Center for Health Statistics, Division of Health Examination Statistics. (in press). *Revised pediatric growth charts for the U.S.* Washington, DC: Author.

Chumlea, W.C., Guo, S.S., & Steinbaugh, M.L. (1994). Prediction of stature from knee height for black and white adults and children with application to mobility-impaired or handicapped persons. *Journal of the American Dietetic Association, 94,* 1385–1388.

Cronk, C.E., Crocker, A.C., Pueschel, S.M., Shea, A.M., Zackai, E., Pickens, G., & Reed, R.B. (1988). Growth charts for children with Down syndrome: 1 month to 18 years of age. *Pediatrics, 81,* 102–110.

Cronk, C.E., & Roche, A.F. (1982). Race- and age-specific reference data for triceps and skinfolds and weight/stature. *American Journal of Clinical Nutrition, 35,* 347–354.

Ekvall, S.W. (1993). Nutritional assessment and early intervention. In S.W. Ekvall (Ed.), *Pediatric nutrition in chronic diseases and developmental disorders: Prevention, assessment and treatment* (pp. 41–76). New York: Oxford University Press.

Food and Nutrition Board, Institute of Medicine, National Academy of Sciences. (1997). *Dietary reference intakes: Calcium, phosphorus, magnesium, vitamin D and fluoride.* Washington, DC: National Academy Press.

Frisancho, A.R. (1981). New norms of upper limb fat and muscle area for assessment of nutritional status. *American Journal of Clinical Nutrition, 34,* 2540–2545.

Garrahie, E.J., Humphrey, K.F., Witschi, J.C., Stephenson, W.P., & Ellison, R.C. (1991). The value of debriefing mothers of 3 to 7 year old children when analyzing children's diets. *Journal of the American Dietetic Association, 91,* 710–715.

Hamill, P.V., Drizd, T.A., Johnson, C.L., Reed, R.B., & Roche, A.F. (1977). *NCHS growth charts for children 0–18 years* (U.S. Vital and Health Services, Series 11, No. 165). Washington, DC: U.S. Government Printing Office.

Hamill, P.V., Drizd, T.A., Johnson, C.L., Reed, R.B., Roche, A.F., & Moore, M.M. (1979). Physical growth: National Center for Health Statistics percentiles. *American Journal of Clinical Nutrition, 32,* 607–629.

Hamill, P.V., Johnston, F.E., & Lemeshow. S. (1973). *Body weight, stature, and sitting height: White and Negro youths 12–17 years, United States.* (U.S. Vital and Health Statistics, Series 11, No. 126 Publication No. HSM 73-1606). Washington, DC: U.S. Government Printing Office.

Hammer, L.D., Kraemer, H.C., Wilson, D.M., Ritter, P.L., & Dornbusch, S.M. (1991). Standardized percentile curves of body-mass index for children and adolescents. *American Journal of Diseases of Children, 145,* 259–263.

Hansman, C. (1970). Anthropometry and related data anthropometry, skinfold thickness measurements. In R.W. McCammon (Ed.), *Human growth and development.* Springfield, IL: Charles C. Thomas Publisher.

Himes, J.H., Roche, A.F., Thissen, D., & Moore, W.M. (1985). Parent-specific adjustments for evaluation of recumbent length and stature of children. *Pediatrics, 75,* 304–313.

Holm, V.A. (1995). Appendix A: Growth charts for Prader-Willi syndrome. In L.R. Greenswag & R.C. Alexander (Eds.), *Management of Prader-Willi syndrome* (2nd ed.). New York: Springer-Verlag New York.

Horton, W.A., Rotter, J.I., Rimoin, D.L., Scott, C.I., & Hall, J.G. (1978). Standard growth curves for achondroplasia. *Journal of Pediatrics, 93,* 435–438.

Johnson, C.L., Fulwood, R., Abraham, S., & Bryner, J.D. (1981). *Basic data on anthropometric measurements and angular measurements of the hip and knee joints for selected age groups, 1–74 years of age, United States, 1971–1975* (U.S. Vital and Health Statistics, Series 11, No. 219. DHHS Publication No. PHS 81–1669). Washington, DC: U.S. Government Printing Office.

Krick, J., Murphy-Miller, P., Zeger, S., & Wright, E. (1996). Pattern of growth in children with cerebral palsy. *Journal of the American Dietetic Association, 96,* 680–685.

Lucas, B.L., & Feucht, S. (Eds.). (1998). *Cost considerations: The benefits of nutrition services for a case series of children with special health care needs in Washington State.* Olympia: Washington Department of Health.

Lyon, A.J., Preece, M.A., & Grant, D.B. (1985). Growth curve for girls with Turner syndrome. *Archives of Disease in Childhood, 60,* 932–935.

Medlin, M.F. (1990). Individual dietary intake methodology, a 50 year review of progress. *Journal of the American Dietetic Association, 88,* 1250–1257.

Morris, C.A., Demsey, S.A., Leonard, C.O., Dilts, C., & Blackburn, B.L. (1988). Natural history of Williams syndrome: Physical characteristics. *Journal of Pediatrics, 113,* 318–326.

Pipes, P.L., & Glass, R.P. (1997). Collecting and assessing food intake information. In C.M. Trahms & P.L. Pipes (Eds.), *Nutrition in infancy and childhood* (6th ed., pp. 68–97). Burr Ridge, IL: WCB/McGraw-Hill.

Pipes, P.L., & Glass, R.P. (1997). Nutrition and special health care needs. In C.M. Trahms & P.L. Pipes (Eds.), *Nutrition in infancy and childhood* (6th ed., pp. 377–405). Burr Ridge, IL: WCB/McGraw-Hill.

Roche, A.F., & Himes, J.H. (1980). Incremental growth charts. *American Journal of Clinical Nutrition, 33,* 2041–2052.

Todd, K.S., Hudes, M., & Calloway, D.H. (1983). Food intake measurement: Problems and approaches. *American Journal of Clinical Nutrition, 37,* 139–146.

Trahms, C.M., & Pipes, P.L. (1997). Growth, development and nutrition. In C.M. Trahms & P.L. Pipes (Eds.), *Nutrition in infancy and childhood* (6th ed., pp. 1–34). Burr Ridge, IL: WCB/McGraw-Hill.

Wodarski, L.A. (1990) An interdisciplinary nutrition assessment and intervention protocol for children with disabilities. *Journal of the American Dietetic Association, 90,* 1563–1568.

Chapter 7

Occupational Therapy Assessment and the Interdisciplinary Team

Katherine B. Stewart and Susan Wendel

Occupational therapists specialize in the assessment and treatment of children who demonstrate performance delays in childhood occupations of self-care, play, and work (i.e., school-related tasks). Examples of young children with performance difficulties who may benefit from occupational therapy assessment include, but are not limited to, a toddler with Down syndrome who is delayed in learning to use a spoon at mealtime (limited in self-care), a preschooler with cerebral palsy who is limited in exploring her physical environment during playtime (limited in play), and a first-grade child with an attention-deficit/hyperactivity disorder who has difficulty adapting to her classroom routine at school (limited in schoolwork).

This chapter describes pediatric occupational therapy assessment of young children with developmental disabilities and illustrates the clinical decision-making process employed by occupational therapists as part of the interdisciplinary team. Specifically, the chapter includes an explanation of the purpose of occupational therapy assessment, the domains of pediatric occupational therapy, the clinical reasoning underlying the assessment process, the challenges occupational therapists face in conducting these assessments, and recommendations for the future.

PURPOSE OF ASSESSMENT

The primary purpose of a pediatric occupational therapy assessment is to provide an in-depth understanding of a child's developmental and functional abilities in occupational performance areas of self-care, play, and school-related tasks. The occupational therapist uses the assessment process to identify the strengths and barriers contributing to the child's successful or limited performance within these functional areas. Case-Smith (1996) proposed two broad goals for occupational therapy assessments: 1) to analyze the child's performance of everyday activities and 2) to assess the reciprocal relationship between the environment and the child.

The first goal, analysis of functional performance, is accomplished by evaluating the child's intrinsic skills and abilities regarding day-to-day tasks that are relevant for the child. For a child to perform a functional task such as putting on shoes, there are myriad underlying component skills (e.g., fine motor coordination and dexterity, perceptual processing, cognitive ability) that enable successful task performance. The occupational therapist employs various assessment techniques to measure the presence, delay, or deficiency of the underlying component skills. It is the identification of the child's intrinsic skills that contributes to an understanding of the child's overall developmental status and functional performance.

The second goal, assessment of the reciprocal relationship between the environment and the child, is met by determining the extrinsic factors contributing to the child's functional performance. Occupational therapists assess and observe the physical and human attributes of the child's environment. It is essential to consider the reciprocal relationship between the child and the environment, as this relationship may either facilitate or limit the child's development. To understand the scope of occupational therapy assessments of young children fully, it is important to become familiar with the domains of occupational therapy practice.

DOMAINS OF PRACTICE

The American Occupational Therapy Association's uniform terminology document (1994) described three basic domains of occupational therapy practice. These areas consist of the individual's performance areas, performance components, and performance context. Figure 7.1 illustrates the relationship among these domains.

Performance Areas

The performance areas represent the core of human functional activity. For children, these functional activities are defined as self-care, play, and early learning or school-related (work) tasks. An important premise of occupational

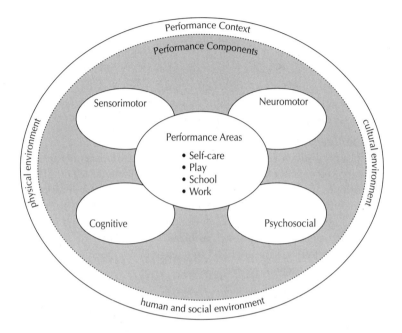

Figure 7.1.   Relationship among the three basic domains of occupational therapy practice.

therapy is that growth and development can be facilitated through the skilled application of activities and relationships within the context of these broad functional areas (Llorens, 1970).

Self-Care Activities
Feeding, dressing, grooming, hygiene, and functional mobility are self-care activities. The establishment of self-care skills follows a developmental sequence toward a child's increasing independence. For example, feeding involves the developmental progression of oral-motor maturity from coordinated sucking and swallowing of liquids to chewing textured foods. Self-feeding requires the maturation of tool use so that the child can use a spoon and fork or drink from a straw. Independent dressing requires following the steps of putting on clothing in an appropriate order, orienting the front and back of clothing, and manipulating the fastenings (e.g., snaps, zippers, shoelaces). Functional mobility is the ability to move independently and negotiate the environment and is used when getting on the school bus and finding the assigned seat or transferring on and off of the toilet.

Play and Leisure Skills
The child's capacity to partake in activity that is motivating, enjoyable, and rewarding depends on play and leisure skills. An infant engages in play by visually

inspecting, mouthing, and manipulating toys. As the child's fine motor and cognitive skills mature, the handling and exploration of objects are refined, enabling a child to build with blocks or to push a button to activate a toy. As more advanced cognitive skills are acquired, the young child expresses his creativity and imagination through make-believe and pretend play. Play also encompasses important social interactions—first, between the infant and the caregiver, then, between the child and his peers. Maturation of motor, cognitive, and social skills also supports success in playing team sports and other games with peers.

School-Related Tasks

The child's performance of school-related tasks (or early learning tasks, if the child is not yet in school) represents important functional accomplishments that contribute to success in school. Examples of school-related tasks include drawing, cutting with scissors, recognizing and matching shapes, comprehending and following verbal directions, developing handwriting, and operating a computer. Personal social skills such as being able to make the transition to a new activity, to follow a routine, and to engage in a cooperative activity with peers also represent school-related tasks.

Performance Components

Performance components form the prerequisite skills required for mastery of the functional tasks in the performance areas of self-care, play, and school, and they encompass specific sensorimotor, cognitive, and psychosocial skills. A summary of these components and abilities is discussed next.

Sensorimotor Skills

Sensory and perceptual processing, neuromusculoskeletal components, and motor skills fall into the category of sensorimotor skills. Sensory processing is the child's ability to register, organize, and understand sensory information. Perceptual processing refers specifically to the organization of sensory material into meaningful patterns. Neuromusculoskeltal components are the underlying foundation of reflexes, muscle tone, range of motion, balance reactions, postural alignment, physical strength, and endurance. Motor skills include gross coordination, fine coordination and dexterity, oral-motor control, visual-motor integration, and praxis (motor planning).

Cognitive Skills

The child's ability to perceive, attend to, and learn from the environment forms the basis of cognitive skills. This domain encompasses problem solving, attention span, and memory, all of which support learning the skills necessary for function in the performance areas. Cognitive skill performance is usually assessed through standardized measures by the psychologist on the interdisciplinary team. Occupational therapists may contribute to the team assessment of a child's cognitive abilities by documenting qualitative aspects of a child's performance. An occupational therapist may note, for instance, a child's poor memory skills, reduced attention span, or difficulty understanding verbal directions during the occupational therapy assessment.

Psychosocial Skills

The abilities necessary for interaction with other children and adults to form friendships and social relationships comprise psychosocial skills. Examples include engaging in reciprocal eye contact, taking turns, sharing a toy or an activity, coping with changes in routine, and producing behavior responses that are socially acceptable. Similar to cognitive performance, the assessment of psychosocial skills is often shared with other members of the interdisciplinary team.

Performance Context

Performance context is the outermost framework in which functional activity is performed. It is represented by the child's physical and social environment, including home, school, and child care. The pediatric occupational therapist plays a central role in evaluating the effects of the environment on the child as well as the child's influence on the environment. For example, the occupational therapist assesses whether physical adaptations made to the home environment will increase independence for a child with a physical disability. In another situation, the occupational therapist may recommend reducing the amount of competing visual stimuli in the classroom to help a distractible child better attend to his or her schoolwork and, in turn, to decrease this child's disruption in the classroom.

The three main aspects of performance context include the human and social environment, the physical environment, and the cultural environment. The social environment is represented by the immediate family members, extended family, and members of the larger community. The physical environment refers to the physical space, including aspects such as the presence of toys and materials, the amount and type of sensory information, and safety factors. The cultural environment is composed of the values, beliefs, rituals, and customs unique to the child's family and their community.

When evaluating a child, the pediatric occupational therapist considers all of the domains of practice: performance areas, performance components, and performance context. Although this initially appears daunting, the experienced therapist realizes that assessing children is an active process that goes beyond the first evaluation session and encompasses ongoing informal observations of the child and family throughout the duration of therapy services (Stewart, 1996). Depending upon the child's and family's immediate needs, the therapist may choose to focus initially on only one of the performance areas and to utilize information from other interdisciplinary team assessments regarding additional performance abilities. A full assessment of all performance domains is best obtained through the collaborative use of information from the family, the therapist's own evaluation of the child, the findings from other professional assessments, and input from other community providers.

REACHING AN INFORMED CLINICAL DECISION

A comprehensive or diagnostic occupational therapy assessment is conducted for three primary reasons: 1) to obtain more in-depth information about the child's developmental and functional status for diagnostic purposes, 2) to determine if a child is eligible for occupational therapy services, and 3) to identify the most appropriate occupational therapy intervention plan for the child. The specific methods and measures used in a comprehensive pediatric occupational therapy assessment vary depending on the purpose of the assessment and the decisions that have to be made regarding the child. Ideally, the primary caregivers, in collaboration with the interdisciplinary team, specify the initial purposes and problems to be addressed (see Section III of this book for case studies).

To assist in the diagnostic process, the occupational therapist uses a combination of standardized norm-referenced measures as well as nonstandardized clinical observations to assess performance areas, performance components, and performance context. The outcome is a greater understanding of the child's functional status and the underlying reasons for performance difficulties in self-care, play, and early learning or school-related tasks. Although there are a number of tools occupational therapists use for assessing underlying performance components in children, fewer tools exist for evaluating performance areas and performance context. Table 7.1 provides a description of selected measures used by pediatric occupational therapists to assess performance areas and performance context. Each assessment tool is summarized in terms of the intended population, purpose, administration method, scoring method, and source.

Selecting the specific assessment tool depends on the purpose of the evaluation. When assessing children to gather information for a diagnosis or to determine occupational therapy services eligibility, standardized, norm-referenced measures are employed to ensure that the test results are reliable and valid. Many public school systems mandate the use of norm-referenced tests by special educators and related personnel (e.g., occupational therapists) when qualifying children for special services. Standardized, norm-referenced instruments are helpful for ascertaining how an individual child's performance compares with age-matched children in the normative sample. Some examples of norm-referenced comprehensive assessment tools commonly used by occupational therapists include the Bayley Scales of Infant Development–Second Edition (BSID-II; Bayley, 1993), the Miller Assessment for Preschoolers (MAP; Miller, 1982), the Peabody Developmental Motor Scales (PDMS; Folio & Fewell, 1983), and the Sensory Integration and Praxis Tests (SIPT; Ayres, 1989). Although standard scores may be required to determine a child's eligibility for an intervention service, these standard scores, when used alone, do not provide complete data on a child. Ideally, a comprehensive assessment includes caregiver interviews and developmental checklists, clinical observation of the qual-

Table 7.1. Selected tools used in occupational therapy assessment of performance areas and performance context

Tool	Ages	Purpose	Administration method	Scoring method	Source
		PERFORMANCE AREA—SELF-CARE			
Behavioral Assessment Scale of Oral Functions in Feeding (Stratton, 1981)	Children and young adults with disabilities ages 10 months–21 years	Assess oral–facial movement and control and chewing, drinking, and swallowing; document function over time	Observation of the child in natural or clinic environment	Performance scored on a five-point rating scale ranging from "passive" to "functional and normal," yielding a profile of oral-motor strengths and weaknesses	Stratton, M. (1981). Behavioral Assessment Scale of Oral Functions in Feeding. *American Journal of Occupational Therapy, 35*(11), 719–721.
Pediatric Evaluation of Disability Inventory (PEDI; Haley, Coster, Ludlow, Haltiwanger, & Andrellos, 1992)	Children with disabilities ages 1 month–7 years	Assess functional skill ability and degree of caregiver assistance in three domains: self-care, mobility, and social function	Interview of the caregiver and/or observation of the child in natural or clinic environment	Norm-referenced standard scores and scaled performance scores calculated for each domain; totals for frequency of task modification levels calculated to describe degree of modifications the child needs	Communication Skill Builders 555 Academic Court San Antonio, TX 78204 1-800-211-8378
Guide for the Uniform Data Set for Medical Rehabilitation for Children (WeeFIM; 1993)	Children with disabilities ages 6 months–7 years	Assess functional status, measure degree of disability and outcomes of intervention in two domains (motor, cognitive) and six subscales (self-care, sphincter control, transfers, locomotion, communication, social cognition)	Interview of caregiver and/or observation of the child in natural or clinic environment	Performance in each subscale scored using a 7-point rating scale, ranging from total dependence to modified dependence to complete independence	Uniform Data System for Medical Rehabilitation State University of New York at Buffalo Buffalo, NY 14241 (716)829-2076 info@udmr.org

(continued)

Table 7.1. *(continued)*

Tool	Ages	Purpose	Administration method	Scoring method	Source
		PERFORMANCE AREA—PLAY			
Revised Knox Preschool Play Scale (Knox, 1997)	Children ages 6 months–6 years	Provide a description of typical play within four dimensions: space management, material management, imitation, participation	Observation of the child in familiar indoor and outdoor play environments, with peers present	Performance scored on a binary scale of occurrence/nonoccurrence of play behaviors Play-age is obtained for each dimension based on majority of play behaviors present and total play-age calculated by determining the mean age of the four dimensions	Knox, S. (1997). Development and current use of the Knox Preschool Play Scale. In L.D. Parham & L.S. Fazio (Eds.), *Play in occupational therapy for children* (pp. 35–51). St. Louis, MO: Mosby.
Test of Playfulness (ToP; Bundy, 1997)	Children ages 18 months–10 years	Describe a child's playfulness by observing the extent (proportion of time engaged), intensity (degree of involvement), and skill (ease and coordination) of play	Observation of the child both in familiar indoor and outdoor environments	Composite scores are not available—tool is currently used to observe and describe playfulness systemically	Bundy, A. (1997). Play and playfulness: What to look for. In L.D. Parham & L.S. Fazio (Eds.), *Play in occupational therapy for children* (pp. 52–66). St. Louis, MO: Mosby.

(continued)

136

Table 7.1. (continued)

Tool	Ages	Purpose	Administration method	Scoring method	Source
		PERFORMANCE AREA—SCHOOL			
School Function Assessment (SFA; Coster, Deeney, Haltiwanger, & Haley, 1998)	Children with disabilities in kindergarten–6th grade	Evaluate and monitor functional performance in the elementary school setting Includes rating of participation in school activity settings, amount of assistance and adaptation for task performance, performance in nine physical task areas and twelve cognitive/behavioral task areas	Observation of the child completed by school personnel familiar with the child's typical school performance	Summary scores yield school participation score, subscale and total task performance scores, scores for assistance and accommodation needed Cutoff points identify typical range of performance of children without disabilities	Communication Skill Builders 555 Academic Court San Antonio, TX 78204 1-800-211-8378
		PERFORMANCE CONTEXT			
Home Observation for Measurement of the Environment–Revised (Caldwell & Bradley, 1984)	Children ages birth–10 years	Assess quality and quantity of social, emotional, and cognitive supports available to identify the developmental stimulation potential in the environment	Caregiver interview and observation in the home	Scored on a binary scale of presence/absence of developmental supports across eight subscales; provides a profile of the home environment	Home Inventory University of Arkansas Little Rock, AR (509)565-7627 lrcoulson@ualr.edu

(continued)

137

Table 7.1. (continued)

Tool	Ages	Purpose	Administration method	Scoring method	Source
		PERFORMANCE CONTEXT			
NCAST Caregiver/Parent–Child Interaction Scales: Feeding and Teaching (Sumner & Spietz, 1994)	Children ages 6–36 months	Rate caregiver and infant interaction, the developmental potential of the environment as observed during a familiar routine (Feeding Scale) and unfamiliar routine (Teaching Scale)	Caregiver interview and observation in the home or clinic environment	Scored on a binary scale of occurrence/nonoccurrence of behaviors to obtain a total descriptive score	NCAST Publications University of Washington CHDD Box 357920 Seattle, WA 98195 (206)543-8528 ncast@u.washington.edu
Family Needs Survey (Bailey & Simeonsson, 1988)	Families who have children with special health care or developmental needs	Assist family and professionals in identifying the family's strengths and needs in caring for the special health care or developmental challenges of the child	Survey completed by the child's primary caregiver(s) and/or extended family members Advised that child's mother and father complete the survey separately	Each of the 35 items rated on a three-point scale of "definitely do not need help with this," "not sure," and "definitely need help with this"; yields a profile of family strengths and needs	Bailey, D.B., & Simeonsson, R.J. (1988). Family Needs Survey. *Journal of Special Education, 22,* 117–127

ity of performance skills in both structured and unstructured situations, and viewing the child in his or her natural environments.

Once it is decided that a child is eligible for occupational therapy services, it is necessary to determine the most appropriate intervention plan. When this is the primary reason for assessment, the occupational therapist considers evaluation methods that include in-depth observations of the child's performance within his or her natural environments (e.g., home, child care, playground) as well as interviews with parents or other adults working with the child. For the purpose of treatment planning, norm-referenced instruments may have limited value. They measure skills that are commonly seen in a typically developing population but do not necessarily measure what is critical for functional performance in children with disabilities. Criterion-based assessments are frequently utilized to establish intervention goals and a treatment plan. Some examples of these assessments include the Hawaii Early Learning Profile (HELP; Parks, 1992), the Revised Knox Preschool Play Scale (Knox, 1997), and the Test of Playfulness (Bundy, 1997). In summary, occupational therapists employ various methods and measures to evaluate the functional and developmental status of the child for making appropriate diagnostic decisions as well as for gathering information regarding further assessment and intervention. Occupational therapists carefully select evaluation methods and measures that best match the specific purpose of the assessment.

Although this chapter focuses on the pediatric occupational therapy comprehensive or diagnostic assessment, as part of an interdisciplinary team, it is important for the reader to appreciate that the process of occupational therapy assessment transcends each stage of the therapeutic relationship with the child and family. Assessment may begin with early screening and proceed through diagnostic evaluation, ongoing intervention, and the evaluation of child progress and parent satisfaction. The following discussion examines the types of clinical reasoning occupational therapists utilize to guide the course of a comprehensive evaluation, and this process is illustrated with a case study.

Clinical Reasoning in Occupational Therapy Pediatric Assessments

Assessment is a fundamental yet complex part of pediatric occupational therapy services for children. This process, due to its complexities and dynamic nature, requires the systematic use of decision-making skills, referred to as *clinical reasoning*. Several critical decision points in the assessment process demand the therapist's careful use of clinical reasoning: "Clinical judgments or decisions are not made on the basis of one or two test scores or an isolated observation, but are determined through the complex process of clinical reasoning" (Hall, Robertson, & Turner, 1992, p. 927).

Clinical reasoning in occupational therapy literature is described in different ways and reflects the evolutionary process of the profession. Rogers, one of the first to describe clinical reasoning, suggested that it is the "[thinking] process through which we [occupational therapists] learn about patients so that we may help them through engagement in occupation" (1983, p. 602). Rogers and her colleagues (Rogers & Holm, 1991; Rogers & Masagatani, 1982) have focused on the prescriptive nature of clinical reasoning, similar to the scientific reasoning commonly used in medicine.

Using another perspective and a different methodology, commonly used in anthropology, Mattingly (1991) advocated the use of narrative reasoning in occupational therapy. She stated that "clinical reasoning in occupational therapy is primarily directed not to a biological world of disease but to the human world of motives and values and beliefs—a world of human meaning" (p. 983). Narrative reasoning is the descriptive notion of clinical reasoning that is a "largely tacit, highly imagistic, and deeply phenomenological model of thinking" (Mattingly, 1991, p. 979). Others recommend that occupational therapists combine different types of reasoning in their clinical practice. For example, Fleming (1991) described clinical reasoning in occupational therapy as a three-track procedure combining scientific reasoning, interactive (narrative) reasoning, and conditional reasoning (a multidimensional process of imagining and integrating images from the child's past, present, and future). Schell and Cervero (1993) suggested another integrative approach to clinical reasoning in occupational therapy that, in addition to scientific and narrative reasoning, includes pragmatic reasoning. Pragmatic reasoning considers important practical issues when making decisions for the child's assessment and intervention, such as reimbursement for services, the expertise of the therapist, and the availability of equipment needed.

Table 7.2 presents the critical decision points within a pediatric occupational therapy evaluation and the types of clinical reasoning employed at each of these points. In addition, the following case study demonstrates the concomitant use of varied clinical reasoning strategies in making decisions during the initial comprehensive assessment process.

Example of Decision Making Through a Case Study

Mui was a 12-month-old girl, born prematurely at 32 weeks' gestation, with a history of medical complications during the neonatal period including anoxia at the time of delivery. Her parents were first-generation immigrants from Vietnam, and Vietnamese was the sole language spoken in the home. Mui's parents were concerned that their daughter was not able to sit alone and that she seemed behind in development compared to other infants her age at the child care center. For this reason, Mui and her family were referred to a developmental clinic for infants at risk in order to obtain a comprehensive interdisciplinary team evaluation. Evaluation by an occupational therapist was included in the team assessment. The parents hoped the assessments would offer some explanation for Mui's developmental delays and would provide the family with suggestions for ways to help Mui.

Table 7.2.   Decision points and clinical reasoning for pediatric occupational therapy assessments

Decision points	Considerations	Types of clinical reasoning
#1 Generate initial and alternative hypotheses	How should the problem be framed? What other ways could this problem be viewed?	Scientific
#2 Select appropriate evaluation methods and measures	What methods and measures should be used to assess the child? What alternative methods or measures might be required?	Scientific Narrative Pragmatic
#3 Conduct the assessment	Who else should be included in the assessment process? How should these individuals be included? How long should the assessment take? Where should the assessment be conducted? Should the test environment, test materials, and test procedures be adapted for the child and family? If so, how?	Narrative Scientific Pragmatic
#4 Interpret assessment data	Should the initial and/or alternative hypotheses be accepted or rejected? How do the assessment results relate to the child's occupational performance areas? How can the assessment data be translated into functional performance terms that are meaningful to the child and caregivers?	Scientific Narrative Pragmatic
#5 Develop recommendations	Does the child need occupational therapy to function effectively in home, school, or community environments? If child does need occupational therapy, what type of service best meets the child's needs? Should the child be referred for other services?	Conditional Pragmatic

The following principles guided the occupational therapist when planning and implementing Mui's assessment:

1. Mui was to be viewed as a whole, unique child.
2. The parents' concerns and needs were considered to be of primary importance and played a central role in Mui's assessment.

3. The influence of Mui's cultural, physical, and family environment was carefully considered.
4. The assessment was directed toward gaining an understanding of Mui's performance abilities in the areas of self-care, play, and early learning.

Generating Initial and Alternative Hypotheses

To prepare for Mui's comprehensive assessment, the occupational therapist used scientific reasoning to generate an initial hypothesis and alternative hypotheses at the first decision point. Rogers and Holm (1991) described this sequence of cognitive activity as diagnostic reasoning. The therapist creates a "clinical image of the patient through cue acquisition, hypothesis generation, cue interpretation, and hypothesis evaluation" (p. 1045). In Mui's case, the therapist looked for pertinent information in birth and medical records and the physician referral letter. The birth records indicated premature birth with the complication of possible anoxia, and the referring physician stated concerns about atypical muscle tone and motor delays. With these cues, the therapist generated the following hypotheses: 1) the neuromotor impairments Mui demonstrated may have been consistent with a diagnosis of cerebral palsy and 2) Mui's motor delays may have been limiting her ability to perform early exploratory play and self-help skills.

Selecting Appropriate Evaluation Methods and Measures

Due to the referral concerns of neuromotor impairments, the therapist decided to examine Mui's presenting problems within the context of a neurodevelopmental frame of reference at the second decision point. This guided the therapist's selection of specific tools to measure Mui's performance component skills (specifically gross coordination, fine coordination and dexterity, and neuromusculoskeletal components). The therapist theorized that problems in these areas may have been directly affecting Mui's ability to engage in functional play skills. The results from the chosen evaluation instruments would enable the therapist to accept or reject the initial hypotheses.

In addition to employing scientific clinical reasoning, the therapist used pragmatic reasoning when selecting the most appropriate evaluation tools. In Mui's situation, there were certain practical considerations that shaped the assessment process. These included 1) her parents' priorities, 2) Mui's corrected age of 1 year, 3) the environment in which the evaluation was to be conducted (a clinical setting, within the context of the clinic procedures), 4) the fact that Mui's managed health care plan had approved only one visit for evaluation, and 5) that the occupational therapy comprehensive evaluation was scheduled to be completed within a 2-hour period.

With all of these considerations in mind, the therapist chose two standardized assessments: BSID-II and the Movement Assessment of Infants (MAI; Chandler, Andrews, & Swanson, 1980). All components of the BSID-II were to be administered, including the Mental Scale, the Motor Scale, and the Behavior Rating Scale. To supplement the formal standardized tests, qualitative data were obtained by the therapist's informal observation of Mui's free play with toys. Using a formal test of play skills was not possible because the available tools required observation of the child in the natural environment of home, child care, or preschool. This was not feasible for the occupational therapist, who was restricted to the clinic setting.

Conducting the Assessment

The therapist began the session with a parent interview facilitated by a Vietnamese interpreter. At this stage, the third decision point, the therapist applied narrative reasoning. The purpose of the first interview was to obtain a clear understanding of the parents' concerns and their specific expectations for the assessment. Mui's parents were also asked to describe Mui's typical day by outlining her daily routine. The interview and verbal exchange with the parents continued throughout the evaluation session, and the ensuing family stories were essential to Mui's comprehensive assessment.

During the course of the assessment, as Mui's abilities and the family narratives unfolded, the occupational therapist continually considered if and how the assessment should be adjusted to obtain the most relevant and accurate information. It is often difficult to develop a realistic and relevant evaluation plan based only on data from the initial referral. Therefore, in most environments (e.g., community-based early intervention centers, public school programs), the initial evaluation plan is revised after the child has been seen at least once by the therapist. In some diagnostic programs, however, such as hospitals and outpatient clinics, the therapist does not have the luxury of evaluating the child over a series of sessions. Thus, adjustments to the assessment plan must be made spontaneously. In this case, Mui's mother stated during the parent interview that she was having some difficulties feeding Mui. The therapist immediately adapted the assessment plan to include time for observing of Mui's oral-motor and feeding skills.

While administering the BSID-II and the MAI, observing Mui's play and feeding skills, and interviewing the parents, the therapist employed scientific, narrative, and pragmatic reasoning. This process guided her decisions about the order of the test items, when to take a break and allow Mui to be comforted by a parent, and how to adjust the assessment plan to meet newly identified needs.

Interpreting the Assessment Data

Once all of the initial assessment information was gathered, the therapist analyzed the quantitative and qualitative data from the standardized tests, the clinical observations of play and feeding, and the parent narratives. Accurate and complete reading of all assessment data, the fourth decision point, is a critical component of the occupational therapist's assessment. Precise interpretation of assessment data allows the therapist to make sound clinical decisions regarding the child's developmental and functional status, eligibility for occu-

pational therapy services, and—if services are indicated—recommendations
for the frequency, duration, and type of therapeutic intervention.

At this stage of the assessment process, the therapist employed a combination of scientific, narrative, and conditional reasoning. Using scientific reasoning, the initial hypotheses were accepted. Mui's performance on the MAI
showed atypical muscle tone distributed asymmetrically (increased tone on the
left side of her body), limitations in joint mobility of the left hip and ankle, and
delayed development of automatic balance reactions. Her performance scores
on the BSID-II were 2 standard deviations below the mean when compared
with other infants 12 months of age, indicating a significant developmental
delay. Qualitative descriptions of performance obtained from the BSID-II Behavior Rating Scale indicated that Mui's attention/arousal and orientation/
engagement were within normal limits while her emotional regulation received
a rating of questionable and motor quality had a nonoptimal rating. Oral-
motor difficulties included poor lip closure for early cup-drinking and the refusal of textured and lumpy foods. Mui's play skills were impaired by factors
such as limited mobility to explore her environment, unstable sitting balance,
and difficulty in reaching for and manipulating toys due to reduced left arm
and hand movements. Mui was alert and interested in toys and was capable of
age-appropriate imitation play; however, her motor delays affected the extent
and quality of her play.

Narrative reasoning was used by the therapist to translate the child's developmental and functional status in terms that would be meaningful to and
relevant for the family. Using conditional reasoning, the therapist interpreted
the assessment data by focusing on Mui's strengths, the known conditions
often inherent to the diagnosis of cerebral palsy, and the family's understanding of cerebral palsy. The therapist used her clinical knowledge of these sets of
interacting elements, and she projected what impact and change might occur
if the child and family were provided with intervention services.

The results of all interdisciplinary assessments were compiled, and the assessment team confirmed the initial hypotheses: Mui's neuromotor impairments were consistent with a diagnosis of cerebral palsy. The occupational
therapist identified that Mui's functional performance for eating and play skills
was impaired secondary to difficulties in gross coordination, fine motor coordination and dexterity, and oral-motor control.

Recommendations

To determine specific recommendations for Mui and her family, the therapist
used both conditional and pragmatic reasoning at the fifth decision point. The
family and the assessment team together agreed that a referral to the community early intervention program would be in the child's and the parents' best
interest. The occupational therapist recommended that Mui receive occupational therapy services to address her play and feeding skills. It was further sug-

gested that the community occupational therapist conduct assessments of the home and child care environments to determine needed adaptations or modifications to support Mui's functional independence.

Mui's story illustrates the complex, and often tacit, procedure of clinical reasoning. The experienced pediatric occupational therapist combines various types of clinical reasoning throughout the assessment process, ensuring attention is given to each of the performance domains. The field of pediatric occupational therapy continues to evolve in its use of functional and ecological assessments and the application of clinical reasoning strategies. The next section explores some issues and challenges in occupational therapy assessment of children with developmental disabilities and suggests some possible solutions.

ISSUES RELEVANT TO OCCUPATIONAL THERAPY AND RECOMMENDATIONS FOR THE FUTURE

Although there are many challenges early childhood professionals face in their quest for providing quality assessments of children with developmental disabilities, four are experienced most commonly by pediatric occupational therapists: 1) overlapping boundaries with other professionals, 2) limited time, 3) the proper selection and use of measures, and 4) the development of measures for assessing performance areas and performance context. These themes are discussed next.

Overlapping Boundaries

Due to the holistic nature of occupational therapy theory and practice, many areas of this field overlap with those of other early childhood professions. For example, occupational therapy shares concerns with physical therapy regarding the child's motor skills, with nutrition regarding feeding skills, with nursing regarding self-help skills, and with psychology regarding cognition and early learning. In addition, some assessment measures employed by occupational therapists and other early childhood professionals may be quite similar. Each discipline, however, uses different frames of reference and theoretical bases when interpreting the assessment data.

Interdisciplinary teamwork requires a flexible, functional approach from each discipline to produce a comprehensive assessment of the child, the family, and the child's environments. The unique contribution of occupational therapy to the interdisciplinary assessment team focuses on addressing the child's occupational performance needs in day-to-day activities that are important to the child and family. Occupational therapists serving on an interdisciplinary team must be highly skilled in the theory and practice of their own discipline and at the same time have a strong working knowledge of the team's other disciplines.

A model of transdisciplinary assessment, referred to as *arena assessment*, promotes interdisciplinary collaboration by replacing the need for individual disciplines to administer separate tests. In an arena assessment, the parent or caregiver and professionals of various disciplines observe and evaluate the child together during a single session. *Transdisciplinary Play-Based Assessment: A Functional Approach to Working with Young Children, Revised Edition* (Linder, 1993), is an evaluation tool that utilizes the arena assessment model.

Limited Time

In reality, there is rarely enough time to assess each area of the child's development within the broad scope of occupational therapy practice. As health care and public education systems demand more cost-effective services, providers must become more efficient. The skilled pediatric occupational therapist realizes that a comprehensive evaluation of the child does not include each and every performance area, performance component, and performance context but instead focuses on the most relevant and critical elements for the child and family at the time of the initial assessment. The experienced therapist recognizes that assessment of children is an ongoing, dynamic process that occurs in different environments. Occupational therapists play a key role in designing and implementing special services for children with developmental disabilities that are well coordinated with other services the child receives, ensuring both quality and continuity of care.

Proper Selection and Use of Measures

Standardized assessments must be administered in a precise and exact manner. An assessment tool administered improperly or used inappropriately, given the context of the situation, results in inaccurate data. This can lead to erroneous decisions regarding diagnosis, program eligibility, or the development of an appropriate intervention plan.

The occupational therapist must be a well-informed consumer of the myriad childhood assessment tools available. This knowledge begins with a thorough review of each assessment measure to become familiar with the tool's purpose and its recommended use, reliability, and validity, as well as its strengths and weaknesses. In most cases, specialized training is required to administer and interpret a standardized test adequately. Occupational therapists need continual comprehensive training regarding the use of standardized measures both at the preservice and in-service training levels. To ensure that standard procedures are followed during child assessments, the therapist should conduct interrater agreement checks with other trained professionals.

When evaluating children from diverse cultural backgrounds, the occupational therapist must also be aware of the cultural limitations inherent in many standardized developmental measures. Some developmental tests are based on restricted norms and, therefore, may not be appropriate measures for children with diverse racial or ethnic backgrounds (Richardson, 1996). In addition, many early intervention personnel, including occupational therapists, may possess limited training in working with families having different cultural backgrounds from their own. Thus, therapists must exercise great caution when interpreting standardized test results and informal observations of children and families.

Similarly, care should be taken when evaluating the cognitive and social components of children with significant motor impairments. Many assessments of early cognition and play skills rely on tasks that require the child to manipulate objects. Severe motor impairments may reduce a child's performance score or make it impossible to administer a standardized measure of cognition. Physical therapists and occupational therapists play an important role in educating other assessment team members about the importance of proper positioning and physical handling of the child to obtain optimal performance on cognitive and social interaction measures.

Development of Measures for Assessing Performance Areas and Performance Context

As mentioned previously, a number of standardized assessments are available to occupational therapists for analyzing a child's performance components. However, only a limited number of reliable and valid measures exist for the assessment of performance areas such as play, self-care, and school-related function. Formal assessment tools that evaluate the child's performance context (i.e., ecological assessments) are even more limited.

Occupational therapy has used measures developed from a variety of different disciplines. Many of these tests are appropriate for the assessment of a child's performance components. However, occupational therapists need to create more tools that measure children's occupational performance within the context of their everyday environments. Occupational therapists are beginning to respond to this challenge. Tools such as the Pediatric Evaluation of Disability Inventory (PEDI; Haley, Coster, Ludlow, Haltiwanger, & Andrellos, 1992), the Early Coping Inventory (Zeitlin, Williamson, & Scezpanski, 1988), the Test of Playfulness (Bundy, 1997), and the School Function Assessment (SFA; Coster, Deeney, Haltiwanger, & Haley, 1998) have been formulated to broaden the understanding of early childhood occupations. Continuing education programs are needed to assist occupational therapists in learning how to utilize these functional assessments in their pediatric practices. Further research, both quantitative and qualitative, is also needed to develop assessment tools for investigating childhood human occupation.

CONCLUSION

Occupational therapy assessments of young children with developmental disabilities focus on the child's performance in day-to-day occupations, including self-care, play, and work. Using different types of clinical reasoning, the occupational therapist selects and adapts a variety of assessment methods and measures, then interprets the evaluation data in light of the child's holistic nature, family priorities, and environmental influences. In collaboration with the family and other interdisciplinary team members, the occupational therapist contributes to decisions regarding the child's diagnosis, the child's eligibility for services, and the development of specific occupational therapy intervention plans. Occupational therapy assessments foster a broader understanding of the child's functional performance on everyday tasks. Thus, the pediatric occupational therapist offers the interdisciplinary team unique frames of reference for viewing the child and family. With specialized training and clinical experience, the therapist effectively blends this knowledge with that of other team members so that child assessments are cost-effective, comprehensive, and coordinated.

REFERENCES

American Occupational Therapy Association. (1994). Uniform terminology for occupational therapy–Third edition. *American Journal of Occupational Therapy, 48,* 1047–1054.

Ayres, A.J. (1989). *Sensory Integration and Praxis Tests (SIPT).* Los Angeles: Western Psychological Services.

Bailey, D.B., & Simeonsson, R.J. (1988). Family Needs Survey. *Journal of Special Education, 22,* 117–127.

Bayley, N. (1993). *Bayley Scales of Infant Development–Second Edition.* San Antonio, TX: The Psychological Corp.

Bundy, A. (1997). Play and playfulness: What to look for. In L.D. Parham & L.S. Fazio (Eds.), *Play in occupational therapy for children* (pp. 52–66). St. Louis, MO: Mosby.

Caldwell, B.M., & Bradley, R.H. (1984). *Home Observation for Measurement of the Environment–Revised.* Fayetteville: The University of Arkansas Press.

Case-Smith, J. (1996). An overview of occupational therapy with children. In J. Case-Smith, A. Allen, & P.N. Pratt (Eds.), *Occupational therapy for children* (3rd ed., pp. 3–17). St. Louis, MO: Mosby.

Chandler, L., Andrews, M., & Swanson, M. (1980). *The Movement Assessment of Infants (MAI): A manual.* Rolling Bay, WA: Authors.

Coster, W., Deeney, T., Haltiwanger, J., & Haley, S. (1998). *School Function Assessment (SFA).* San Antonio, TX: The Psychological Corp.

Fleming, M.H. (1991). The therapist with the three-track mind. *American Journal of Occupational Therapy, 45*(11), 1007–1014.

Folio, M.R., & Fewell, R.R. (1983). *Peabody Developmental Motor Scales and Activity Cards (PDMS).* Itasca, IL: The Riverside Publishing Co.

Guide for the Uniform Data Set for Medical Rehabilitation for Children (WeeFIM; Version 4.0). (1993). Buffalo: State University of New York at Buffalo.

Haley, S.M., Coster, W.J., Ludlow, L.H., Haltiwanger, J.T., & Andrellos, P.J. (1992). *Pediatric Evaluation of Disability Inventory (PEDI).* San Antonio, TX: Therapy Skill Builders.

Hall, L., Robertson, W., & Turner, M.A. (1992). Clinical reasoning process for service provision in the public school. *American Journal of Occupational Therapy, 46*(10), 927–936.

Knox, S. (1997). Development and current use of the Knox Preschool Play Scale. In L.D. Parham & L.S. Fazio (Eds.), *Play in occupational therapy for children* (pp. 35–51). St. Louis, MO: Mosby.

Linder, T.W. (1993). *Transdisciplinary play-based assessment: A functional approach to working with young children* (Rev. ed.). Baltimore: Paul H. Brookes Publishing Co.

Llorens, L.A. (1970). Facilitating growth and development: The promise of occupational therapy. *American Journal of Occupational Therapy, 24,* 93–101.

Mattingly, C. (1991). What is clinical reasoning? *American Journal of Occupational Therapy, 45*(11), 979–986.

Miller, L.J. (1982). *Miller Assessment for Preschoolers (MAP)*. San Antonio, TX: The Psychological Corp.

Parks, S. (1992). *Inside HELP: Hawaii Early Learning Profile administration and reference manual*. Palo Alto, CA: VORT Corporation.

Piper, M.C., & Darrah, J. (1994). *Alberta Infant Motor Scale*. Philadelphia: W.B. Saunders Company.

Richardson, P.K. (1996). Use of standardized tests in pediatric practice. In J. Case-Smith, A.S. Allen, & P.N. Pratt (Eds.), *Occupational therapy for children* (pp. 200–224). St. Louis, MO: Mosby.

Rogers, J.C. (1983). Eleanor Clarke Slagle Lectureship—1983; Clinical reasoning: The ethics, science and art. *American Journal of Occupational Therapy, 37*(9), 601–616.

Rogers, J.C., & Holm, M.B. (1991). Occupational therapy diagnostic reasoning: A component of clinical reasoning. *American Journal of Occupational Therapy, 45*(11), 1045–1053.

Rogers, J.C., & Masagatani, G. (1982). Clinical reasoning of occupational therapists during the initial assessment of physically disabled patients. *Occupational Therapy Journal of Research, 2*, 195–219.

Schell, B.A., & Cervero, R.M. (1993). Clinical reasoning in occupational therapy: An integrative review. *American Journal of Occupational Therapy, 47*(7), 605–610.

Stewart, K.B. (1996). Occupational therapy assessment in pediatrics: Purposes, process, and methods of evaluation. In J. Case-Smith, A.S. Allen, & P.N. Pratt (Eds.), *Occupational therapy for children* (pp. 165–199). St. Louis, MO: Mosby.

Stratton, M. (1981). Behavioral Assessment Scale of Oral Functions in Feeding. *American Journal of Occupational Therapy, 35*(11), 719–721.

Sumner, G., & Spietz, A. (1994). *Nursing Child Assessment Satellite Training (NCAST) Caregiver/Parent–Child Interaction Scales*. Seattle, WA: NCAST Publications.

Zeitlin, S., Williamson, G.G., & Sczepanski, M. (1988). *Early Coping Inventory*. Bensenville, IL: Scholastic Testing Service.

Chapter 8

The Role of Pediatric Physical Therapy in the Interdisciplinary Assessment Process

Mary E. Tatarka, Marcia W. Swanson,
and Kathleen A. Washington

Pediatric physical therapy addresses a child's capacity for functional movement, often referred to as *motor development* or *motor performance*. *Functional movement* implies that the activity is purposeful, goal-directed, and meaningful (Campbell, 1994). For a young child, the purpose of movement is mobility, and the goal is exploration and manipulation of the environment. Through physical investigation, growing children learn about their world and discover how they can influence and modify conditions within their environments in order to achieve personal objectives.

Movement is the product of the dynamic interaction of multiple factors and systems. The characteristics of a specific motor skill are shaped by the individual child's neuromotor composition and personal motivation in combination with the physical and social environment (see Figure 8.1). The biological structures and physiology underlying motor function are determined primarily by an infant's genetic endowment and health status. During maturation, the pace and quality of motor development are influenced by the child's own temperament and cognitive ability, the conditions of the home and parenting environment, and the various types and levels of sensory stimulation processed by the child. Consequently, the optimal physical therapy assessment is conducted within the context of the child's natural environment and evaluates motor skills that are functional and meaningful in the life of that particular child. Although "the emphasis on assessing relevant functional behaviors in naturalistic settings should be the cornerstone of the physical therapy motor assessment in young infancy" (Haley, Baryza, & Blanchard, 1993, p. 231), this is not always possible given the restrictions of the physical environment of the interdisciplinary assessment team's clinic and the constraints of standardized assessment tools. Nevertheless, the observations, conclusions, and recommendations of the pediatric physical therapy assessment need to be interpreted within the framework of the individual child's personal needs and unique social and physical environment.

The pediatric physical therapist evaluates a motor impairment in relation to the age of the child and considers the role of movement in the developmental tasks of that particular age level. Within the first 12 months of life, the major

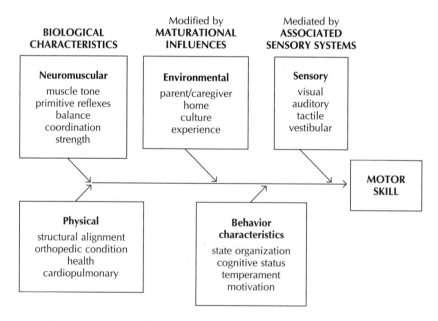

Figure 8.1.   The characteristics that shape a specific motor skill.

motor task is the acquisition of upright posture and the development of reciprocal motion. The emergence and refinement of stance, balance, and antigravity
movement are key components of this maturational process. From 1 to 3 years
of age, while the young child's ambulatory skills mature with running and stair-
climbing, the self-help skills of feeding, dressing, and toileting also develop. Between 4 and 5 years of age, the motor skills necessary for school readiness are
maturing, including visual-motor coordination and fine motor skills. For the
school-age child of 6 years and older, independence in self-care skills is essential
for social integration; mature gross motor skills—characterized by speed, agility,
and coordination—are necessary for participation in recreational sports.

A movement disorder can disrupt this developmental process in a variety
of ways depending on the nature, severity, and chronological timing of the disorder. To assess the full impact of a movement disorder on a young child, it is
helpful to utilize the National Center for Medical Rehabilitation Research's five-
dimensional model of disablement (National Institutes of Health, 1993). In this
model, the five dimensions are not hierarchical but, rather, interact synergisti-
cally to conceptualize the rehabilitation process for a person with a disability.

The model begins with *pathophysiology*, the damage at the cellular or tissue
levels that can result in an impairment. An intraventricular hemorrhage in a
premature infant is an example of pathophysiology. The second dimension is
impairment, indicating loss or abnormality of an organ or physiological system,
such as impairment of muscle function, balance, sensorimotor control, or coordination. *Functional limitations*, the third dimension, are inadequate or atypical
motor skills that result from physical impairments. A gait problem (e.g., decreased velocity) is an example of a functional limitation. In this model, *disability* means that the child is unable to perform activities that are necessary for independent function, such as mobility or self-care. The fifth dimension, *societal
limitation*, refers to a child's inability to participate in school, sports, or social activities due to societal barriers, as in policies that limit accessibility. The pediatric physical therapy assessment typically focuses on the dimensions of impairment, functional limitations, and disability. However, in conjunction with
other interdisciplinary team members, the therapist considers observed motor
dysfunction in relation to any known or suspected pathophysiology. In addition, the child's functional needs must be evaluated within the context of existing societal limitations that restrict his or her life or activities. Several advocacy
strategies that can be employed by pediatric physical therapists to address
societal limitations were proposed by Shaw in 1997.

PRINCIPLES OF ASSESSMENT

Three basic principles underlie the process of pediatric assessment and guide
the therapist throughout planning and implementation. These three principles
inform the assessment process, guide the information gathering, and ensure
the social validity of the findings.

The first of these principles dictates that the assessment must be ecologically valid. In an ecological model of child development, the reciprocal interaction between the child and the many levels of the environment within the developmental process is recognized (Bailey & Wolery, 1992; Bronfenbrenner, 1977). The child has an effect on the environment which, in turn, influences the child's development. Guided by this model, the therapist examines and interprets the child's developmental skills relative to the child's own milieu. This includes the child's proximate social environment, such as the caregivers, siblings, and extended family. It also encompasses the more remote environments of the early intervention or school environment, and the broad social, cultural, and institutional factors that influence the family system.

A related but distinct principle is that of an holistic view of the child (Cherry, 1991). In the context of pediatric physical therapy assessment, holism is the perspective that the child's motor development interrelates with other organ systems and developmental processes. In the assessment of the "whole child," the therapist considers how motor abilities interact with other organ systems (e.g., sensory, cardiopulmonary) and processes (e.g., cognitive, social). Holism will also guide the assessment process itself in determining the most important aspects of functional movement that are required to achieve individual movement goals. For example, the assessment of a toddler with both cerebral palsy and a severe respiratory disorder might include direct measures of endurance and respiratory function so that full and independent participation in preschool can be attained. Following the assessment, the therapist interprets the findings and formulates recommendations relative to the child's strengths and needs in all organ systems and in all dimensions of the child's functioning, including psychosocial and cognitive domains.

Legislation that governs the provision of special education for infants and children with special needs, which encompasses related services such as physical therapy, also drives the assessment process. In the United States, the Individuals with Disabilities Education Act (IDEA) of 1991 (PL 102-119) provides guidelines for the assessment and intervention of infants, toddlers, and preschoolers who have established disabilities or who are at risk for disabilities. A basic principle of legislation is that the assessment must be family centered or family driven. Caregiver and family considerations have priority in all steps of the assessment process, including the focus of the assessment, the preferred environment, and the sharing of information. The evaluating therapist often assumes a role of child and family advocate in assisting the family with the coordination of resources, communicating with community service providers, and obtaining educational services in the least restrictive environment (Effgen, 1994). Pediatric therapists need a thorough understanding of legislation and its ramifications for young children and their families.

Given these principles, the interdisciplinary assessment team process includes the parents or caregivers, as well as individuals who can provide background regarding the child's other environments and professionals with expertise in different developmental domains. Adherence to these three principles will enable the therapist to provide an assessment that is broad-based and socially valid.

PURPOSES AND EXPECTED OUTCOMES OF PEDIATRIC PHYSICAL THERAPY ASSESSMENT

The purposes of the physical therapy assessment are 1) to identify atypical development, impairment, or delay in the young child's motor function; 2) to determine the neuromuscular basis for observed deviations from typical motor function; 3) to assess the level of impairment, functional limitation, or disability; and 4) to provide recommendations for management and therapeutic intervention. Together, this information contributes to the broader issues of the interdisciplinary team process. The objectives of the pediatric physical therapy assessment are explored in the following discussion.

Establish a Relationship with Family and Caregivers

Establishing a relationship of communication and collaboration with the child and his or her family or caregivers is a primary goal of the evaluation. The assessment provides the therapist with the opportunity to learn from the parents or caregivers and to hear their concerns and priorities for their child. The therapist has the responsibility to inform the family of the purpose and format of the assessment and the activities and domains to be tested and to explain the procedures that will be used to evaluate the child. Throughout the assessment process, the therapist can increase the parents' understanding of their child's motor function by identifying the child's specific movement activities and by indicating how particular components of movement, such as balance, coordination, or muscle tone, are contributing to the child's movement skills or difficulties. Caregiver education should be an integral part of every phase of the assessment.

Determine Developmental Level of Motor Skills

Determining the child's developmental level of gross and fine motor function is another objective of the physical therapy assessment. Specific quantitative information regarding a child's level of motor ability relative to other children of the same chronological age is often required for formulating a clinical decision or for gaining access to therapeutic services. The therapist distinguishes between a generalized delay reflected in multiple areas of motor function (e.g., a delay of ambulation, hand use, and oral-motor skills) and delay or immaturity in only one aspect of motor function (e.g., a delay in stair-climbing, hopping, and other skills requiring balance on one foot). When motor function is delayed in more than one area, recognizing variations in the extent of delay in different areas can be important for determining the underlying causes of the motor dysfunction and for developing intervention strategies and priorities.

Identify Underlying Impairments

The physiological and structural components of movement are evaluated in the physical therapy assessment to detect the neuromuscular impairments that may be the underlying cause of delayed or dysfunctional motor skills. This information is necessary to understand the nature of a child's motor problem and to determine the appropriate focus and therapeutic approach for intervention. Orthopedic, muscular, neurological, sensory, and vestibular systems are evaluated depending on the child's developmental history and performance on tests of motor function. Quantitative measures, such as range of motion of joints and scores on neuromotor examinations as well as qualitative observations of atypical movements and specific movement strategies, are incorporated into the assessment process.

Recognize Strengths of Child

Identifying and describing the child's areas of personal strength and capabilities are additional aims of the assessment process. Recognition of a child's abilities is essential for a child's personal development as well as for the formation of a therapy plan to deal with disabilities. The impact of a motor impairment (e.g., gross motor dysfunction) can be minimized when the child can capitalize on skills in other areas (e.g., fine motor dexterity). A muscle tone abnormality that restricts a child's movement may be partially compensated by the child's intact motor planning skills and the ability to control his or her movements to minimize the effects of spasticity. A child's enjoyment of movement, tolerance for physical handling, or responsiveness to sensory stimulation can greatly enhance the benefit of therapeutic intervention. For a child with limited motor ability, personal characteristics such as motivation, curiosity, and persistence are traits to be valued and supported.

Assess Functional Abilities

Assessing the extent to which motor function enables or restricts the child's ability to perform in other arenas (e.g., communication, cognitive tests, activities of daily living) is also a part of the physical therapy assessment. This information will assist other team members as they form conclusions about the child's capabilities and difficulties in their domains of interest.

Develop Intervention Plans and Recommend Areas for Additional Evaluation

A major objective of the assessment is to ascertain priority areas for therapeutic intervention and to develop recommendations for intervention strategies that are specific to the individual child and family situation. The therapist considers the unique contributions and the goals of each child and family in making recommendations. The therapist also indicates domains requiring more comprehensive investigation or concerns to be referred to specialists not on the interdisciplinary team. Children may need additional evaluations for diagnosis or treatment based on findings from the initial assessment, such as orthotic, ophthalmologic, or orthopedic evaluations.

DIMENSIONS ASSESSED BY THE PHYSICAL THERAPIST

The physical therapy assessment is a multidimensional process that enables the physical therapist to detect and describe a movement disorder, to determine the neuromuscular impairments that are the basis of the disorder, and to evaluate the functional implications of a disability in the context of the child's personal environment. The individual dimensions that are discussed in the following section are often assessed sequentially using instruments or methods specifically designed to evaluate one aspect of development. For example, the pediatric physical therapist may initially administer a standardized test of gross and fine motor skills to ascertain motor delay and particular areas of disability. This could be followed by an examination of muscle tone or muscle strength, or by an assessment of balance reactions and reflexes, to identify the neuromotor impairments that contribute to the motor delay. The therapist may conclude with an interview of the child's parents to discern any child-rearing practices or conditions in the home that might affect the child's motor behavior. In actual clinical practice, multiple dimensions are assessed simultaneously. While administering a test of motor skills, the therapist observes qualitative aspects of the child's movements and attends to the parents' comments and interactions with their child. The dimensions to be assessed in the physical therapy evaluation are discussed in the next section.

Neurodevelopmental History

Neurodevelopmental history is usually obtained from a review of medical records supplemented by an interview with the parents or caregivers. Components of a comprehensive history are the child's birth and medical history; chronology of developmental milestones; previous neuromotor problems, delays, or concerns; and information about the nature and frequency of previous therapeutic interventions. Particular attention is given to reports of medical conditions that could restrict or influence the sequence, pace, or quality of motor development, such as chronic lung disease, physical immobilization, or nutritional deficiency.

Developmental Level of Gross and Fine Motor Skills

Standardized tests are often used to document the child's level of functioning. In addition to quantitative results, areas of relative strength and limitation can be described. For example, a child may be functioning at age level in dynamic activities that involve mobility and propulsion while performing below age level in activities that require static balance. Other children excel at manipulation tasks and demonstrate reliable sitting balance yet have limitations in locomotor or ambulatory activities.

Functional Skills

Abilities to be assessed in this area include self-help skills, perceptual-motor function, and feeding or oral-motor function. In addition to describing the child's capabilities and limitations, all adaptations and equipment required for performance of skills are noted. Adaptive tools for dressing or fine motor skills, seating modifications, and assistive equipment for mobility are documented. Gait may be assessed by a wide range of methods from clinical observations to videographic or kinematic assessment.

Quality of Movement

Qualitative aspects of movement are evaluated by clinical observations made either during the administration of standardized motor tests or during the child's spontaneous play and movement. Components of typical movement, such as rotation, symmetry, and coordination, are evaluated for their presence and degree of maturity within the child's motor repertoire. Atypical patterns of movement; compensatory movements; and deviations such as tremors, jerkiness, or apraxia are noted and described. The child's motor planning skills and ability to initiate and to organize skilled volitional movement are assessed in both spontaneous and goal-directed tasks.

Physical Structure

Quantitative measurements as well as nonstandardized clinical evaluations are typically used to evaluate the physical structures that provide the foundation for motor function. Areas assessed include joint flexibility and range of motion, spinal alignment and posture, and orthopedic conditions, including deformities and contractures. Particular attention is given to areas of asymmetry, such as a muscle imbalance or a leg length discrepancy, that may lead to further impairments.

Neuromuscular Components of Movement

Clinical observations, systematic evaluations, and functional tests are used to assess the neuromuscular components of movement. These include muscle tone, muscle strength, balance, and equilibrium reactions. Primitive reflexes are assessed relative to the child's maturational age and to the extent to which the reflexes may interfere with functional movement.

Associated Systems

The physical therapy assessment may include a screening of nonmotor systems that influence the quality and competency of motor function. These include the sensory systems of vision; hearing; and response to tactile, vestibular, and proprioceptive stimulation. Although other disciplines may obtain comprehensive evaluations of cognitive ability and communication, the physical therapist often needs to determine the child's general level of function in these domains so the assessment of motor function will be geared to the child's language comprehension, interests, and motivations.

Child's Behavior

The child's motivation, attention span, and temperament affect his or her responsiveness to testing and may alter the validity of test results. For assessment of motor function, it is essential to gain an understanding of the child's orientation to movement. Is the child fearful, apprehensive, and insecure, or is he or she reckless and unrestrained in motor activity with apparent insensitivity to the risk of injury? The child's overall activity level and degree of compliance with requests by the therapist and by the parents influence how the assessment is conducted. The therapist observes how the child responds to different methods of evaluation so the most effective approaches can be identified and recommended. For example, some children respond best to structured, task-oriented environments in which they are given clear, specific directions. For other children, their best performance is elicited by indirect engagement in activities through play and games.

Family and Caregiver

The home environment can be assessed by a parent interview or questionnaire completed by the parent or primary caregiver. For the physical therapist, the information to be gathered includes the physical setting of the home; potential hazards; opportunities for physical exploration and mobility; and environmental factors such as stairs, an infant walker, or an infant jumper that might affect the child's motor development. The therapist also gathers information about the child's daily experience, including the positions and activities in which the child is engaged throughout the day. During the interview and observations of the parent–child interaction, it may be evident whether the home environment is restrictive or permissive, organized or unstructured. The cultural practices of the home may also affect motor development. For example, infants who have been in homes in which the typical parenting style is to hold or carry the child throughout the day may be less mature in floor activities such as pushing up in prone. The therapist also inquires about other environments and individuals significant in the life of the child, such as child care providers, relatives and siblings, school, and therapy facilities.

MAJOR CHALLENGES TO ACCURATE ASSESSMENT

The major challenges to accurate physical therapy assessments of young children relate to the measurement devices used, the assessment environment, and the many diverse factors that influence a child's motor behavior. The assessment tools are often limited by deficiencies in their reliability and validity as well as by their linear approach to developmental assessment of motor function and the acquisition of motor skills. The cultural biases of most assessment tools are also a problem. These issues are discussed in greater detail subsequently in this chapter.

The typical setting of an interdisciplinary team assessment presents a major challenge to the pediatric physical therapist. The clinic environment is a foreign space to the child and the parents, and they may feel inhibited and apprehensive. Consequently, the child may not demonstrate his or her full range of skills and abilities. This is a particular concern for a child with spasticity because the muscle tone may increase when the child is anxious or nervous. Moreover, it is impossible for a pediatric therapist to evaluate the child's functional capabilities fully in a clinic setting that is different from the home or school environment. A child who can ambulate on the smooth floor of the clinic may have difficulty at home where there are carpets, uneven surfaces, narrow hallways, and varying outdoor terrain. Although the child may be able to ascend and descend stairs that are standard measurements in the clinic, stairways at home or school that have different stair depth or height, no handrails, and angled landings may not be negotiable. Functions that can be performed in the isolation and calm of a quiet clinic environment may not be possible at home or in public where distractions and the presence of other children may heighten anxiety and increase muscle tension so that movement is impaired. Hence, the therapist could overestimate or underestimate a child's functional ability based on a clinic assessment that is not conducted in a naturalistic environment.

The administration and interpretation of a pediatric physical therapy assessment are also complicated in that many factors in addition to neuromotor status determine a child's motor function. A child's ability to perform a task on a standardized test is influenced by prior experience with the test materials, which may reflect home environment, cultural identity, or parenting style. For example, many tests of fine motor skills include use of a crayon or scissors. Some children are given these tools at very young ages, but other children may not be exposed to these materials until preschool or kindergarten. Ethnic variations, the presence of other children in the home, preschool or child care attendance, and safety concerns on the part of the family can determine a child's prior experience and, consequently, how well he or she performs with these materials. Stairs in the home or school environment will similarly influence how a child performs the task of negotiating stairs.

Racial variations in acquisition of motor skills, as well as different caregiving practices such as sleep position and use of an infant walker, may influence the performance of young children on tests of motor function (Allen, 1990; Caputo, Shapiro, Palmer, Ross, & Wachtel, 1985; Cintas, 1988; Jantz, Blosser, & Fruechting, 1997; Thein, Lee, Tay, & Ling, 1997). The therapist can also affect a child's performance during an assessment. By skillful handling and positioning of a child with hypertonia or an infant with an immature neuromotor system, a therapist may unintentionally enable a child to accomplish a skill that is not typically performed independently at home or at school.

Additional challenges to accurate assessment are related to the age of the child. For example, a young child of 8–10 months of age often demonstrates stranger anxiety and will not tolerate physical handling by the therapist. A 2-year-old child is typically very active and may be resistant to sitting at a table and performing requested fine motor tasks.

REACHING AN INFORMED CLINICAL DECISION

The assessment of motor dysfunction in children poses many challenges for even experienced pediatric physical therapists. In each case, the therapist must be thoughtful, well prepared, and able to modify the assessment based on the individual needs and responses of children and family members. Ideally, the assessment process should be the first step in a intervention approach that is family centered and facilitates achievement of functional outcomes. Several elements of clinical decision making, including a conceptual model, are described next for guidance.

Factors that Influence the Assessment Process

As the therapist prepares for the physical therapy assessment, preliminary consideration of several factors will optimize the session and assist with delineating assessment goals. In all cases, the assessment process is individualized to respond to the particular child, the caregivers, the facility or institution, and the therapist. At the outset, the stated reason for the child's referral and the purpose of the assessment will guide the therapist in planning for the assessment. Caregiver preferences and the family's concerns should take precedence over other factors. Medical and developmental history as well as the caregiver's reports of the child's behavioral state and sensitivity to environmental circumstances often dictate the pace and setting of the assessment. Children who are medically fragile or premature may need many breaks during the assessment or may require testing over more than one session. Light, noise, and other distractions in the environment may have to be reduced or minimized for a child who is hypersensitive or highly distractible. If the child has a known condition, the therapist will consider this in the choice of the environment and materials. For example, adaptive seating equipment can be provided for a child who lacks sitting balance. The therapist will consider the child's behavioral history and reported cognitive level in developing a plan for establishing rapport with the child and for gaining the child's attention and cooperation.

A major factor that influences the design of the physical therapy assessment is the therapist's interdisciplinary role within the agency or facility. When the therapist is a member of a large multidisciplinary team, the physical therapy assessment can focus on specific neuromotor aspects of a child's development. In other situations, the therapist may be required to extend the assessment to include transdisciplinary testing or screening. For instance, the physical therapist may perform a more comprehensive test of fine motor or perceptual function if there is no occupational therapist on the team. In some cases, the physical therapist may assume more responsibility for cognitive or behavioral testing of a young child. In the case of a child with significant motor delays, the team may decide that the physical therapist can best determine how neuromotor impairments compromise performance on a cognitive evaluation. Due to managed health care and cost containment policies, the pediatric physical therapist may be required to provide a broad screening test of multiple areas of development in addition to the dimensions of motor performance that are typically assessed. The results of this screening would then be used to determine the need for further comprehensive assessment in other functional domains.

A final factor that influences the assessment process is the degree to which the child and the family already know the therapist. When the child is well known to the therapist or is receiving intervention with the evaluating therapist, the family and the therapist may prefer a less formal assessment process that is integrated into the child's ongoing treatment sessions. Whenever possible, the stressful aspects of prolonged testing should be avoided.

Specific Assessment Strategies and Instruments

The therapist may choose from a number of methods or measurement strategies. These include interviews, chart review, naturalistic observations, and standardized clinical assessments, and they are examined in greater detail in the following section.

Interviews

Caregivers, community services providers, and extended family can provide information about functional skills in different environments and in response to varying levels of structure and stimulation. Interviews may be standardized parent report measures, such as the Pediatric Evaluation of Disability Inventory (PEDI; Haley, Coster, Ludlow, Haltiwanger, & Andrellos, 1992), or may be nonstructured conversations with caregivers. It is helpful to include a few open-ended questions at the outset of an evaluation to elicit information from the caregiver about the family's general impression of the child's functional skills and specific concerns. When appropriate and feasible, a direct interview with the child should also be included to understand his or her perspective, motivations, and preferences.

Chart Reviews

Important information regarding the child's birth, neonatal, medical, and developmental history is found by chart reviews. Summaries of past interdisciplinary assessments and physical therapy evaluations are another source of information. The therapist may then decide to select an assessment tool that was previously administered to obtain longitudinal data on a child's development or to use a different instrument that would augment and refine the child's prior evaluations.

Naturalistic Observations

Nonintrusive behavioral and functional assessments of the child during spontaneous activities are known as naturalistic observations. They include standardized evaluations of movement as well as the therapist's incidental observations of dimensions such as gait, postural alignment, functional range of motion, use of adaptive equipment, or play behavior. Behavioral and interactive traits are also readily observed using a naturalistic approach.

Standardized Assessments

Measures that adhere to a formal protocol for test administration and scoring are standardized assessments. Neuromotor components, such as range of motion, muscle tone, postural responses, reflex integration, functional motor skills, or developmental milestones, may be assessed by either criterion-based or norm-referenced standardized instruments. *Criterion-referenced*, or judgment-based, assessments evaluate an individual child's motor ability relative to a performance standard that has been operationally defined. Assessments such as the Movement Assessment of Infants (MAI; Chandler, Andrews, & Swanson, 1980) or the Gross Motor Function Measure (GMFM; Russell et al., 1993) and its companion, the Gross Motor Performance Measure (GMPM; Boyce et al., 1991), are criterion-referenced instruments. *Norm-referenced* developmental tests evaluate a child's performance of a motor skill relative to a normative sample, and results are reported in standard scores. These instruments provide the therapist with a measure of the child's acquisition of motor skills compared with typically developing children. Tests such as the Bayley Scales of Infant Development–Second Edition (BSID-II; Bayley, 1993) and the Peabody Developmental Motor Scales (PDMS; Folio & Fewell, 1983) are examples of instruments in this category.

Although norm-referenced tests are frequently used by physical therapists, these measures should not be used exclusively when the goals of the assessment are both to identify or quantify the developmental problem (i.e., diagnostic goal) and to propose objectives for remediation and intervention (i.e., prescriptive goal). Criterion-referenced measures are more meaningful for prescriptive purposes, whereas norm-referenced testing will provide diagnostic information and normative scores that may be used to qualify a child for intervention services.

Choosing an Assessment Tool

The number of assessment instruments available to the pediatric physical therapist increased dramatically during the 1990s. The choice of assessment tool will depend upon the purpose of the assessment, the age of the child, the hypothesized or known diagnosis, and the usefulness of the findings in providing diagnostic or prescriptive information. The therapist will also be guided by his or her own theoretical framework and specialized training as an examiner. Many instruments require formal training or guided practice in order to be administered in a standardized fashion. Therapists are advised to establish interrater agreement with a trained or experienced examiner prior to using a given instrument. Periodic testing of typically developing infants and young children will improve the therapist's ability to interpret the findings from developmental assessments accurately and will minimize the likelihood of systematic examiner bias.

In some communities, local standards or preferences for various instruments will determine the choice of the instrument. Individual states and school districts may have their own requirements to qualify a child for services. In all situations, the therapist should choose instruments with well-established and sound psychometric properties, including documented reliability and validity. The American Physical Therapy Association has published guidelines for the ethical and psychometrically valid use of assessments (Task Force on Standards for Measurement in Physical Therapy, 1991). These guidelines apply to pediatric assessment as well as to assessment in adult rehabilitation.

Although it is beyond the scope of this chapter to review the myriad assessment instruments available to the physical therapist, Table 8.1 provides a partial listing and a review of selected assessments. The instruments presented are described as to their content, age range, and purpose. Resultant information and scoring, as well as the instruments' clinical and psychometric strengths and limitations, are briefly noted. Textbooks of pediatric physical therapy and reviews in professional journals, plus the test manuals themselves, should be consulted for comprehensive information about specific instruments. In addition, development of a number of promising instruments began in the 1990s. Among them are the Test of Infant Motor Performance (TIMP; Campbell, Kolobe, Osten, Lenke, & Girolani, 1995), the Chandler Movement Assessment of Infants Screening Test (Chandler, 1990), and the Harris Infant Neuromotor Test (HINT; Harris & Daniels, 1996). Therapists may find that some of these newer tests are better suited to specific clinical populations, uses, environments, or theoretical frameworks.

Clinical Decision-Making Models

Conceptualization and documentation of clinical decision making in pediatric physical therapy has become increasingly important. Historically, many physical therapy evaluations were specific tests ordered by physicians. With the advent of "direct access," wherein the physical therapy practice mandates of many states allow physical therapists direct access and intervention with clients without referral from a physician, therapists are more autonomous in their assessment and treatment plan and have greater responsibility for the decisions that influence the lives of the children in their practice. Managed health care has also had a significant impact on the physical therapy practitioner in terms of clinical decision making. Third-party payers expect that health care professionals will provide objective documentation of the purpose and outcomes of their interventions.

Several models for clinical decision making have been described in the physical therapy literature, including clinical decision analysis (Watts, 1989), problem-knowledge coupling (Weed & Zimny, 1989), and the Hypothesis-

Table 8.1. Review of selected pediatric physical therapy assessments

Assessment	Type/content	Age range	Purpose	Scoring/results	Strengths	Limitations
Alberta Infant Motor Scale (AIMS; Piper & Darrah, 1994)	Norm-referenced screening test; gross motor and postural control	Birth–independent walking	Identification of delayed or typical motor development	Pass/fail; percentile ranks relative to normative group	Extensive normative data; brief administration time (15 minutes)	New assessment; clinical use limited to date
Bayley Infant Neurodevelopmental Screener (BINS; Aylward, 1995)	Norm-referenced measure of neuropsychological competence	3 months–24 months	Identifies optimal neurological function in five areas: 1) intactness (tone, reflexes), 2) receptive (visual, hearing, verbal), 3) expressive (fine, gross, and oral motor), 4) higher-order functions (memory, problem solving), and 5) mental activity (goal-directedness, attention)	Optimality scores are used for delay or nondelay designation at 3, 6, 9, 12, 18, and 24 months of age	Brief administration time; plans to develop age equivalencies; identifies functional areas for further assessment	Newer test; not widely used clinically
Bayley Scales of Infant Development (Motor Scale)–Second Edition (Bayley, 1993)	Norm-referenced; motor milestones	Birth–42 months	Quantification of motor development relative to normed group	Pass/fail based upon strict criterion; derived psychomotor developmental index (mean = 100; SD = 15)	Widely used; large normative, representative samples; wide age range and companion Mental Scale allow broad interpretation	Examiner training recommended; developmental quotients not predictive
Bruininks-Oseretsky Test of Motor Proficiency (Bruininks, 1978)	Norm-referenced test of gross motor and fine motor proficiency	4½ years–14½ years	Assesses running speed and agility, balance, bilateral coordination, strength, upper-limb coordination, response speed, visual-motor control, and upper-limb speed and dexterity	Derived standard scores for each of eight subtests, including developmental indices, percentile ranks, age equivalents, and stanines	Well standardized; good reliability and validity; short form available	Difficult to administer to younger children and to those with delays; long administration time

(continued)

165

Table 8.1. *(continued)*

Assessment	Type/content	Age range	Purpose	Scoring/results	Strengths	Limitations
Gross Motor Function Measure (GMFM; Russell et al., 1993)	Gross motor function in children with disabilities	Children within gross motor developmental range of birth–5 years	Designed to measure change over time in children with cerebral palsy	Quantification of five dimensions of motor behavior: lying and rolling; sitting; crawling and kneeling; standing; walking, running, and jumping	Designed for evaluating effects of treatment; measure of functional movements; has a companion test of postural control (GMPM)	Test not normed; relatively new test; measures only achievement of functional skills, not quality of movement
Gross Motor Performance Measure (GMPM; Boyce et al., 1991)	Gross motor movement quality	Children within gross motor developmental range of birth–5 years or children with cerebral palsy from 5 months–12 years	Designed to measure quality of movement in children with motor disabilities	Quality of performance of tasks scored for postural alignment, selective control, coordination, stabilization, and weight shift	Designed for evaluating effects of treatment; measure of functional movements; has a companion test of functional skills (GMFM)	Relatively new test; little supportive research as of 2000; does not assess all qualities of movement (e.g., speed, effort, efficiency)
Miller Assessment for Preschoolers (MAP; Miller, 1982)	Norm-referenced assessment of sensory and motor abilities, cognitive abilities, and complex tasks	2 years, 9 months–5 years, 8 months	Identification of children with mild to moderate "preacademic problems"	Percentile ranks	Strong psychometric data; good reliability and predictive validity for primary school performance	Not designed for moderate to severe developmental delays; not diagnostic
Movement Assessment of Infants (MAI; Chandler, Andrews, & Swanson, 1980)	Standardized test of neuromotor capability	Birth–1 year	Quantification of muscle tone, primitive reflexes, automatic reactions, and volitional movement	Ordinal scoring of all items yields risk scores for 4-, 6-, and 8-month-olds	Assesses quality of movement; adequate predictive validity	Limited normative data; examiner training recommended

(continued)

166

Table 8.1. (continued)

Assessment	Type/content	Age range	Purpose	Scoring/results	Strengths	Limitations
Peabody Developmental Motor Scales (PDMS; Folio & Fewell, 1983)	Norm-referenced and criterion-referenced; gross and fine motor scales	Birth–83 months	Identification of developmental levels for fine motor skills (grasping, hand use, eye-hand coordination, manual dexterity) and gross motor skills (reflexes, balance, nonlocomotor, locomotor, and ball skills)	Derived scores for each skill category, including z- and T-scores, motor quotients, and percentile ranks	One of few standardized tests of motor performance; can be used for children with disabilities	Some scoring criteria unclear; relatively small normative sample; not recommended for children younger than 5 months of age
Pediatric Evaluation of Disability Inventory (PEDI; Haley, Coster, Ludlow, Haltiwanger, & Andrellos, 1992)	Standardized and norm-referenced caregiver report measure of activities of daily living	6 months–7½ years or within that developmental range	Designed to assess functional skill development and level of independent performance	Functional skills, caregiver assistance, and modification scores as percents of items passed; summary standard scores and scaled scores are norm-referenced	Comprehensive; based on child's function in typical environment; caregiver report involves family; comparable school measure available; sound psychometrics	Relatively new test; not recommended for children younger than 1 year of age or 5- to 7-year-old children with minimal disability

SD = Standard deviation.

Oriented Algorithm for Clinicians described by Rothstein and Ecternach (1986). Key features of clinical decision analysis are the use of decision trees, the estimation of successful outcome probabilities for each possible approach, and making cost-effectiveness comparisons after considering available resources. In the problem-knowledge coupling method, specialized computer software is used to link individual patient findings with relevant clinical knowledge from the literature to determine a range of possible diagnostic and management strategies. The Hypothesis-Oriented Algorithm for Clinicians focuses on the relationship between the examination of the patient and treatment planning, and it attempts to assist the physical therapist in individualizing the treatment to the particular problems of the patient. This approach emphasizes the physical therapist's generation and revision of hypotheses (i.e., testable ideas) that relate to the cause of functional limitations.

A model that is specific to the treatment of children was proposed by Embrey, Guthrie, White, and Deitz (1996). They identified and described the clinical decision-making processes that experienced and novice pediatric physical therapists employ in the treatment of children with cerebral palsy. A qualitative methodology using videotaped therapy sessions and retrospective think-aloud procedures identified the following four characteristics of clinical decision making: 1) movement scripts, based on previous clinical experience that helped the therapists apply clinical information; 2) psychosocial sensitivity, which enabled the therapists to meet the emotional and social needs of the child; 3) procedural changes, or the rapidity with which therapists changed the position, activity, or environment; and 4) self-monitoring, or the therapists' reflections regarding their own clinical performance. Differences in the frequency with which experienced and novice therapists demonstrated the above four characteristics were also determined.

According to Magistro (1989), clinical decision making during the initial evaluation is the cornerstone of a well-developed, appropriate treatment program. Yet the preceding clinical decision-making models are not fully applicable to the pediatric physical therapy assessment process within an interdisciplinary team setting for several reasons. First, models such as clinical decision analysis (Watts, 1989) are specific to treatment instead of the assessment component of an intervention program. Second, feedback from a child that suggests distress or pain is typically not as salient as the verbal feedback provided by adult clients. The physical therapist must be sensitive to the child's subtle, nonverbal cues of stress and should incorporate parental report of the child's responses and tolerance into decision making. Time constraints are a third factor limiting the application of models that require multiple opportunities for reassessment. Within the interdisciplinary clinic setting, the child is commonly seen only once by each discipline for an assessment and then referred to another facility for treatment. Thus, the physical therapist in this environment must be able to reach an informed decision regarding a child's functional motor status in a relatively brief period of time.

Because no clinical decision-making models specific to the assessment process for pediatric physical therapists were found in the field's literature, the authors of this chapter propose such a model, illustrated in Figure 8.2. This model incorporates the hypothesis generation and testing components of the Hypothesis-Oriented Algorithm for Clinicians and involves a sequence of alternating Action Steps and Decision Points. Key features of the model include collaboration between parents and the other team members throughout the assessment process and a perspective that views a child's motor functioning within the context of the family, the environment, and other aspects of his or her development. It should be emphasized that clinical decision making is a complex process with overlapping steps; thus, Figure 8.2's linear sequence of decision making is not fully representative of the process. For example, the experienced clinician may begin generating hypotheses relative to a child's functional limitations while obtaining the child's history or assessing muscle tone, thereby intermingling decision points with action steps. However, for the less experienced physical therapist, a step-like approach to clinical decision making during the assessment process will reduce the possibility of omitting any key components. The next section outlines the model components and is followed by a case study illustrating the action steps and decision points.

A Clinical Decision-Making Model for Pediatric Physical Therapy Assessment

The following clinical decision-making model is outlined in Figure 8.2. Action Step 1 in Figure 8.2 is the process of obtaining a relevant history of the child. The therapist pays particular attention to information from the referral source that indicates parental concerns, biological insult or environmental vulnerability, delayed motor milestones, atypical movements (e.g., tremors, asymmetry), or the child's inability to participate in functional activities at home or at school. Specific referral information is augmented by 1) medical background, such as birth history and health status; 2) developmental history, including motor milestones, adaptive skills, and possible delays in other domains, such as language or cognition; 3) social information relating to family support, cultural background, and parental perspectives; and 4) environmental information describing the child's functional abilities at home as well as at school or a child care center. Methods for gathering this information have been described previously in this chapter.

Decision Point 1 consists of the physical therapist's generation of an assessment plan, including selection of the most appropriate tools, measurement strategies, and evaluation setting. The purpose of the assessment is a primary consideration in this phase of clinical decision making and will influence the choice of evaluation tools. Examiner expertise and time and space constraints are also considered in test selection. The choice of measurement strategies (e.g., parent interview, standardized testing, clinical observations) will be influenced by family members' priorities and preferences. A parental concern may be better addressed by clinical observation of the parent and child engaged in

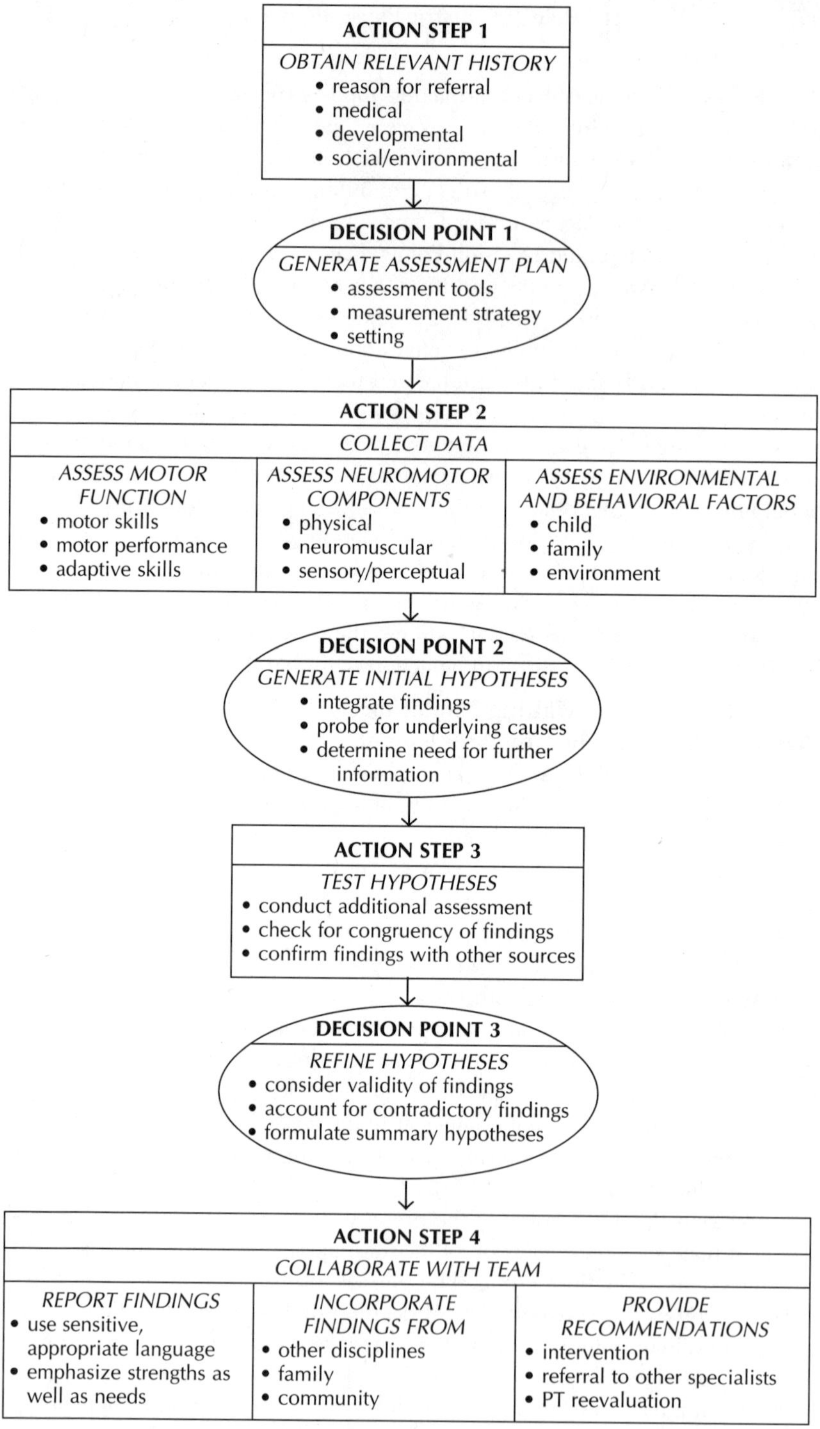

```
┌─────────────────────────────────────┐
│            ACTION STEP 1             │
├─────────────────────────────────────┤
│     OBTAIN RELEVANT HISTORY          │
│       • reason for referral          │
│       • medical                      │
│       • developmental                │
│       • social/environmental         │
└─────────────────────────────────────┘
```

DECISION POINT 1

GENERATE ASSESSMENT PLAN
 • assessment tools
 • measurement strategy
 • setting

ACTION STEP 2

COLLECT DATA

ASSESS MOTOR FUNCTION	*ASSESS NEUROMOTOR COMPONENTS*	*ASSESS ENVIRONMENTAL AND BEHAVIORAL FACTORS*
• motor skills	• physical	• child
• motor performance	• neuromuscular	• family
• adaptive skills	• sensory/perceptual	• environment

DECISION POINT 2

GENERATE INITIAL HYPOTHESES
 • integrate findings
 • probe for underlying causes
 • determine need for further information

ACTION STEP 3

TEST HYPOTHESES
 • conduct additional assessment
 • check for congruency of findings
 • confirm findings with other sources

DECISION POINT 3

REFINE HYPOTHESES
 • consider validity of findings
 • account for contradictory findings
 • formulate summary hypotheses

ACTION STEP 4

COLLABORATE WITH TEAM

REPORT FINDINGS	*INCORPORATE FINDINGS FROM*	*PROVIDE RECOMMENDATIONS*
• use sensitive, appropriate language	• other disciplines	• intervention
• emphasize strengths as well as needs	• family	• referral to other specialists
	• community	• PT reevaluation

Figure 8.2. A clinical decision-making model for pediatric physical therapy assessment.

a specific activity, such as dressing, than by a standardized assessment tool. Attention is given to the potential effects of the physical environment on the child (e.g., visual distractions, lighting, temperature, noise). Supplemental data collection conducted in natural environments, such as home and school, may be considered a necessary adjunct to the clinic evaluation.

Action Step 2 is the data collection process that involves assessment of the child's motor function, the underlying neuromotor components of movement, and the behavioral and environmental framework of his or her motor function. Depending on the referring concerns, different aspects of motor skills (e.g., gross or fine motor), motor performance (e.g., coordination, dexterity, motor planning), and adaptive skills (e.g., self-help abilities, use of assistive technology) may be evaluated. A typical physical therapy assessment combines administration of standardized testing procedures with clinical observations of physical structures and neuromuscular parameters of motor function. During test administration, the physical therapist must be flexible and remain open to the possibility of changing to a more appropriate tool for a given child. For instance, if suspected cognitive delays prevent a child from comprehending the verbal directions necessary to complete test items, an instrument that allows demonstration of test items by the examiner may provide a more valid assessment of the child's capabilities. The therapist evaluates the child's use of sensory systems (e.g., visual, tactile, auditory, vestibular) and his or her other perceptual skills to assess their role as associated factors that could contribute to motor delay. Throughout the assessment, the physical therapist observes the influence of the child's behavior, temperament, attention span, and motivation on motor performance. Evaluation of family and cultural influences through observation of the caregiver–child interaction and discussion of home routines will assist the physical therapist in determining the degree to which the home environment may facilitate or restrict the child's motor development.

Decision Point 2 involves generating initial hypotheses regarding the child's functional motor status. At this time, the physical therapist integrates findings from the previous steps of the assessment and determines the need for further information. When the testing indicates delayed or abnormal motor function, the therapist identifies specific limitations in motor skills and considers possible underlying impairments (e.g., musculoskeletal, sensory). The physical therapist decides what additional testing and information gathering are needed to confirm initial hypotheses. It is possible that the child's motor function is within the expected range for his or her age. In this case, the therapist would consider other possible reasons for the parents' concerns and observations. The therapist may decide to have further discussions with the family and professionals from other disciplines or to conduct additional testing to identify subtle neuromotor abnormalities that might be present but do not affect the child's performance on a standardized test of motor skills.

Action Step 3 involves the use of one or more strategies to substantiate the initial hypotheses through additional data collection and gathering of information. This may require administering another standardized test; assessing a specific neuromotor component such as muscle tone in greater detail; or more interviewing of the child's caregiver, teacher, child care provider, or other individuals who are familiar with the child's daily activities. Checking for congruency of findings established during the assessment (e.g., the presence of left-sided spasticity) with medical information (e.g., documentation of a right intraventricular hemorrhage by cranial ultrasound) is one strategy used in hypothesis testing. Confirmation of findings with others (e.g., a follow-up interview with family members following assessment of the child) can also provide confirming or conflicting evidence for initial hypotheses. If a sensory impairment or medical condition, such as a visual impairment or seizure disorder, is hypothesized to be a factor in the child's motor limitations, consultation with another professional may be indicated.

Decision Point 3 involves refinement of the hypotheses and consideration of which aspects of the initial hypotheses are best supported by the findings. To confirm the hypotheses, the therapist verifies the validity of the assessment results. This involves considering the appropriateness of the selected assessment tools, the optimality of the testing environment, and ways in which the child's behavioral state may have influenced motor performance. The child's attention span, temperament, health, fatigue, anxiety, and communication skills may affect performance of motor tasks. In the same manner, conditions of the assessment setting may similarly affect test results. For example, environmental distractions, such as noise or the presence of observers during the assessment, may be overly stimulating for a particular child and could be a negative influence.

An additional step in hypothesis refinement involves accounting for contradictory findings, including those obtained directly from the test procedures as well as findings from other sources. For instance, if previous testing indicated normal motor functioning in a child who now is demonstrating delays, the physical therapist should address possible reasons for this discrepancy. If school personnel have expressed concerns about a child's tendency to fall and yet there is no evidence of a balance problem, further exploration of this inconsistency is warranted. Similarly, if caregivers are worried about poor attention and a high activity level, the structured procedures of the test-taking environment may have masked a child's inability to organize play independently and to focus attention. After considering the validity and relevance of all of the assessment findings, the physical therapist formulates summary hypotheses and conclusions.

Action Step 4 is the process of reporting the assessment results and conclusions, sharing information with other team members, jointly interpreting findings, and setting collaborative goals. The therapist summarizes his or her assessment in a written report and in oral communication with the child's caregivers and other team members. The physical therapist's findings are presented within the context of functional abilities to facilitate understanding by the family and other disciplines; the use of professional jargon is avoided. Emphasis on a child's strengths as well as limitations provides meaningful information for family members and is helpful for planning intervention goals. Variables that may have negatively influenced a child's performance (e.g., timing of testing during child's usual nap time) are included in the written summary, in addition to all deviations from standardized testing procedures. At the team meeting, the physical therapist hears team members from other disciplines describing the child's performance in different domains.

Before formulating final recommendations for the child, family preferences and priorities are reviewed by the team members. Resources such as time, energy, finances, and social support, as well as the level of involvement the family desires, will influence the recommendations. Input from community personnel, such as a child's teacher, and the availability of community resources are also considered. The provision of recommendations is a crucial step in the assessment process for family members. As one parent indicated on an anonymous feedback form, "We're not bringing our child for evaluation to find out what he can and cannot do—we're very aware of that. We want to know why and what we can do about it." Team members need to be able to inform families about community resources and to give them information and strategies for gaining access to and utilizing local services.

The child with suspected motor impairment may require evaluation by specialists not present on the initial team (e.g., a neurologist, an ophthalmologist) prior to the final determination of the diagnosis or formulation of specific intervention goals. If intervention is indicated for a child, service frequency, setting, and preliminary intervention goals should be jointly determined by the team and family members. If the child does not need regular therapeutic intervention, the therapist can give the caregivers recommendations for ways to enhance their child's emerging skills. Periodic monitoring of motor development or a comprehensive reevaluation may be recommended as well.

Example of Decision Making Through a Case Study

The following case study illustrates the action steps and decision points the pediatric physical therapist encounters during assessment.

Obtain Relevant History

Eddie was referred by his pediatrician for an interdisciplinary team assessment at 19 months corrected age (adjusted for prematurity). The primary reasons for referral were delayed gross motor milestones and possible growth retardation. Because Eddie was born out of state, birth information was limited. At Action Step 1, the physical therapist reviewed the medical chart, which indicated that Eddie was born at 32 weeks' gestational age at a birth weight of 1,590 grams. His problems in the neonatal period included mild respiratory distress and possible intrauterine drug exposure. Eddie's developmental, social, and environmental history were obtained from a caregiver questionnaire that was completed by his adoptive parents prior to the assessment. Eddie lived with his biological parents for the first 6 months of life and then was placed in foster care. He was adopted at 12 months of age and resided with his adoptive parents and his 3-year-old half-sister at the time of this assessment. He received child care in his home while his mother worked.

Generate Assessment Plan

Based upon the developmental history, caregiver concerns, and referral information, Eddie was scheduled by the service coordinator to see the following disciplines as part of the interdisciplinary assessment: nutrition, psychology, pediatrics, and physical therapy. The purpose of the physical therapy assessment was to verify Eddie's gross motor delay, to determine the underlying impairments that limit functional skills, and to identify other possible areas of motor dysfunction. At Decision Point 1, the physical therapist selected a norm-referenced test, the PDMS, to provide a quantitative measure of his motor development relative to other children his age and to document his need for therapy services if necessary. She chose to use the MAI, a criterion-referenced assessment, to evaluate muscle tone, reflexes, and automatic reactions for potential areas of neuromotor impairment that might be contributing to his delays. The physical therapist planned to observe Eddie's attention, motor planning, play skills, and language during his spontaneous play and social interactions with his parents and the examiner. She would interview his parents to learn about Eddie's routines and activities at home.

Collect Data

Eddie was initially shy and hesitant when he entered the testing room. During the second action step, the physical therapist used this opportunity to ask his parents about their specific concerns. They reported that he had made some progress since he had been in their home but that he seemed weaker in the legs than the arms and was still not walking. Eddie's mother indicated that although he used a spoon and a cup independently and had no difficulty chewing and swallowing, he did not seem to gain weight. Eddie's performance on the PDMS Fine Motor Scale was within normal limits for his age. However, the therapist noted that he did show tremulousness in his upper extremities during some tasks. On the PDMS Gross Motor Scale, Eddie was significantly delayed, with skills comparable to those of a 10-month-old child. He sat alone but tended to W-sit, with his legs behind him and his hips internally rotated and adducted. Eddie crept reciprocally on his hands and knees and, with effort, could creep up four stairs by pulling up with his arms. He was not able to support his weight through his legs when placed in a standing position. Using the MAI, the physical therapist documented marked hypotonia (low muscle tone) of the legs and trunk, with mild hypotonia in the arms. Eddie had complete equilibrium reactions in sitting and had fully developed protective reactions of the arms when his balance was displaced. Gross sensory testing indicated intact sensation.

Generate Initial Hypotheses

Based on the test results, the physical therapist concluded at the second decision point that Eddie's primary motor problem was delayed gross motor skills. She hypothesized that this delay was due to hypotonia because she saw no evidence of spasticity, ataxia, incoordination, or atypical movement patterns. Because of Eddie's alert state, his ability to follow directions, and the comprehension he demonstrated, particularly in performance of the PDMS fine motor tasks, she felt that his delay was not due to cognitive impairment or lack of motivation. Based on his mother's report that Eddie had made some progress since coming to her home, the therapist hypothesized that Eddie's motor delay was not due to a progressive muscular condition, such as muscular dystrophy or Werdnig-Hoffman disease, but further investigation was required. The therapist felt that she needed more information about Eddie's present home and the foster home setting to rule out environmental deprivation as a contributing factor in Eddie's developmental delay. Finally, she hypothesized that although Eddie was small and undergrown, his delay and hypotonia were not due to nutritional deficiency. She based this on her observations of Eddie's alert and active state, his ability to move and to exert himself physically, and his feeding skills, which she observed incidentally while he was having a snack break. The therapist decided on the following plan of action: 1) interview his mother to gain additional information about Eddie's history and home environment; 2) conduct further evaluation of Eddie's neuromuscular status; and 3) as available, briefly discuss findings with other disciplines involved in the assessment—pediatrics, psychology, and nutrition.

Test Hypotheses

At the third action step, the physical therapist evaluated Eddie's neuromuscular condition more thoroughly with some modified muscle-testing techniques and careful observation of the quality of his spontaneous movement. She concluded that the upper extremity tremor she observed during fine motor tasks was due to lack of stability in the proximal shoulder musculature because of hypotonia. The therapist asked Eddie's mother more detailed questions about his daily activities and the physical environment of his present home and previous placements. From the mother's descriptions, the therapist concluded that Eddie's home environment during the last 12 months had been sufficient to promote typical gross motor development.

After completing Eddie's assessment, the physical therapist talked briefly with the pediatrician who had seen Eddie earlier in the day. The physician was also concerned about the possibility of a degenerative muscle disease, such as muscular dystrophy, and had requested that blood samples be drawn to test for this condition. The psychologist and nutritionist had not yet completed their assessments of Eddie, so the physical therapist could not yet discuss findings and questions with them. The therapist reviewed Eddie's medical chart again to assess the congruency between her findings and hypotheses and Eddie's medical and developmental history.

Refine Hypotheses

The physical therapist, at the third decision point, reflected on her assessment to determine the validity of her findings. Given Eddie's cooperation during testing and his willingness to perform requested motor skills, even when they required considerable effort (e.g., when he pulled himself to a standing position to retrieve a toy from a low table), she felt that she had seen his full capabilities. Eddie did show some fearfulness when he was tipped on the ball to test his equilibrium reactions, but he was not at all hesitant when attempting to climb the stairs. He had completed one assessment earlier in the day, but he did not seem to be fatigued. Eddie had a snack during the physical therapy assessment so it seemed unlikely that hunger compromised his test performance. His mother confirmed that his performance during the assessment was consistent with his typical abilities at home. The test used was the PDMS, which is a standardized assessment that was appropriate for Eddie's age and ability level. Overall, the therapist considered her assessment to be a valid measure of Eddie's motor function.

The therapist's finding of general hypotonia, more pronounced in the lower extremities, was consistent with the observed gross motor delay. On one hand, the report that described Eddie as a "floppy baby," and the history of slow but steady development with no regression or loss of skills, supported the therapist's hypothesis of a static neuromuscular disorder rather than a progressive muscle disease. On the other hand, Eddie's failure to thrive was not a typical component of congenital hypotonia. This aspect of Eddie's condition required further assessment by the nutritionist to rule out a syndrome or metabolic disorder of which hypotonia is just one characteristic.

Collaborate with Team

The physical therapist reported her findings at the team conference during the fourth action step. She recommended that Eddie receive physical therapy services. As Eddie had mild delays in cognitive and language functioning, the team recommended a comprehensive developmental program that would include both individual therapy and group learning. Following an explanation of the purpose of physical therapy and other early intervention services, Eddie's parents were asked whether they were interested in obtaining these services for him. They indicated that they were eager for Eddie to receive therapy but were concerned about the financial cost. Because of the extent of his gross motor delay, Eddie would qualify for state-supported services at a developmental center that was close to his home. The team also recognized the need to establish regular channels of communication between the center personnel and Eddie's parents so that they could support the therapy program with activities at home. The nutritionist, who was the service coordinator for Eddie, agreed to coordinate the intervention program with personnel at the developmental center as well as to monitor with Eddie's mother the child's health and weight gain. The physical therapist planned to discuss her recommendations with the center therapist and to call the family after Eddie had been receiving services for a month to ascertain their satisfaction with the program. The team recommended that Eddie be reevaluated in 1 year.

The Art of Assessment

The proposed model outlines strategies for clinical decision making during pediatric physical therapy assessment. In addition to these steps, what other factors contribute to the complex "art" of assessment? First, communication skills, particularly active listening, are essential for successful collaboration between therapists and family members. Research by Harris in 1994 suggested that parents are often accurate in estimating the developmental status of their children. Information gathered during a parent interview can provide the physical therapist with insights into a child's areas of strengths and limitations that may not be observable during formal testing. In addition, verifying with family members whether the child's performance during the formal assessment is typical of motor performance in the home environment is useful in interpreting findings. The ability to communicate assessment findings in clear, descriptive, functional terms for parents and to articulate the rationale for recommendations are also necessary skills.

A second factor that contributes to the clinical decision-making process is professional experience. Magistro (1989) described how the role of intuition may influence clinical decision making and showed that intuition is likely derived from both theoretical knowledge and practical experience. Research examining how experienced physical therapists solved clinical problems during the initial evaluation demonstrated that they intermingled the steps of data collection, problem list formation, and treatment planning during the evaluation (Payton, 1985). Research on the clinical-reasoning process of physicians during diagnostic evaluations lends further support to the value of experience in clinical problem solving. Schmidt, Norman, and Boshuizen (1990) proposed that experienced physicians rely on a knowledge structure referred to as *illness scripts*, which emerge from continuous exposure to patients and are the result of extended clinical practice. These scripts contain relevant information about disease, its consequences, and the context in which it develops. This theory presupposes that physicians use the memories of previous patients while diagnosing a new case. Embrey and others (1996) described therapists' use of *movement scripts*, or cognitive schema, that represent typical movement patterns of children with spastic diplegia. Experienced physical therapists reported use of movement scripts much more frequently than novice therapists, suggesting a benefit of experience in treating children with neuromotor impairments. Further research comparing the clinical reasoning skills of experienced and less experienced clinicians will be necessary to elucidate the role that experience plays in clinical decision making in physical therapy.

ISSUES PARTICULARLY RELEVANT TO PHYSICAL THERAPY

For the physical therapist to use assessment tools properly and to interpret the findings correctly, he or she must be aware of several measurement issues relating to the assessment of infants and young children. First, the predictive validity of many assessments of infants and young children is highly variable (McCune, Kalmanson, Fleck, Glazewski, & Sillari, 1990). That is, a child's performance on standardized tests of early development may have a low probability of predicting the individual child's later performance on similar or future criterion measures. Likewise, some early diagnostic tests may indicate motor delays in children who later perform within the normal range. Therapists' understanding of both sensitivity (the test's ability to correctly identify children with developmental problems) and specificity (the ability to correctly identify children who do not have developmental problems) as they apply to each instrument will assist with more accurate interpretation (Campbell, 1990).

Caregivers may assume that standard scores of motor or adaptive function reported for young children are comparable to cognitive or intelligence quotients derived from tests of older children. When standardized scores are included in evaluation summaries or reports, the meaning and implication of the scores relative to the specific test should be clearly explained to the caregivers. Therapists should frame their reports of standard scores with explanations that clarify possible misconceptions and that emphasize functional skills rather than test scores. For example, successful performance of many items on the Mental Scale of the BSID-II requires fine motor competency, such as the ability to stack blocks, put pegs into the pegboard, or pick up beads. When a child's standard score on the Mental Scale is compromised by a fine motor impairment, it is important that caregivers understand that the score is not a valid indicator of the child's "mental" capabilities.

Test–retest reliability, or the replication of the findings over successive tests, is a third area of concern. Consistency across testing sessions is often poor, especially with young children who are tested in strange environments by unfamiliar adults. The therapist can minimize some of these effects by attempting to control the factors that might mediate a child's responsiveness or diminish the optimality of the child's performance. Timing of the assessment to match the child's sleep–wake and feeding schedules, allowing for feeding and rest breaks, or multiple testing sessions may be necessary. The therapist who is seeing a child for the first time must be cautious in the interpretation of the findings. Checking with the caregiver or with other providers about the typicality of the child's performance during the assessment, relative to other familiar environments, will minimize the risk of misinterpretation.

During the 1990s, researchers and clinicians began to reevaluate earlier models of child development that were based on a linear or hierarchical organization to motor skill acquisition. New systems models were proposed that view a child's development within a more complex array of interrelated factors (Foundation for Physical Therapy, 1991). Both the model of child development depicted in Figure 8.1, as well as the ecological model of child development described previously in this chapter, are examples of a systems perspective, wherein multiple factors contribute to and influence the child's development. In general, the majority of motor assessment tools are based upon earlier models of child development and were created and validated using these models. Some assessments formulated in the 1990s, such as the PEDI and measures of postural stability (see Wescott, Lowes, & Richardson, 1997), embody a systems approach to developmental skills and consider the many factors that influence motor behavior. The knowledgeable evaluator will take these limitations into account in the choice of assessment tools and in the interpretation of the findings.

Delay or deviation in motor development may be the first indication of a neuromotor condition such as cerebral palsy or generalized developmental delay. Consequently, the physical therapist may be the first of many professionals whom family members will encounter as they initiate early intervention services for their child. To ensure a positive entry into the early intervention system, physical therapists must incorporate the principles of family-centered care into practice. Guidelines for fostering family-centered, integrated services within the context of the initial assessment (Shelton, Jeppson, & Johnson, 1987) include the following:

- Family decisions should be a primary consideration in how assessment and intervention services are planned and provided.
- The integration of an ecological perspective means that the assessment process should incorporate input from multiple naturalistic environments in which the child typically functions.
- Awareness of community resources (e.g., recreational, educational, medical) is necessary to guarantee appropriate referral when necessary.

RECOMMENDATIONS FOR THE FUTURE

Until the late 1980s, motor assessment tools were limited in the psychometric rigor under which they were developed. With greater awareness among practitioners and the growing need for objective measures to improve treatment accountability, there has been an increase in new pediatric assessments for the physical therapist. Two instruments have been specifically developed to be sensitive to changes in control and movement that result from physical therapy intervention (Boyce et al., 1991; Russell et al., 1993). Reliable and valid instruments that incorporate the newer models of motor learning, dynamic systems theory, and motor control are necessary (see Foundation for Physical Therapy, 1991). Existing assessments require further scientific inquiry and refinement to increase their reliability and validity.

The format of pediatric physical therapy assessment is beginning to change in response to changes in health care delivery, parent preferences, educational models of intervention, and systems models of development. These new formats allow therapists to move out of the more traditional medical models of assessment and to redefine their roles on the interdisciplinary team. Examples of these roles in pediatric assessment are found in transdisciplinary, arena, and play-based assessments. Using the transdisciplinary assessment method, the physical therapist alone may assess a child in multiple domains or may "release" his or her role to a professional from another discipline who conducts the motor assessment (Effgen, 1994). In arena assessments, the entire team observes the child engaged in a wide variety of developmental activities and simultaneously conducts individual disciplinary assessments (Effgen, 1994). Motor performance is evaluated in the natural context of the child at play during play-based assessments (Couch, 1996).

One of the most significant factors affecting the provision of early intervention services is that of the changing demographics in many countries. For example, by the year 2000, it is estimated that 38% of children in the United States younger than 18 years of age will be nonwhite (Research and Policy Committee of the Committee for Economic Development, 1987). As the number of children from a variety of cultures who require services increases, physical therapists will need to demonstrate cultural sensitivity in their choice of assessment tools and practices. The collection of additional normative data on children from various ethnic backgrounds will strengthen the validity of assessment tools. Until these data are available, interpretation of standardized tests should be made with extreme caution when assessing children from cultures underrepresented in the norming sample.

Training for physical therapists at the preprofessional level should provide opportunities for the development of communication skills. Active listening, negotiation, collaboration, and team building are necessary skills for interdisciplinary promotion of family-centered services. Enhanced specialty training in pediatric assessment for physical therapists will be necessary to ensure the appropriate use and interpretation of new tests. Further refinement of a clinical decision-making model specific to pediatric physical therapy will assist practitioners in assessment, diagnosis, and treatment planning, and it will promote the delivery of improved services for children and their families.

REFERENCES

Allen, M.C. (1990). Gross motor milestones in preterm infants: Correction for degree of prematurity. *Journal of Pediatrics, 116*, 955–959.
Aylward, G. (1995). *Bayley Infant Neurodevelopmental Screener.* San Antonio, TX: The Psychological Corp.
Bailey, D., & Wolery, M. (1992). An ecological framework for early intervention. In D. Bailey & M. Wolery (Eds.), *Teaching infants and preschoolers with disabilities* (pp. 63–94). New York: Merrill.

Bayley, N. (1993). *Bayley Scales of Infant Development–Second Edition*. San Antonio, TX: The Psychological Corp.

Boyce, W., Gowland, C., Rosenbaum, P., Lane, M., Plews, N., Goldsmith, C., Russell, D., Wright, V., Potter, S., & Harding, D. (1991). Gross Motor Performance Measure: Validity and responsiveness of a measure of quality of movement. *Physical Therapy, 75*(5), 603–613.

Bronfenbrenner, U. (1977). Toward an experimental ecology of human development. *American Psychologist, 32*, 513–531.

Bruininks, R. (1978). *Bruininks-Oseretsky Test of Motor Proficiency*. Circle Pines, MN: American Guidance Service.

Campbell, S. (1990). Using standardized tests in clinical practice. *Topics in Pediatrics, Lesson 11*. Alexandria, VA: American Physical Therapy Association, Education Department.

Campbell, S. (1994). The child's development of functional movement. In S. Campbell (Ed.), *Physical therapy for children* (pp. 3–38). Philadelphia: W.B. Saunders Company.

Campbell, S., Kolobe, T., Osten, E., Lenke, M., & Girolani, G. (1995). Construct validity of the Test of Infant Motor Performance. *Physical Therapy, 75*(7), 585–596.

Caldwell, A.J., Shapiro, B.K., Palmer, F.B., Ross, A., & Wachtel, R.C. (1985). Normal gross motor development: The influences of race, sex, and socioeconomic status. *Developmental Medicine and Child Neurology, 27*, 635–643.

Chandler, L.S. (1990). Neuromotor assessment. In E.D. Gibbs & D.M. Teti (Eds.), *Interdisciplinary assessment of infants: A guide for early intervention professionals* (pp. 45–61). Baltimore: Paul H. Brookes Publishing Co.

Chandler, L., Andrews, M., & Swanson, M. (1980). *The Movement Assessment of Infants*. Rolling Bay, WA: Author.

Cherry, D.B. (1991). Pediatric physical therapy: Philosophy, science, and techniques. *Pediatric Physical Therapy, 3*(2), 70–76.

Cintas, H.M. (1988). Cross cultural variation in infant motor development. *Physical and Occupational Therapy in Pediatrics, 8*, 1–20.

Couch, K. (1996). The use of the Preschool Play Scale in published research. *Physical and Occupational Therapy in Pediatrics, 16*, 77–84.

Effgen, S.K. (1994). The educational environment. In S. Campbell (Ed.), *Physical therapy for children* (pp. 847–872). Philadelphia: W.B. Saunders Company.

Embrey, D.G., Guthrie, M.R., White, O.R., & Deitz, J. (1996). Clinical decision making by experienced and inexperienced pediatric physical therapists for children with cerebral palsy. *Physical Therapy, 76*, 20–33.

Folio, M.R., & Fewell, R. (1983). *Peabody Developmental Motor Scales and Activity Cards*. Itasca, IL: The Riverside Publishing Co.

Foundation for Physical Therapy. (1991). Contemporary management of motor control problems. *Proceedings of the II Step Conference*. Alexandria, VA: Author.

Haley, S.M., Baryza, M.J., & Blanchard, Y. (1993). Functional and naturalistic frameworks in assessing physical and motor disablement. In I.J. Wilhelm (Ed.), *Physical therapy assessment in early infancy* (pp. 225–256). Philadelphia: Churchill Livingstone.

Haley, S.M., Coster, W.J., Ludlow, L.H., Haltiwanger, J.T., & Andrellos, P.J. (1992). *Pediatric Evaluation of Disability Inventory (PEDI)*. San Antonio, TX: Therapy Skill Builders.

Harris, S.R. (1994). Parents' and caregivers' perceptions of their children's development. *Developmental Medicine and Child Neurology, 36*, 918–923.

Harris, S.R., & Daniels, L. (1996). Content validity of the Harris Infant Neuromotor Test. *Physical Therapy, 76(7)*, 727–737.

Individuals with Disabilities Education Act Amendments of 1991, PL 102-119, 20 U.S.C. §§ 1400 *et seq*.

Jantz, J.W., Blosser, C.D., & Fruechting, L.A. (1997). A motor milestone change noted with a change in sleep position. *Archives of Pediatric and Adolescent Medicine, 151,* 565–568.

Magistro, C.M. (1989). Clinical decision making in physical therapy: A practitioner's perspective. *Physical Therapy, 69,* 525–534.

McCune, L., Kalmanson, B., Fleck, M., Glazewski, B., & Sillari, J. (1990). An interdisciplinary model of infant assessment. In S. Meisels. & J. Shonkoff. (Eds.), *Handbook of early childhood intervention* (pp. 219–245). New York: Cambridge University Press.

Miller, L.J. (1982). *Miller Assessment for Preschoolers (MAP).* San Antonio, TX: The Psychological Corp.

National Institutes of Health. (1993). *Research plan for the National Center for Medical Rehabilitation Research.* (NIH Publication No. 93-3509, p. 34). Bethesda, MD: Author.

Payton, O.D. (1985). Clinical reasoning process in physical therapy. *Physical Therapy, 65,* 924–928.

Piper, M., & Darrah, J. (1994). *Alberta Infant Motor Scale (AIMS).* Philadelphia: W.B. Saunders Company.

Research and Policy Committee of the Committee for Economic Development. (1987). *Children in need: Investment strategies for the educationally disadvantaged.* New York: Committee for Economic Development.

Rothstein, J.M., & Ecternach, J.L. (1986). Hypothesis-oriented algorithm for clinicians: A method for evaluation and treatment planning. *Physical Therapy, 66,* 1388–1394.

Russell, D., Rosenbaum, P., Gowland, C., Hardy, S., Lane, M., Plews, N., McGavin, H., Cadman, D., & Jarvis, S. (1993). *The Gross Motor Function Measure Manual: Second Edition.* Hamilton, Canada: McMaster University.

Schmidt, H.G., Norman, G.R., & Boshuizen, H.P.A. (1990). A cognitive perspective on medical expertise: Theory and implications. *Academic Medicine, 65,* 611–621.

Shaw, M. (1997). *Advocacy and pediatric physical therapy in educational environments: Lessons from the past, strategies for the future.* Unpublished manuscript.

Shelton, T.L., Jeppson, E.S., & Johnson, B.H. (1987). *Family-centered care for children with special health care needs.* Alexandria, VA: Association for the Care of Children's Health.

Task Force on Standards for Measurement in Physical Therapy. (1991). Standards for tests and measurements in physical therapy practice. *Physical Therapy, 71,* 589–662.

Thein, M.M., Lee, J., Tay, V., & Ling, S.L. (1997). Infant walker use, injuries, and motor development. *Injury Prevention, 3,* 63–66.

Watts, N.T. (1989). Clinical decision analysis. *Physical Therapy, 69,* 569–576.

Weed, L.L., & Zimny, N.J. (1989). The problem-oriented system, problem-knowledge coupling, and clinical decision making. *Physical Therapy, 69,* 565–568.

Wescott, S.L., Lowes, L.P., & Richardson, P.K. (1997). Evaluation of postural stability in children: Current theories and assessment tools. *Physical Therapy, 77,* 629–645.

Chapter 9

Psychological Assessment and the Interdisciplinary Team

Anne Hay and Amy G. Breiger

The purpose of a psychological assessment in an interdisciplinary team of child specialists is to provide information on children's developmental functioning in a number of areas, including cognition, adaptive functioning, behavior, and social and emotional status. Psychologists can also assess language abilities as well as fine and gross motor skills in cases in which specialists from those areas are not involved. Moreover, psychologists gather background material concerning the child's family and environment, which is used to help interpret all other data.

The type of psychological assessment a particular child receives is driven by the purposes of the evaluation. Questions raised by the parents or another referral source help focus the assessment. For example, for very young children, cognitive development is often the primary focus. However, if difficult behavior is one of the concerns at the time of referral, assessments of behavior and social and emotional functioning as well as an evaluation of family factors are also crucial. Sometimes the child may have received a recent cognitive assessment through his or her school district, and the psychologist may be asked to address diagnostic issues such as autism, socioemotional status, or specific learning difficulties.

Psychologists determine strengths and weaknesses in the aforementioned areas and identify what additional information is necessary to make a thorough psychological evaluation. At times, a center-based assessment provides relatively little material in some domains, especially those related to school behavior or family interactions. When the center-based evaluation is incomplete, contact with the schools and local community mental health centers, home observation, or questionnaires supply important collateral or follow-up information.

In addition, psychological assessments yield results crucial to establishing diagnoses within an interdisciplinary framework. Diagnoses in young children for which psychologists play a key role include developmental delay, autism, and attention-deficit/hyperactivity disorder (ADHD). Psychologists contribute to diagnoses of mental retardation and learning disabilities in older children. Additional diagnoses that professionals from other disciplines determine using psychological assessment material are genetic syndromes, language disorders, and fetal alcohol syndrome (FAS). Yet the type of information supplied by psychology can vary according to the diagnosis sought. For instance, a basic standardized assessment of cognitive development is essential for a diagnosis of developmental delay. In cases in which factors such as behavior disorders or other psychopathology are involved, however, a low cognitive score may not provide the best estimate of intellectual abilities and must be read with caution. A psychologist both administers the test and comments on the best interpretation of a given child's test results.

Psychological assessments are typically broad-based, and psychological assessment across many domains is often critical. The need to look across domains is usually obvious, as when psychologists assess the adaptive behavior and cognitive status of a child who may have a developmental disability. In some cases, several areas are evaluated to distinguish among possible diagnoses. Assessing the specific domains of a child's abilities is also important within a general concept such as intelligence. Most intelligence tests developed since the late 1980s distinguish between verbal and performance skills, for instance, the Wechsler Preschool and Primary Scale of Intelligence–Revised (WPPSI-R; Wechsler, 1989) and the Wechsler Intelligence Scale for Children–Third Edition (WISC-III; Wechsler, 1991). Some tools yield other types of area scores (e.g., the fourth edition of the Stanford-Binet Intelligence Scale [Stanford-Binet-IV; Thorndike, Hagen, & Sattler, 1986], the Kaufman Assessment Battery for Children [K-ABC; Kaufman & Kaufman, 1983]). At times, the presenting problem indicates that the psychologist should test more specific abilities. For example, a psychologist would test short-term memory when assessing for learning disabilities, which entails the use of several different assessment tools. See Table 9.1 for a list of frequently used psychological assessments.

Suggestions for an appropriate diagnosis or recommendations for more detailed interventions are made after considering patterns of strengths and

Table 9.1.   Frequently used psychological assessment tools for children ages 1–5 years

Assessment tool	Type/content	Ages	Scoring/results
Cognitive development			
Bayley Scales of Infant Development (BSID): a. 1st edition (Bayley, 1969) b. 2nd edition (Bayley, 1993)	Cognitive and motor development	a. 0–30 months b. 0–42 months	Standard score, age-equivalent
Differential Ability Scales (DAS; Elliot, 1990)—preschool battery	Cognitive development: verbal, nonverbal	2 years, 7 months–6 years	Standard score: general and verbal; nonverbal clusters
Kaufman Assessment Battery for Children (K-ABC; Kaufman & Kaufman, 1983)	Cognitive development	2 years, 6 months–12 years	Standard score; intelligence and achievement
Stanford-Binet Intelligence Scale (4th ed.; Thorndike, Hagen, & Sattler, 1986)	Cognitive development: verbal, visual, quantitative, short term memory	3 years and older	IQ score; four area scores
Wechsler Preschool and Primary Scale of Intelligence—Revised (Wechsler, 1989)	Cognitive development: verbal, performance	3–7 years	IQ score; verbal and performance IQ scores
Leiter International Performance Scale a. 1979 (Leiter) b. 1997 (Roid & Miller)	Nonverbal cognitive development (useful for nonverbal children)	3–12 years	Nonverbal IQ score equivalent
Other aspects of development and learning			
Peabody Picture Vocabulary Test—Revised (Dunn & Dunn, 1981)	Receptive vocabulary test (pointing response, no speaking)	2½–10 years	Standard score (receptive language)
Test of Early Reading Ability, Second Edition (TERA-2; Reid, Hresko, & Hammill, 1989)	Many aspects of early reading	4 years and older	Reading quotient and percentile; profile component reading skills
Test of Early Mathematics Ability–Second Edition (TEMA-2; Ginsburg & Baroody, 1990)	Early number skills	4 years and older	Math quotient and percentile; profile types of math skills
Developmental Test of Visual-Motor Integration (VMI; 3rd revision; Beery, 1989)	Drawing of geometric shapes	3 years and older	Standard score (visual-motor integration)

(continued)

Table 9.1.   *(continued)*

Assessment tool	Type/content	Ages	Scoring/results
Vineland Adaptive Behavior Scales (VABS; Sparrow, Balla, & Cicchetti, 1984)	Interview of parents, teachers; four domains: communication, daily living, social, motor	Infancy and older	Standard scores; age equivalents (for each domain and composite)
Child Behavior Checklist and Youth Self-Report (Achenbach & Edelbrook,1986)	Rating scale filled out by parents, teachers; more than 100 typical behavior problems listed; opportunity to list strengths	2 years and older	Profile of seven behavior domains
Conners' Rating Scales (CRS; Conners, 1989)	Rating scale filled out by parents, teachers; typical behavior problems listed	3 years and older	Profile of five behavior domains (useful for attention-deficit/ hyperactivity evaluations)
Barkley questionnaires (Barkley, 1998)	Checklist filled out by parents, teachers		Profile of behavior
The Childhood Autism Rating Scale (CARS; Schopler, Reichler, & Renner, 1988)	Rating scale filled out by evaluator during evaluation and interview	2 years and older	Ranking on scale of autism
Bracken Basic Concept Scale (Bracken, 1984)	Measure of preschool concepts	2½–8 years	Profile of kindergarten readiness

weaknesses in every area assessed by the interdisciplinary team. Such recommendations are often formulated by representatives of each discipline individually but are refined and modified in conjunction with the other team members. Regardless of the diagnoses determined by the team of professionals, recommendations for intervention are dependent on the child's developmental level and learning patterns. Thus, a child at a preschool-age developmental level might benefit from play therapy while a younger child or one having more severe delays would not; a child with a weakness in verbal skills might best learn from visual or kinetic teaching methods but a child with autism would need additional training and support for communication and social skills.

It is also necessary to consider cross-cultural issues and general issues of family functioning when interpreting assessment findings and recommending interventions (McGoldrick, Giordano, & Pierce,1996). Exposure to what might be considered standard American child-rearing techniques; expectations for early learning; and the availability of social experiences, toys, and other materials can vary greatly, and these variations can influence a child's performance on a normed evaluation tool. In terms of designing appropriate interventions, the family and their community are even more crucial. Suggesting reading material and asking them to contact national organizations may be quite helpful for some families. For others having difficulties coping, supports such as group therapy may be more important in helping them to help their child. Furthermore, families from some ethnic groups easily accept professional advice while those from other ethnic groups may feel strongly about perceived interference in private family matters from professionals.

CHALLENGES TO ASSESSMENT

A center-based setting holds many advantages for psychological assessment but also poses significant challenges. It is often difficult to determine whether the behavior or the level of functioning demonstrated during formal testing is representative of the broader scope of behavior. From a single assessment, only a snapshot of the child's behavior is obtained—other family members' interactions with the child may not be seen, and knowledge of the child's functioning in a particular child care or school environment is not always available. After traveling long distances or waking at unaccustomed hours, a child may not exhibit optimal behavior or cognitive functioning. If the child is evaluated under stressful conditions (e.g., feeling tired, interacting with unfamiliar adults, being in an unfamiliar environment), as is often the case, the performance may be typical of the child under stress but may be well below the child's actual abilities. For other children, such as those with ADHD, the quiet, highly structured testing situation is optimal and one that they may never encounter at home or at school. Behavior in a one-to-one setting may be quite different than that at school or at home. The psychologist must consider the characteristics of the test environment and how it compares to the child's experience in order to judge the degree to which the behavior is representative. It is also necessary to consider how this behavior, however optimal, will generalize to other situations. In addition, the psychologist must attempt to determine what the behavior predicts for future functioning or how it will interact with proposed interventions. An ideal assessment includes observation of the child at home and at school and over several visits, which gives a much more accurate picture of the child and improves the ecological validity of the assessment. Collateral information such as questionnaires filled out by parents, child care providers, and school personnel can be helpful when extensive observation is not possible (Harris, 1994; Kim, O'Connor, McLean, Robson, & Chance, 1996). At the very least, it is crucial to evaluate the child when he or she is well rested, well fed, and experiencing a minimal level of stress. If these conditions cannot be obtained, the effect of assessment circumstances must be clearly integrated into any conceptualization of the child.

Another challenge is the variable reliability and validity of standardized psychological instruments. In addition, the assessment measures do not cover all areas of interest or provide a complete profile of the child's strengths and weaknesses. Tests that have been used for many years may also come to have outdated norms. Of note, there are 10 or more points difference between different versions of the WISC or between the first and second editions of the

Bayley Scales of Infant Development (Bayley, 1969, 1993). Furthermore, *floor effects* (when a child does not succeed on the required basal number of items at the beginning of a test) are often seen when testing children who function at lower levels. *Ceiling effects* (when a child does not fail on the required number of items to determine a stopping point at the upper end of a test) may occur when a child's developmental level is above that expected for a particular test. Both floor and ceiling effects emerge when testing children at the borders of any tool's age range (Anastasi, 1988).

Some children cannot be accurately tested using any standardized measure available at the end of the 20th century. Sensory or motor skills difficulties or behavior problems may preclude accurate assessment of other domains. Cerebral palsy or other motor involvement, if severe, can interfere with adequate intellectual assessment. Children who are blind or deaf are not well served by the more common measures of intelligence, and there are few alternatives designed for specific use for children with sensory impairments (Anastasi, 1988; Sattler, 1992). In addition, attention problems can mask problem-solving skills. When a psychologist must evaluate a child for whom standardized procedures in commonly used tests will not work, it is crucial to clarify the essential assessment question. Modifications of testing procedures or materials will allow better performance, but the test cannot then be considered standardized. If it is necessary to determine how a child will perform in a typical school environment, then standard tests, however imperfect, may be the best choice. Criterion-referenced tests can also be used but must be individualized to the child's school program. Nonetheless, if psychologists want to "tease out" the child's optimal abilities, then adapted or nonstandardized assessments may be more appropriate.

THE ASSESSMENT PROCESS

Material available before the assessment allows the psychologist to make an informed hypothesis regarding the type of assessment needed and the instruments to use. The first step in making such decisions is to establish what is already known or believed about the child. The results of parent questionnaires (see the Appendix at the end of this book) obtained prior to the assessment include the child's developmental history and current concerns. School records, which may provide information about previous testing and classroom behavior, are also crucial. Psychologists also employ teacher comments on the child's skills in the areas of cognition, communication, and social skills—as well as fine and gross motor skills—to assist in determining the appropriate tests to use. They may also comment on ways to work with the child effectively. For example, by suggesting techniques that work or possible reinforcers for a given child, school personnel can help the center-based assessment go more smoothly.

The referral questions will indicate the domains that should be evaluated. Families, teachers, and other referral sources will often say what they anticipate from the evaluation. If they do not state what they expect in preassessment materials, it is important to ask directly at the beginning of the evaluation. However, family and school staff are not always in agreement about their assessment expectations. For instance, the school may ask how to manage difficult behavior and the family may want to find appropriate schooling. In such a case, there may be more than one assessment question, and each should be addressed.

A psychologist on an interdisciplinary team usually evaluates cognitive development unless it has been recently tested elsewhere. An assessment of cognitive level provides a framework for the interpretation of the child's behavior. In addition, suggestions for appropriate interventions depend on the child's cognitive level. The choice of which other areas to evaluate (e.g., behavior, emotional issues) depends on referral questions (see Figure 9.1). Assembling information about the child's age, reported skills, and developmental history will aid in choosing the standardized instruments or other assessment techniques and constitutes the first step in the decision-making process (see Figure 9.1). Yet it is very important to note that the circumstances of the actual assessment or factors discovered during the evaluation can render these initial guesses inappropriate. The other members of the interdisciplinary team can provide valuable material in these situations, allowing the psychologist to prepare appropriate testing instruments and to compare the child's behavior across different environments. For example, if a pediatric evaluation occurred earlier and a lower-than-expected cognitive level is indicated, the psychologist can prepare to alter the planned psychological assessment. It is very common to have to switch testing methods or tools unexpectedly during the assessment and as each situation demands. Thus, it is crucial that psychologists remain flexible and have a broad-based knowledge of what can be done or what tools can be used in the wide variety of situations encountered during assessments.

Types of assessment tools are shown in Table 9.1. They include clinical child interviews, behavior observation, parent–child play sessions, child play observations, parent interviews, structured and standardized parent interviews (e.g., the Vineland Adaptive Behavior Scales [VABS; Sparrow, Balla, & Cicchetti, 1984]), parent report checklists (e.g., Achenbach Child Behavior Checklist [CBCL; Achenbach & Edelbrook, 1986]), teacher interviews and checklists, and standardized testing (e.g., IQ tests). When testing a child with established or likely developmental disabilities or behavior problems, a psychologist must weigh the value of adhering to standardized procedures as opposed to using more optimal procedures. Assessment techniques such as testing of limits, when coupled with standardized tests, can provide valuable information (Sattler, 1992, p. 111). Testing of limits involves altering standard procedures to determine under which circumstances a child might succeed at a task. Methods might include providing additional cues, changing modalities (e.g., reading an item to a child who would otherwise read it him- or herself), eliminating time limits, or asking probing questions.

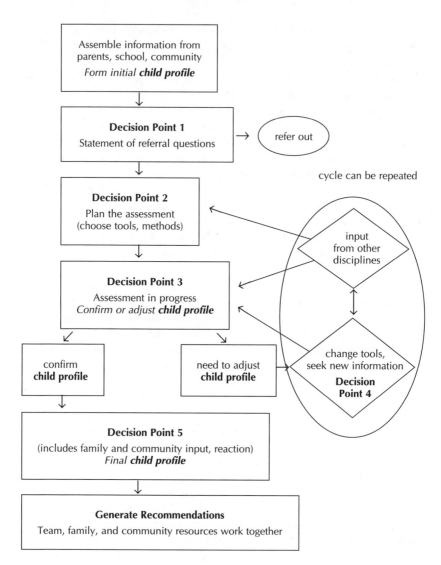

Figure 9.1.   Flow of decision making.

The purpose of the assessment should remain constantly in focus. For example, if the evaluation goal is qualifying the child for school services, it is important to know that only certain tests are accepted by school districts or states for program availability. If the aim is to determine developmental progress and a child has been assessed before, using the same test battery can make it possible to recognize true gains. If the purpose is to gather information that will be used for a legal case, more careful consideration of psychometric data supporting the test and how commonly it is used would be warranted. When a child has been assessed elsewhere recently and the purpose is a broader perspective on the child, much can be accomplished by viewing abilities differently or assessing various domains of competence; therefore, a less common test may be a better choice. If educational planning is the intent of the assessment, a more naturalistic observation or criterion-referenced test may be required to establish patterns of strengths or weaknesses in learning.

For children who cannot be assessed using standardized procedures, it is possible to adapt a tool, as in using only the sensorimotor tasks for a child with severe language delays. An instrument may not have an adequate floor for a child with delays. For example, a child in the age range for the Stanford-Binet-IV or WPPSI-R may be developmentally capable only of the Bayley Scales of Infant Development–Second Edition (BSID-II; Bayley, 1993). With children who function at very low levels, one can use instruments grounded in developmental theory (e.g., Piagetian developmental stages) to create a skill profile, such as object constancy or responses to visual, aural, or tactile stimulation (Sattler, 1992). Regarding these decisions, a psychologist makes an informed guess about the child's developmental level and probable skills in advance of actual testing. When tests are adapted or nonstandard testing has been conducted, it is crucial to note that one is no longer using standardized, norm-referenced instruments. The purpose of such an assessment is to provide a developmental profile analysis of a child's skills and abilities.

REACHING AN INFORMED CLINICAL DECISION

Decision making occurs at five primary points in a psychological assessment. During each step of the decision-making process, a profile of the child is being defined and refined. The first step occurs while reading the referral information and any other material available before the child is seen. Typically this includes the parent report about current skills, development, and the reasons that prompted the request for an assessment. It may also involve information from physicians or teachers suggesting areas of concern. This initial material allows the interdisciplinary team to determine the basic referral question or questions, the first decision point of the process. When these questions have been ascertained, the team or the designated service coordinator decides if the child is an appropriate candidate for an interdisciplinary assessment or whether the child should be referred elsewhere for help. For children who will be seen by the interdisciplinary team, the team or service coordinator must then choose which disciplines will participate in the assessment and which aspect of the child will be considered by each discipline. Next, at the second decision point, the psychologist needs to review the preassessment information to establish what types of psychological assessment testing instruments should be used.

The third decision point occurs during the testing session itself, when the psychologist must determine if the assessment as originally planned can yield a clear profile of the child or if adjustments need to be made in the assessment process. It often happens that new information obtained during testing indicates that the original testing method and instruments are not appropriate. In that case, it is necessary to change methods based on the new situation or information; this is the procedure's fourth decision point. After the assessment results are reviewed, the psychologist can confirm or adjust the child's profile. At that time, the psychologist may consider a tentative diagnosis or address the presenting issues and generate a set of recommendations. Even then, a psychologist may discover that more information is needed, either from another member of the interdisciplinary team or from outside sources. The fifth decision point occurs when a final child profile and a set of recommendations are concluded in conjunction with the entire interdisciplinary team.

Example of Decision Making Through a Case Study

Fred was 3 years and 6 months old and lived with his paternal aunt and her four older children. The child and his aunt were Hispanic. Fred's aunt spoke fluent English, but both Spanish and English were spoken at home. Fred lived with his mother for the first 2 years of his life and was in a foster home for a few months before being placed with his aunt. His mother was a substance abuser in jail in another state. Little was known about Fred's early history, although it was suspected that his mother used crack cocaine and alcohol while pregnant and received little or no prenatal care. When Fred arrived at his aunt's house a year before the assessment, he did not speak or attempt to play with the older children. At the time of assessment, Fred was reported to speak using single words or two-word combinations, both in English and Spanish. He played with others sometimes but often fought with and bit his cousins. In addition, his aunt reported that he had a favorite cousin but disliked strangers. His aunt was also worried because Fred was loud and destructive with toys and did not respond to her requests. The child was very active but clumsy and fell down often. His aunt tried to place him in child care so she could work, but Fred was not toilet trained and the child care center could not handle him. His pediatrician made the referral to the interdisciplinary team, citing concerns about Fred's development and activity level.

Determine Referral Questions and Initial Profile

At the first decision point, the initial referral question involved Fred's cognitive development, adaptive skills, emotional functioning, and behavior. These questions were within the scope of the interdisciplinary team, so the decision was made to assess the child. It was planned that Fred would be seen by the pediatrician, the occupational therapist, the speech-language pathologist, and the psychologist, and Fred's aunt would be interviewed by the social worker. The team decided that an interpreter was not necessary because Fred's aunt spoke English well and because Fred was said to know English as well as Spanish. Based on this information, Fred appeared to be a child with prenatal (maternal substance abuse) and environmental (early separations, unpredictable home environments) risk factors. He seemed to be exhibiting possible language delays, adaptive skill impairments, motor concerns, emotional issues, and behavior problems.

Psychologist Plans the Assessment

At the second decision point, the psychologist planned an assessment that would evaluate Fred's cognitive development, adaptive skills, emotional functioning, attention, and behavior. The social and emotional situation in the home was also of concern. In the case of a typically functioning child of 3 years and 6 months of age, a test such as the Stanford-Binet-IV or the WPPSI-R might be appropriate. However, given Fred's probable delays and likely difficult behavior, the demands of the customary tests would be too great, and he probably would not complete them. The BSID-II could also be used, but Fred's age was at the upper limit of the BSID-II's age range. Also, based on the initial referral questions, the psychologist was interested in distinguishing between verbal and nonverbal domains. The psychologist chose to use the Differential Ability Scales (DAS; Elliot, 1990), a tool that can give verbal and nonverbal domain scores and has a wide age range.

The VABS interview was used with Fred's aunt to look at Fred's adaptive skills at home. The psychologist noted Fred's late language development and his difficulties with social interaction and decided to have the Childhood Autism Rating Scale (CARS; Schopler, Reichler, & Renner, 1988) available in case it seemed appropriate. To further evaluate behavioral and emotional concerns, the psychologist would also interview Fred's aunt to ascertain the effect of parenting skills as well as the antecedents of problem behaviors. In addition, the psychologist planned to observe Fred during free play, structured interaction (i.e., the testing), and adult–child interactions to help identify possible emotional issues as well as his level of social skills.

More information would be available from other disciplines at the team conference. In particular, the psychologist hoped the social worker would gain more background about the family situation, the stability of the aunt's home, and Fred's early history. The speech-language pathologist would gather important information about Fred's language skills and determine whether the child was truly bilingual. The psychologist relied on the team pediatrician to look at possible neurological concerns and general health. All professionals were to note Fred's social adaptive skills and behavior.

Assessment

The third decision point occurred with Fred's assessment by the psychologist. This was his second assessment that morning, and he had to get up 2 hours earlier than usual to come to the clinic. Fred's aunt said that they had not had breakfast and that Fred was cranky, so they were sent to the cafeteria for food and a break. They returned half an hour later. Once in the testing room, Fred seemed wary and sat in his aunt's lap with his back to the psychologist. While talking to the aunt about general issues, the psychologist placed two toy cars on the table and scooted them around in an attempt to help Fred relax. (Although the psychologist also wanted to observe play, it is difficult to begin formal testing after free play.) After a few minutes, Fred became interested in the toy cars and the psychologist, and the two of them took turns moving the cars back and forth to each other. Fred then seemed at ease and was smiling and laughing at the car game. From this brief interaction, it became clear that Fred was able to understand turn-taking, an important social skill. After a few minutes of this play, formal testing was attempted. The DAS blocks were presented to assess nonverbal reasoning and imitation skills. With some encouragement, Fred built an eight-block stack. However, he did not copy the other block patterns. It was the psychologist's impression that Fred did not understand the directions of the task (i.e., to copy a model block design). On the second task, which tested language comprehension, Fred was able to point to body parts on the teddy bear. He identified several toys by name but resisted giving up toys to go on to the next item. He hid in his aunt's lap when asked to follow one-step directives. On the third task, a measure of visual analysis and nonverbal concepts, he matched only the first two picture cards with considerable coaching then slid under the table and would not get back up. Fred's aunt appeared upset and told Fred to be a good boy so they could get ice cream later. This incentive did not bring Fred out from under the table.

During these three tasks, Fred had succeeded on too few test items, and the psychologist had heard only three one-word utterances. At that point, it seemed likely that Fred was functioning below the 2-year and 7-month basal required on the DAS, so further assessment with that tool was terminated. The BSID-II was opened, and the most engaging toy was placed on the table. The psychologist began to ask Fred's aunt the VABS interview questions until Fred approached the toys. The BSID-II Mental Scale assessment continued without much difficulty, although Fred often got down from the table and needed to be redirected. However, he responded well to reinforcement and could be distracted from undesirable behaviors by presenting a new, interesting toy. When observed in a play session later, Fred did not engage interactively with the adults in the room. He made stacks of toys and knocked them over, threw toys, and wanted to leave the room. Fred's aunt seemed embarrassed and frustrated by his behavior. She had difficulty with limit-setting but handled him with affection and some patience. When he did cooperate, Fred's aunt appeared relieved but talked to the evaluator rather than attending to Fred.

The behavior and skills the aunt described during the interview were generally below those expected for Fred's age. Among the noteworthy behaviors were a fear of strangers, throwing tantrums when demands were placed on him, not using silverware when eating, and taking his food into a corner to eat in seclusion. The psychologist noted some concerns regarding Fred's social skills but, based on his social responsiveness and the delayed but not atypical language development described in his aunt's interview, autism was ruled out. Therefore, the CARS was not used.

After the Assessment

The results of the evaluation were then analyzed, comprising the fourth decision point. On the Bayley Mental Scale, Fred achieved a developmental age of 28 months for a Mental Development Index of 63. He had a Psychomotor Development Index of 80, although the psychologist was not sure whether Fred understood the directions for the more complicated items. His lowest cognitive domain was language. These scores indicated that Fred's cognitive skills were developing below the range expected for his age, in the range consistent with a developmental delay. In addition, gross motor skills were in the low-average range. Adaptive behaviors measured by the VABS were low (scores in the 60s) in the areas of Communication, Daily Living Skills, and Socialization. His VABS motor score was also borderline. Overall, he was socially responsive, and his attention and activity level were not out of line with his low developmental level. A profile suggesting a global developmental delay was formed, with language as a primary concern. Questions remained about the extent of early deprivation, early separations, and current family stability.

Team Process

At the fifth decision point, the team worked together to use the assessment outcomes. The other team members concurred with the diagnosis of developmental delay, especially in the area of language and fine motor skills. The pediatrician noted that Fred was healthy, and the pediatrician did not suspect any syndromes (e.g., FAS). In the area of language, the speech-language pathologist described a significant speech delay, above and beyond general cognitive problems. Bilingualism did not appear to contribute significantly to the delay. To provide additional understanding of Fred's emotional functioning and behavior, the social worker added that Fred's early history indicated that neglect was certain and abuse was possible. The child's aggression, food hoarding, and difficulty with strangers could have been related to this neglect and possible abuse. Fred's mother was going to be in jail for 3 more years, but Fred's aunt seemed to be doing her best to provide a stable home. Nevertheless, the family's financial situation was difficult. In addition, she had a hard time coping with the needs of five children. Three of Fred's cousins appeared to be doing well in school. However, the oldest boy had been diagnosed with ADHD and was experiencing problems at school and at home, requiring much of the aunt's energy. Furthermore, although Fred's aunt was affectionate and patient, she seemed to have difficulty with parenting skills such as limit-setting and positive reinforcement for appropriate behavior. The pediatrician observed a long tantrum in response to frustration when Fred could not make a toy work. This demonstrated Fred's trouble with emotion regulation and showed one antecedent of his tantrums (i.e., frustration with cognitive challenges).

Recommendations

The team decided to refer Fred to a developmental preschool through his school district, where he would be able to receive speech-language services. Consultation by a specialist in English as a second language was also suggested to the school district. Therapeutic child care for Fred was recommended to provide more structure and to help Fred work through emotional issues related to early neglect and his separation from his mother. Further behavior analysis to determine antecedents and consequences of his difficult behavior was suggested as well. Fred had a Child Protective Services caseworker, who would be asked to provide more support services (e.g., respite care, parenting classes) for the family. Several questions remained, including to what degree Fred's early deprivation and possible abuse contributed to his delay and behavior problems. The team asked to have Fred return in a year for reevaluation. At that time, motor skills would be assessed and the social situation would also be a focus. The team hoped to see marked improvement after a year of receiving services and living in a supportive, nurturing home environment.

PSYCHOLOGICAL ASSESSMENT IN AN INTERDISCIPLINARY TEAM

As a member of an interdisciplinary team, the psychologist is expected to make a series of complex decisions about the assessment process and appropriate recommendations for the child. All of these decisions will be driven by the initial referral questions for each child, as interpreted by the entire team. Assessment and recommendation conclusions will also be made in conjunction with the assessment decisions of other team members. Choices made as a team member may be different than those made as an individual professional (Bailey, Buysse, Simeonsson, Smith, & Keyes, 1995). The psychologist is likely to take responsibility for assessing one or more particular domains of the child's development while considering the potential interactions of any one domain (e.g., cognition) with other domains that may be assessed by another discipline (e.g., language and communication skills, family social and cultural factors). Sharing among team members at every step of the process assists in ensuring that potential interactions among domains of development are not overlooked.

In the year 2000, challenges for psychology as a discipline include learning more about the multiple domains of the child's experience and competence and the way these elements might interact. Some developmental domains are closely related and interact with each other. For example, it is known that language and some aspects of cognition are linked. Cognition itself is a multifactorial concept, although psychologists typically assess, at best, only verbal and performance (visual/spatial) domains on standardized intelligence

tests. A child's social responsiveness and social skills and the social environment in which he or she lives are separate aspects of psychological development, but they also interact with cognitive factors. A child's adaptive behavior
and life skills are other areas that must be considered. In older children, the
issue of academic skills and the type of schooling the child receives generally
comes into play. As of 2000, there are no formalized ways to determine the interactions of the various domains or their relative contributions to a child's developmental status.

In the future, psychologists hope to have access to additional and better
instruments for assessing children so that their assessments can be more accurate and objective. There are standardized assessment tools to consider cognition, academic skills, and—to some extent—adaptive skills and socioemotional
issues, but many of these tools have flaws. In other areas, there are no reliable
tests. Children with sensory or motor disabilities are not well served by these
instruments. It is also difficult to find appropriate assessment instruments for
preschoolers who function at lower levels and are too old for the infant evaluations but cannot attend to or succeed on the tests designed for typical preschoolers. For older children, it would be helpful to be able to assess more domains of skills, such as social competence, and to be sure that the domains are
reliably differentiated. In sum, much work needs to be done to enhance standardized assessment tools.

Improving the ecological validity of assessments is another concern for
psychologists. Conducting formal testing in an unfamiliar environment may
have limited relevance to the child's functioning at home or school. Discussions
with the family, as well as questionnaires they fill out, can help the team focus
on important issues in the child's home environment. Background material
from teachers, therapists, child care providers, and other community members
can help the team as well. Furthermore, home visits and school observations
provide important insights into how the child functions in his or her home environment. Conducting such observations and obtaining more information will
improve the ecological validity of the assessment process, therefore increasing
the ability to make realistic recommendations for each child.

The formulation of appropriate, constructive suggestions for children is
the desired end product of an interdisciplinary team assessment. These recommendations flow naturally from the initial referral question as it has been interpreted by the team. Each team member makes deductions based on their particular discipline's assessment, and then the team as a group combines these
into a coherent set of conclusions or a diagnosis, if appropriate. The recommendations that are made should deal with each conclusion individually. For
example, if a cognitive delay was determined for the child, the team can suggest
educational services to address cognitive skills. It is at this stage when the family and community members become crucial. With each aspect of the child's
development assessed by the team, it is necessary to ensure that recommenda-

tions can be implemented realistically in the child's home environment. For example, many communities provide developmental preschools to help a child overcome a cognitive delay. However, one child's community may not have a developmental preschool, or another child may have reasons (e.g., physical illness) preventing him or her from participating in an early childhood program. If the implementation of the "ideal" recommendation is not possible, then the team members can generate alternate ways—in this case, home-based services—for the child to receive the needed help. In many cases, a suggestion to return in the future for an assessment of the child's progress is also made.

Psychologists will find that functioning as a member of an interdisciplinary team can be exceptionally rewarding. Through communication with other professionals and sharing information within the team, the psychological assessment becomes increasingly accurate and valid. In addition, the team's recommendations may more appropriate than those made by the psychologist and other professionals in isolation. This benefits not only the children and their families but also the professionals involved.

REFERENCES

Achenbach, T.M., & Edelbrook, C.S. (1986). *Child Behavior Checklist and Youth Self-Report.* Burlington, VT: Author.

Anastasi, A. (1988), *Psychological testing* (6th ed.). New York: Macmillan Publishing USA.

Bailey, D.B., Buysse, V., Simeonsson, R.J., Smith, T., & Keyes, L. (1995). Individual and team consensus ratings of child functioning. *Developmental Medicine and Child Neurology, 37,* 246–259.

Barkley, R.A. (1998). *Attention-deficit hyperactivity disorder: A handbook for diagnosis and treatment* (2nd ed.). New York: The Guilford Press.

Bayley, N. (1969). *Bayley Scales of Infant Development.* San Antonio, TX: The Psychological Corp.

Bayley, N. (1993). *Bayley Scales of Infant Development–Second Edition.* San Antonio, TX: The Psychological Corp.

Beery, K.E. (1989). *Developmental Test of Visual-Motor Integration (VMI)* (3rd revision). Itasca, IL: The Riverside Publishing Co.

Bracken, B.A. (1984). *Bracken Basic Concept Scale.* San Antonio, TX: The Psychological Corp.

Conners, C.K. (1989). *Conners' Rating Scales (CRS).* North Tonawanda, NY: Multi-Health Systems.

Dunn, L.M., & Dunn, L.M. (1981). *Peabody Picture Vocabulary Test–Revised.* Circle Pines, MN: American Guidance Service.

Elliot, C.D. (1990). *Differential Ability Scales.* San Antonio, TX: The Psychological Corp.

Ginsburg, H.P., & Baroody, A.J. (1990). *Test of Early Mathematics Ability, Second Edition (TEMA-2).* Austin, TX: PRO-ED.

Harris, S.R. (1994). Parents' and caregivers' perceptions of their children's development. *Developmental Medicine and Child Neurology, 36,* 918–923.

Kaufman, A.S. (1994). *Intelligent testing with the WISC-III.* New York: John Wiley & Sons.

Kaufman, A.S., & Kaufman, N.L. (1983). *Kaufman Assessment Battery for Children (K-ABC).* Circle Pines, MN: American Guidance Service.

Kim, M., O'Connor, K.S., McLean, J., Robson, A., & Chance, G. (1996). Do parents and professionals agree on the developmental status of high-risk infants? *Pediatrics, 31,* 676–681.

Leiter, R.G. (1979). *Instruction Manual for the Leiter International Performance Scale*. Wood Dale, IL: Stoelting Co.

McGoldrick, M., Giordano, J., & Pierce, J. (1996). *Ethnicity and family therapy* (2nd ed.). New York: The Guilford Press.

Reid, D.K., Hresko, W.P., & Hammill, D.D. (1989). *Test of Early Reading Ability, Second Edition (TERA-2)*. Austin, TX: PRO-ED.

Roid, G.H., & Miller, L.J. (1997). *Leiter International Performance Scale–Revised* (Leiter-R). Wood Dale, IL: Stoelting Co.

Sattler, J. (1992). *Assessment of children* (Rev. 3rd ed.). San Diego, CA: Author.

Schopler, E., Reichler, R.J., & Renner, R. (1988). *The Childhood Autism Rating Scale (CARS)*. Los Angeles: Western Psychological Services.

Sparrow, S.S., Balla, D.A., & Cicchetti, D.V. (1984). *Vineland Adaptive Behavior Scales (VABS)*. Circle Pines, MN: American Guidance Service.

Thorndike, R.L., Hagen, E.P., & Sattler, J.M. (1986). *Stanford-Binet Intelligence Scale for Children* (4th ed.). Itasca, IL: The Riverside Publishing Co.

Walker, C.E., & Roberts, M.C. (Eds.). (1992). *Handbook of clinical child psychology* (2nd ed.). New York: John Wiley & Sons.

Wechsler, D. (1989). *Wechsler Preschool and Primary Scale of Intelligence–Revised*. San Antonio, TX: The Psychological Corp.

Wechsler, D. (1991). *Wechsler Intelligence Scale for Children–Third Edition*. San Antonio, TX: The Psychological Corp.

Chapter 10

The Role of Social Work with Families that Have Young Children with Developmental Disabilities

Douglas S. Cook

Families face unique challenges when they have young children with atypical patterns of growth and development. This chapter presents social work practice with these families as part of an interdisciplinary team that provides assessments and community referrals. Information is included on social work roles, interview content, the assessment process, and expected outcomes.

Social workers interview families in order to gain an understanding of the broader family's history, their current concerns, the impact of the child on the family, and resources that might be useful. These professionals work with very diverse families. Single parents, two-parent families, foster families, grandparents raising their grandchildren, and relatives who have taken in young children from their extended families use the services of the interdisciplinary clinic.

Refugees are also seen. Some of these families have caregivers who are gay or lesbian. A few children's parents have cognitive impairments themselves.

When a child is diagnosed with a developmental delay, whether at birth or later in childhood, the family is almost always stunned. They often have to work through the grief of lost expectations for the child. A sense of assumed guilt may stay with caregivers, especially mothers, even after assurance by professionals that they did nothing that would have caused the syndrome or condition. Families frequently do not know where to turn for more information about resources that offer parent support or help them promote their children's development.

Sometimes extended family members blame the caregivers for the child's slow progress, and fathers who are not primary caregivers may not be able to see the child's impairments. Immediate family members also may have to endure denial from friends or extended family that anything is wrong with the child. Many mothers with children who have developmental delays report that other family members, friends, and professionals attempted to reassure them, saying the child would "grow out of it." Furthermore, siblings may resent that a sister or brother is treated differently or demands most of a caregiver's attention. Friends and relatives may pull back from the family as their children take different developmental paths. Occasionally a couple will divorce as a result of the stress that accompanies parenting a child with developmental delays, although it is seldom that the child is the only factor.

Parents must learn to accommodate their children with special needs within the broader needs of the whole family. Often it is helpful for them to learn new coping mechanisms and to identify new resources that better support the family. At some point almost all families bond with and cherish their children with disabilities. They see hope where there is hope. They enjoy the gains their children make and appreciate the gifts they bring to the family. In fact, over time, most families with children with disabilities adjust well if they have appropriate supports and services. One source of support and services is contact with an interdisciplinary group of professionals who try to respond to family concerns. The purpose of this chapter is to highlight how the practice of social work within the interdisciplinary team can assist in providing support to these families.

SOCIAL WORK ROLES AND EXPECTED OUTCOMES

In broad terms, the role of social work is to assess, to support, and to empower the child's family so they have the understanding, the resources, and the initiative to maximize their child's growth and development. For the first outcome, assessment, it is necessary to learn about the family's daily routines, interactions, and current issues. This is usually accomplished through a face-to-face interview with the child's caregivers. Other family members or support people can participate in the interview if the caregivers so desire. In the case of separated or divorced parents, the parents are asked whether they want to meet with the social worker together or separately.

It is critical that the assessment interview be primarily driven by the family's agenda and needs. This means social workers must listen carefully and take the family's input seriously. It is usually helpful to use an ethnographic interviewing style that attempts to understand how people see and express their perceived reality (Rubin & Babbie, 1997). This model uses open-ended questions to elicit information about the child's strengths, the impact of the child's condition on family members, the resources they have and those they may need, and concerns about their child's present and future. This process, when carried out respectfully and thoroughly, usually brings to light the family's beliefs about their child and the interaction patterns among family members; it assists family members in teaching social workers about their ecological framework. Working from this ethnographic, or ecological, framework helps ensure that the assessment is conducted in a family-centered context.

Providing family support, the social worker's second role, includes giving positive verbal feedback to the family and identifying the family's strengths. It also includes identifying potential resources and making referrals requested by the family, such as birth-to-3 programs, parent-to-parent programs, and a wide variety of other early intervention and community services. Support can also mean helping caregivers foster a more positive view of themselves and of their child with a disability. This outcome is achieved through establishing rapport with the family and making referrals that match the caregivers' perceived needs for the child as well as for themselves.

Family empowerment, the third outcome, focuses on helping families take charge of their own lives with respect to their child with a disability. This framework is based on the assumptions that families need to be at the center of decision making for their young children (see Table 10.1) and that they are or can become adept at identifying, finding, and utilizing needed resources. Families have the most information about their child, and social workers need to interact as peers with the caregivers in the evaluation and recommendation processes to achieve the best possible outcome for the child. Almost always, it is the family members who ultimately decide—by the beliefs they hold and the actions they take—the resources to which their children will have access. Simply put, children with developmental delays require ongoing oversight and advocacy by a committed and knowledgeable caregiver if they are to obtain the needed short- and long-term resources.

Social work professionals must take what they have learned about the family from the family's own perspective and seek ways for the family to build on its current strengths. For example, caregivers might join a parent group where they learn self-advocacy strategies or come to realize that they can make needed telephone calls rather than relying on a professional to do it for them. Long-term empowerment usually includes joining with other caregivers who

Table 10.1.   Summary of elements of family-centered care

1. Recognition that the family is the constant in the child's life while the service systems
    and personnel within those systems fluctuate.
2. Facilitation of parent/professional collaboration at all levels of health care:
    —care of an individual child;
    —program development, implementation, and evaluation; and
    —policy formulation.
3. Sharing of unbiased and complete information with parents about their child's care
    on an ongoing basis in an appropriate and supportive manner.
4. Implementation of appropriate policies and programs that are comprehensive and
    provide emotional and financial support to meet the needs of families.
5. Recognition of family strengths and individuality and respect for different methods
    of coping.
6. Understanding and incorporating the developmental needs of infants, children, and
    adolescents and their families into health care delivery systems.
7. Encouragement and facilitation of parent-to-parent support.
8. Assurance that the design of health care delivery systems is flexible, accessible, and
    responsive to family needs.

Reprinted with permission of the Association for the Care of Children's Health, P.O. Box 25707, Alexandria, VA 22313 from Shelton, T.L., Jeppson, E.S., & Johnson, B.H. (1987). *Family-centered care for children with special health care needs* (p. 71). Alexandria, VA: Association for the Care of Children's Health.

are fighting similar battles. This broader focus may involve working to change administrative policies, influencing legislative action, or acquiring needed services from community providers. This third outcome results in caregiver and family advocacy for the child and often for other children with developmental disabilities as well.

This outcome paradigm can be perceived in a linear fashion (see Figure 10.1), although the process itself tends to be circular. Individual issues emerge one after the other, are incorporated into the growing picture of family life, and are revisited in light of additional shared information. The process usually requires the social worker to elicit the family's knowledge of its important issues and values, especially those concerning the child being evaluated and the family's interactions with the child. A successful assessment leaves the social worker with an accurate view of the family's issues from the family's perspective. It also encourages the family members to become aware of their major stresses and how they are currently coping with those issues.

During the interview the social worker must also determine the strengths that have allowed the caregivers to raise their child and maintain their family, and these observations should be shared with the family. The process is most effective when the family's strengths can be utilized in gaining needed resources. For instance, if a single parent has learned to ask her immediate relatives to care for the child when she needs to run errands, she may also be willing to ask them or other friends for help when she needs time for herself. Successful support results in the ability of the family and the social worker to identify strengths and

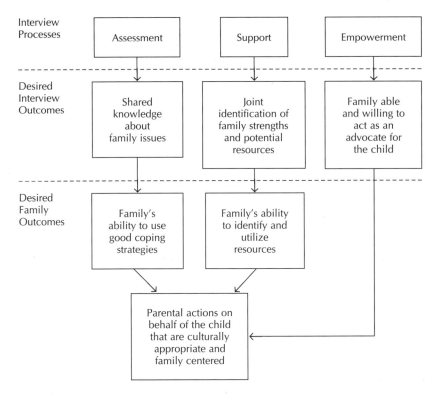

Figure 10.1.   A social work advocacy model for early intervention.

potential resources mutually. As a result of the relationship, the family should have an increased ability to obtain and manage needed resources.

Empowerment of the family occurs when all of its members, aware of their stresses, coping strategies, and management abilities, can obtain the culturally appropriate and family-centered advocacy needed by the child. Families may employ current resources or create new ones for themselves and others. The proliferation of parent-to-parent groups in the late 1990s, often started by one caregiver, is a good example of growing family self-advocacy. The goal is for the family to acquire an awareness of and access to community resources, thereby decreasing the need for a social worker's services.

Realistically, in an hour interview with the interdisciplinary team, it is impossible to cover the three foci fully with any family. Two additional constraints limit the social worker's scope of information. First, only one family member is often available for interviewing and that person must convey information about the rest of the family. Second, follow-up is not routinely provided after the family conference. Social workers may contact families regarding resources that could not be identified at the time of the family conference or those that may have a difficult time obtaining needed resources. However, given the short interview time, the social worker must be skilled in establishing rapport, able to discern and stay focused on the family's issues and values, and conversant with available resources.

INTERVIEW CONTENT

Krauss and Jacobs (1990) identified three general content areas that continue to be the major foci of social work family assessments relevant to early intervention arenas: 1) caregiver and family stress, 2) coping strategies and resources, and 3) the family home environment. Each of these areas is explored in detail in the following sections.

Stress: A Window into the Family Environment

Self-reported family stress has become the major framework for assessing the difficulties families face when they have a child with a developmental disability. There are at least three major reasons self-reported stress is useful in these evaluations. A wide variety of research shows that, in the absence of good social support, high levels of family stress are related to poor family functioning (Dunst & Trivette, 1990). These studies include families coping with a child who has a developmental disability or a chronic medical condition (Solomon & Draine, 1995). Because self-reported stress has been correlated with the level of family functioning, social workers can gather information about family difficulties through face-to-face interviews. In addition, the experience of stress is generally accepted as an inescapable part of life and often carries little negative valence. Hence, it is relatively easy for many caregivers to speak of their stresses without feeling self-conscious. In a child evaluation clinic where families are seldom seen more than once a year, and commonly only once if ever, this face-to-face assessment focus offers relatively quick insight into the family situation without creating great turmoil for the family.

When caregiver or family stressors are evaluated, it is important to consider stress based on child characteristics, caregiver characteristics, environmental stresses, and life changes. Each of these categories is multidimensional and open ended. Table 10.2 identifies a range of items in each category that have been identified as family stressors. Most of these items are taken from published reports (Hodapp, Dykens, & Masino, 1997; Murata, 1994; Newby, 1996; Parkerson, Broadhead, & Tse, 1995; Patterson & Garwick, 1994; Pianta & Lothman, 1994; Short & Johnson, 1997), and some of the listed stresses have been identified by caregivers who have actually attended clinics.

Although it is necessary to be aware of the range of potentially stressful issues, it is critical to be sensitive to matters that especially affect families with a child who has a developmental disability. These include learning of the child's diagnosis, parental worries about having caused the condition, negotiating an

Table 10.2.   Examples of potential sources of stress

Child characteristics	Family characteristics	Environmental issues
Premature Birth	*Composition*	Lack of cross-culturally
Long neonatal intensive	Single parent	trained professionals
care unit stay	Blended family	Poverty or financial
Sick as well as premature	Grandparent care	difficulty
High risk of death	provider	Insufficient/inadequate
Death of a prior child who	Parent(s) with mental	housing or
was born prematurely	retardation	homelessness
One twin dies	*Family constructs*	Birth-to-3 early
Still on oxygen, feeding	No place for a person	intervention program
tube, and so forth when	with a disability in	not easily available
sent home	cosmology	Three-to-6 early
Diagnosis of syndrome or	No personal awareness	intervention program
neurological condition	of other people with	not easily available
Higher stress with some	disabilities	Lack of medical coverage
diagnoses	No awareness of	Lack of transportation
Prader-Willi syndrome	options for adults	resources
Degenerative conditions	with disabilities	Unsafe neighborhoods
Disability with little	Fear that the parents	Life changes
likelihood of change	may have caused	New roommate(s)
Fetal alcohol syndrome	the disability	Losing a job
Mental retardation	Belief that a limited	Changing jobs
Multiple disabilities	child is refusing to	Marriage
Autism	walk, talk, and so	Separation
Difficult behavioral issues	forth	Divorce
Destructive behaviors	*Parental dysfunction*	Moving to a new house
Hitting, pushing, biting	Social isolation	Immigrating to the U.S.
Destroying siblings' toys	Lack of time for spouse	Out of home placement
and so forth	or partner	of child(ren)
Hurting pets	Lack of individual time	Birth of another baby
Setting fires	for siblings	Death of a significant
Attentional difficulties	Depression	person
Can't stop moving	Mental health	
Awake most hours of	diagnosis	
the day	Serious medical issues	
Needs constant super-	Illegal drug use	
vision for safety	Alcohol abuse	
Autistic behaviors	Domestic violence	
Lack of eye contact	Criminal activity	
Rejection of touch or	Sexual predation	
holding	*Parental response to*	
Frustration with	*diagnosis*	
communication	Parent overwhelmed	
Sexual behaviors	by diagnosis	
Inappropriate touching	Parent denies needed	
of others	early intervention	
Masturbation in public	services	
places		

appropriate educational plan with birth-to-3 or 3-to-6 early intervention programs, and coping with the stigma and exclusion that still exist in late 20th
century society. Important but more general issues include the impact of poverty on a family's resources and the stress that results from caregiver depression, drug use, alcohol abuse, or domestic violence. In addition, interviewers
must be competent and sensitive to issues of family-centered practice and cultural issues if the family and clinician are to benefit fully from the interview.

Coping and Resources: Reducing Stress

Coping has been defined as a multidimensional process that refers to the ways
in which people deal with stress (Lazarus & Folkman, 1984). Many different
frameworks have been created to measure it. The ones mentioned here have
been used with families that have children with developmental disabilities or
other neurological conditions. The Coping Health Inventory for Parents (CHIP;
McCubbin et al., 1983) was one of the earlier attempts to integrate a number
of coping strategies. The three coping patterns identified were 1) maintaining
family integration, cooperation, and an optimistic definition of the situation;
2) maintaining social support, self-esteem, and psychological stability; and 3) understanding the medical situation through communication with other parents
and medical staff. The presence of each of the factors contributed to better family coping.

A second major effort, using the third iteration of The Ways of Coping
questionnaire, compared the efficacy of *palliative coping* versus *adaptive coping*
(Thompson, Zeman, Fanurik, & Sirotkin-Roses, 1992). In palliative coping,
the caregiver utilizes avoidance, wishful thinking, and self-blame to maintain a
comfortable level of feeling or emotion. In adaptive coping, the caregiver utilizes problem-solving strategies such as cognitive restructuring and seeking resources and social support.

Research studies of caregivers who have children with developmental delays or other chronic medical conditions have identified a number of factors
that are thought to predict positive or negative adjustment to high levels of
stress. Factors believed to buffer stress are getting information from professionals; joining associations of caregivers who have children with a similar diagnosis (Hymovich & Baker, 1985); having personal resources; being efficacious on
one's own behalf; creating a high level of social support for the family; increasing network density; participation in a family support group; and having a
broad, affirming social support network (Solomon & Draine, 1995). Factors believed to result in poor adjustment are high levels of daily stress, decreased family supportiveness, and reliance on palliative coping strategies (Thompson, Gill,
Burbach, Keith, & Kinney, 1993).

Clinically, this picture suggests that helping caregivers and other family
members with high levels of stress requires a variety of resources. Social workers need to be knowledgeable regarding, for instance, parent-to-parent groups.

Introducing parent-to-parent services is especially crucial when working with parents who have a child who has been recently diagnosed with a developmental disability. Caregivers almost always report that finding someone who "really understands" what they are dealing with and what they are feeling means finding a caregiver with a child similar to their own. Other outreach programs with which social workers must be familiar are groups for caregivers of color; disability-specific associations; fathers' groups; new mothers' groups; multiple-birth groups; and county, state, or federally funded parent initiatives. A growing number of caregivers now use e-mail and Internet resources, so social work professionals must know these also.

Family Environment: A Glimpse of Family Context

Historically, social work assessments of family environments meant making a home visit to determine whether the house was safe and functional for the family, whether developmentally appropriate toys were available, and whether caregivers interacted well with each other and the children in the home. Interdisciplinary evaluation teams, however, have generally chosen to see children and their families in centralized hospitals or clinics. This has made it much more efficient to conduct multiple evaluations but more difficult to assess the day-to-day home environment correctly, as both children and family members may be shy, uncomfortable, or intimidated in the clinical, often medical, environment. When working with the family, the social worker must elicit an understanding of the family's home environment. This generally includes a sense of the child's, caregivers', and other family members' experiences of their life together, as well as the beliefs held by family members. Some initial questions that produce glimpses of the everyday family environment include

1. How does the child's condition appear to affect his or her life presently? How does it affect caregivers and other family members?
2. How do family members interact with each other and with the child? What is the frequency, tenor, and outcome of these interactions (e.g., supporting, ignoring, blaming)?
3. Does the child have toys appropriate for his or her developmental level? Are there safe places to play both inside and outside of the home?
4. Is the home in a safe neighborhood for caregivers and children?

Explorations of the family's understanding of current stresses, coping strategies, needed resources, and the home environment provide a multidimensional framework for understanding the family's current life experience and to suggest potentially useful strategies and resources. In addition, what is learned from the family helps guide the team to approach evaluation concerns and recommendations using the family's beliefs, values, and experiences. This framework can be identified as an advocacy model that uses three processes to help families take a proactive role in their child's care (see Figure 10.1). When it is used well, families themselves are empowered to take actions on behalf of their children that are culturally appropriate and family centered. Social workers may continue to provide resources that the family finds useful, but the family actually is in charge of what is happening to their child.

TWO UNIQUE ISSUES FOR SOCIAL WORK

Caregivers come to a clinic in order to obtain a detailed developmental assessment of their child or to address a specific set of developmental concerns. Unless they have been to the clinic before, they do not anticipate also being asked about family stress, sources of support, and their construction of meaning about their child's condition. Although many caregivers welcome a chance to talk about these issues, some are hesitant, and a small percentage decline the offer of social work services. Some caregivers who have had contact with Child Protective Services (CPS) are afraid to talk with a social worker. They may blame social workers for losing custody of other children or be fearful that the social worker might report them to CPS. Some caregivers assume that social workers are long-term therapists and, therefore, do not want their services. The largest group is comprised of people who have had only minimal contact with social workers in interdisciplinary arenas and, consequently, do not have a clear idea of what social workers actually do. People living in rural areas or recent immigrants may not have ever encountered professional social workers and so do not easily understand the help these professionals can offer. To minimize this uncertainty, social workers must announce their purpose when first meeting with a family, saying something such as "Although the other disciplines in our center evaluate your child, we want to learn how you and your family are doing. We also may know resources that you or your family might find useful. Perhaps you could begin by telling us how you heard about the clinic and what you hope to gain from your child's evaluation."

A second issue for social work is that the child may need to be in the room during the caregiver interview. With very young children (e.g., from birth to 1-year-old), this is not usually a problem, as they seldom follow the discussion. They can, however, sense a caregiver's feelings during the interview and respond to them. With older children who do not need a caregiver to be present during their evaluation, the social worker may interview the caregiver while another discipline is evaluating the child. Sometimes another sibling has accompanied the caregiver to the evaluation or the child being evaluated requires the caregiver to be present physically at each evaluation. What is important is that neither the child nor the caregiver feel uncomfortable because of the need to have children present. Thus, the social worker may have an attenuated interview if everything appears to be fine, or he or she can schedule a telephone meeting to complete sensitive items that would not be appropriate for children to hear. Occasionally another team member, with the caregiver's permission, may play with the child in the interviewing room while the social worker interviews the caregiver in the observation room. This way, the caregiver can monitor the child's activities without the child hearing the conversation.

ASSESSMENT PROCESS

The assessment process begins by gathering information from the family as well as from medical, school, and other professionals who have evaluated the child. A good assessment requires the social worker to be skilled at interviewing family members and able to think analytically about his or her interactions with them. The interview must focus on listening to the family, supporting their strengths, and encouraging them to begin or to continue their advocacy on behalf of the child. One important issue requires special attention. If a child appears to need protection from the caregiver, it is best addressed in a sensitive way that allows the social worker to obtain legal protection for the child while still supporting the parent. This requires great skill and can be very helpful for the family.

Gathering Information for the Interview

The first source of family information is a parent questionnaire (see the Appendix at the end of this book). This is sent to all new families by the clinic coordinator and returned prior to the clinic visit. Returning families are asked to complete a one-page update on the family (see Appendix). The parent questionnaire details the family's composition and its members' ages, employment, marital status, and residence. With this information, the social worker becomes familiar with the family demographically and anticipates potential socioeconomic issues. Some topics will need to be handled differently depending on the age and marital status of the caregiver. Teenage parents often need child care so they can return to school. They may also be struggling with estrangement from their own parents while still living with them. Grandparents who have taken over the care of their grandchildren generally have different issues. They may have to give up anticipated travel following their retirement or lose long-time friends who do not have the stamina for or interest in constantly watching young children. These and other issues need to be raised by the social worker if the family does not first identify them.

The parent questionnaire also asks the family to list concerns about the child and the desired outcomes of the evaluation. This information usually provides initial clues about how the family sees the child. Caregivers who want a diagnosis are working with different concerns than those who want to "cure" the child or those who want to know what to expect when their child becomes a young adult. It is important that the social worker and the caregiver spend some time exploring these issues so the interdisciplinary team has information about the family's perception of the child. Talking about how a family sees a child can sometimes help caregivers enlarge their vision of what is possible. For instance, families that take on intensive therapy and teaching roles sometimes neglect making time to enjoy their children. Similarly, being able to talk with other caregivers of preadolescent children who have disabilities can be very helpful. Hearing about young adults who are living with community support services, who have jobs supported by a job coach, or who are considering marriage can provide long-term hope for families that do not know older children with special needs.

The clinic coordinators also request input from medical providers, school personnel, and other professionals who have seen and assessed the child. This is a second source of information. In addition to the historical insight into the child's condition, there is information about the family's involvement with teachers, therapists, and other professionals. This material may be helpful in anticipating how the family will respond to clinic evaluations. For instance, if the parent routinely volunteers in the classroom and has implemented some of the school's behavior interventions at home, the social worker can anticipate that the caregiver is very knowledgeable about his or her child's daily school routine.

The third source of family information prior to the interview is a child and family services questionnaire sent out with the parent questionnaire (see the Appendix at the end of this book). This sheet asks whether the child is currently receiving services from a primary care physician, Supplemental Security Income (SSI), the state's Division of Developmental Disabilities, a public health nurse, or a special education program. Questions also focus on basic services that families use such as Temporary Aid to Needy Families (TANF); the Special Supplemental Nutrition Program for Women, Infants, and Children (WIC); respite care; caregiver support groups; or counseling. The completed list helps quickly identify services that are in place and potential additional services that might be useful to the family. Information from all of the above sources is entered on a social work family assessment form (see Appendix at the end of this book), which is used as a guide for the interview.

Often, a fourth source of information, feedback from a discipline that has already seen the child, is available prior to the social work interview. This input is usually passed on in short, private conversations between team members and addresses the family's perceived strengths and issues as well as any concerns the prior evaluator had about the family. Knowing that a family is worried about finances or that each caregiver sees their child differently assists the social worker in focusing more quickly on an area important to the family. It also may save the caregivers from having to retell their story to each professional assessing their child.

Skills Needed for Interviewing

Two types of skills are needed for social workers to work best with families. The first is to have a broad set of interviewing skills, based on the ability to empathize, that help families demonstrate their strengths, values, and needs. An interviewing schema that has been shown to be clinically useful with parents of children with disabilities (Davis & Rushton, 1991) comes out of Kelly's (1963) personal construct theory. This is elaborated in Davis's (1993) book *Counselling Parents of Children with Chronic Illness or Disability*. Personal construct theory assumes that everyone sees the world differently and that there are a variety of ways to perceive anything that happens. Davis identifies five "fundamental attitudes" (respect, humility, genuineness, empathy, and quiet enthusiasm) and five "basic skills" (attending to others, active listening, prompting, demonstrating empathy, and exploration) as necessary for the caregiver interviewing process to go forward (1993, pp. 53–69). These skills allow the social worker to ask questions that deepen knowledge about the family while also building the family–social worker relationship. Although Davis also identifies a more advanced set of "challenging skills," these are not as useful for interdisciplinary clinical assessment because they rely on a high level of client trust that usually does not emerge in initial interviews.

The second skill needed is the ability to think analytically. This requires employing observation, inference, and reasoning skills to generate judgments that reflect information from the family rather than interviewer biases. Nurius and Gibson (1990) listed the constraints that often bias clinical judgments in direct practice. It is critical that social workers understand and continue to evaluate their thinking processes when they interview families. Although the subject is beyond the scope of this chapter, social work professionals must acknowledge that processing information requires utilizing short cuts to handle the vast amount of material available even in a 1-hour session. Each social worker comes to the interview with his or her own beliefs, values, and theories regarding parents with cognitive disabilities raising children, gay or lesbian caregivers who adopt children with special health care needs, or caregivers who decide whether they want to bear children on the basis of ultrasounds (which provide diagnoses for some children with disabilities in utero). The interviewer may also identify with a caregiver and then assume that this person has the same values. When searching for an understanding of the caregiver's perceptions, most people are prone to make quick decisions. Therefore, an acute awareness of one's own biases is crucial for making accurate family characterizations. It is from this perspective that social workers should continually monitor their own work as well as utilize consultation with other professional staff.

The Interview Process

The interview actually starts when approaching the family in the waiting room. Both the social worker and the family are visually assessing the other. After introductions, the social worker indicates the direction of the interview room and begins moving toward it. It is helpful to walk side by side to the interview room so that the process of reciprocal communication can begin. If the parent does not initiate talking at the start of this walk, it is helpful for the social worker to introduce an innocuous subject that can be either agreed upon or laughed about and then dropped (e.g., the weather, traffic, newspaper headlines). When people do not know each other, it is wise to make these first communications "low-risk" offerings. If these go well, caregivers begin to assume that they can discuss more personal issues with clinic professionals. It is generally not useful to start talking about the family or their child until everyone is in the privacy of the interviewing room.

The social worker explains his or her role and, unless the family member begins talking, asks broad questions such as "What are you hoping for from this evaluation?", "What impact does Matt's condition have on you and your partner?", "Where would you like to start?", or "Will you tell me about your daughter?" The initial answer to any one of these questions almost always elicits additional queries before the caregiver's stress and sense of the child emerge. In this early stage, social workers rarely suggest resources even if they might be helpful. Rather, it is important to build rapport with the family members first by listening carefully, being empathetic, validating family perspectives, and reflecting their affect. The following case exemplifies an early interaction that would build rapport:

Tom's father was asked, "What is the main thing you and your family want from Tom's evaluation?" The father responded that Tom had always been "a little slow" and had been in a birth-to-3 early intervention program for 2 years. However, he had never been formally evaluated or diagnosed. The family talked with the birth-to-3 center staff, who suggested bringing Tom to the interdisciplinary clinic for an evaluation. The boy's father then became teary-eyed. The social worker responded by saying, "You have some feelings about your son's evaluation," and Tom's father stated that he had always known something was not right but did not want to think about it. After a short pause, the social worked quietly asked, "Being here makes it more real that Tom has some problems?" Tom's father agreed and then fell silent. Then, with warmth and understanding, the social worker said that this experience must be difficult. Tom's father replied, "Yes—but we really do want to find out what is going on and whether we should be doing something else besides the birth-to-3 program to prepare him for a preschool program." The social worker then suggested that it might be scary to find a possible problem but that doing so would help the child in the future, and the father agreed.

At this point the social worker might ease into asking questions more systematically, which would deepen his or her understanding of how the family views the child. Questions might include the following:

- "Are there any other ways a diagnosis might be helpful for your family?"
- "Do you see any downside to Tom's receiving a diagnosis?"
- "When did the family first notice Tom's possible impairment?"
- "Has anyone ever put a name to that?"
- "In what ways is he behind?"
- "What are Tom's strengths?"
- "Who is involved in his life?"

It is especially important to keep asking questions on one topic until arriving at a sense of what is important about it to the family. Once that is achieved, the social worker should briefly say what he or she believes was learned from the exchange and ask whether it is right. A summary of the last set of questions sounds as follows: "I am impressed that your whole family has talked about this, and you have really prepared yourselves to help Tom be as ready as possible for preschool. That's really great support for him!"

Skipping quickly from one topic to another, whether initiated by the social worker or the family member, does not provide the depth needed for good assessments. The social worker needs to build rapport with the family through eliciting information methodically, listening very carefully to the caregivers, and checking to be sure he or she understands the family's relationship to and view of the child. As the interview progresses, the same technique is used with each new topic that seems important to the family. If the social worker still does not have adequate insight, he or she needs to seek more information and then try a new summary. In this way, the social work professional learns about the family and begins to determine the resources they might find useful.

Interviewing works best when one is genuinely interested in those being interviewed. To do that, the interviewer should be honestly open and respectfully curious, and he or she must use questions and statements that support people. However, this does not mean that difficult questions should be avoided, including topics such as alcohol or other drug abuse, domestic violence, or child abuse. These queries are usually best left to the later part of the interview, but they should not be the last topic discussed. This allows the social worker to generate as much rapport with the caregiver as possible before approaching these formidable issues. If the interactions are very confrontational, it is helpful to get as much mutual closure with the caregiver as possible by acknowledging the difficulty of the matter and the social worker's appreciation of the caregiver's perspective.

At the end of the interview, the social work professional usually talks about potential resources the family might find useful. These will be revisited and are often revised during the team's conference with the family at a later point in the interdisciplinary process. If the family has not identified any needed resources during the interview, it is helpful to ask them if there are specific resources that they need. Once their self-identified needs have been explored, they should also be told about specific resources that the social worker believes might be useful. It is helpful to find out how families perceive different potential resources and for caregivers to be able to anticipate suggestions. This information helps guide case conference recommendations because it identifies resources families have already learned to use, resources they would like to employ but do not know how to obtain, and those that do not seem useful to them. It is always families that make the decision to pursue or ignore a suggestion, and it usually is within the caregiver's rights to use or reject a recommended resource. Thus, working from within the family's point of view is critical for making effective referrals.

The general exception to this guideline is if an infant or a child appears to require protection. In these cases, by law, one must make a CPS referral or a police report. If this happens, the need to make the referral must be explained to the family. It is usually helpful to offer condolence to the family and express sadness at this turn of events. Caregivers respond much better and social workers are more likely to continue being useful to the family if these difficult actions are handled by offering verbal and concrete support to the caregiver.

A word of caution is needed here because social workers often fall back on trying to "fix" things as soon as they think they might know what to suggest. As a result, they may move to problem solving before gathering enough information to understand the family's perceptions. This usually results in a poor match between what the social worker and the family think would be helpful. When differences in perceptions are not well recognized, it can lead to the social worker blaming the caregiver for not following his or her suggestions rather than realizing that more input was needed from the family. In addition, it can create family guilt for not following through with the recommendation (Hepworth, Rooney, & Larsen, 1997). For example, a traditional Hispanic woman, whose two teenage daughters were having a hard time getting along with their brother who had a disability, was interviewed. When the social worker said that he thought her daughters might benefit from a sibling workshop, she smiled and nodded without replying directly. The social worker assumed that the mother desired the referral. However, when her husband joined the interview a bit later, it became apparent that the family did not want their daughters away from trusted adults for a 3-hour period. Knowing this was a traditional Hispanic family should have led the social worker to anticipate that such activities might not be seen as appropriate.

PUTTING IT ALL TOGETHER

This chapter provides guidelines for social work practice with families who bring their young children to an interdisciplinary clinic that focuses on developmental assessments and community referrals. Social workers must skillfully integrate the family's hopes with their strengths, stresses, coping abilities, and resource needs. This requires mature interviewing skills and excellent analytical reasoning. Given the time constraints, social workers must focus on the family's most important issues, their emotional support (both during the interview and from their community), and their ability to be advocates for their children. This is a daunting task. To be carried out successfully, social workers and family members must honor each other as equal partners in the search for knowledge, care, and understanding. Children deserve nothing less.

REFERENCES

Davis, H. (1993). *Counselling parents of children with chronic illness or disability*. Leicester, United Kingdom: The British Psychological Society.

Davis, H., & Rushton, R. (1991). Counselling and supporting parents of children with developmental delay: A research evaluation. *Journal of Mental Deficiency Research, 35*, 89–112.

Dunst, C.J., & Trivette, C.M. (1990). Assessment of the social support in early intervention programs. In S.J. Meisels & J.P. Shonkoff (Eds.), *Handbook of early childhood intervention* (pp. 326–349). Cambridge, United Kingdom: Cambridge University Press.

Hepworth, D.H., Rooney, R.H., & Larsen, J.A. (1997). *Direct social work practice: Theory and skills*. Pacific Grove, CA: Brooks/Cole Publishing Co.

Hodapp, R.M., Dykens, E.M., & Masino, L.L. (1997). Families of children with Prader-Willi syndrome: Stress, support and relations to child characteristics. *Journal of Autism and Developmental Disorders, 27*(1), 11–24.

Hymovich, D.P., & Baker, C.D. (1985). The needs, concerns and coping of parents of children with cystic fibrosis [Special Issue: The family and health care]. *Family Relations: Journal of Applied Family & Child Studies, 34*(1), 91–97.

Kelly, G.A. (1963). *A theory of personality: The psychology of personal construct*. New York: W.W. Norton & Company.

Krauss, M.W., & Jacobs, F. (1990). Family assessment: Purposes and techniques. In S.J. Meisels & J.P. Shonkoff (Eds.), *Handbook of early childhood intervention* (pp. 303–325). Cambridge, United Kingdom: Cambridge University Press.

Lazarus, R.S., & Folkman, S. (1984). *Stress, appraisal, and coping*. New York: Springer Publishing Co.

McCubbin, H.I., McCubbin, M.A., Patterson, J.M., Cauble, A.E., Wilson, L.R., & Warwick, W. (1983). CHIP—Coping Health Inventory for Parents: An assessment of parental coping patterns in the care of the chronically ill child. *Journal of Marriage and the Family, 45*(2), 359–370.

Murata, J.E. (1994). Family stress, social support, violence, and son's behavior. *Western Journal of Nursing Research, 16*(2), 154–168.

Newby, N.M. (1996). Chronic illness and the family life-cycle. *Journal of Advanced Nursing, 23*(4), 786–791.

Nurius, P.S., & Gibson, J.W. (1990). Clinical observation, inference, reasoning, and judgement in social work: An update. *Social Work Research & Abstracts, 26*(2), 18–25.

Parkerson, G.R., Jr., Broadhead, W.E., & Tse, C.K. (1995). Perceived family stress as a predictor of health-related outcomes. *Archives of Family Medicine, 4*(3), 253–260.

Patterson, J.M., & Garwick, A.W. (1994). Levels of meaning in family stress theory. *Family Process, 33*(3), 287–304.

Pianta, R.C., & Lothman, D.J. (1994). Predicting behavioral problems in children with epilepsy: Child factors, disease factors, family stress, and child–mother interaction. *Child Development, 65*(5), 1415–1428.

Rubin, A., & Babbie, E. (1997). Qualitative research methods. In A. Rubin & E. Babbie (Eds.), *Research methods for social work* (3rd ed., pp. 371–418). Pacific Grove, CA: Brooks/Cole Publishing Co.

Shelton, T.L., Jeppson, E.S., & Johnson, B.H. (1987). *Family-centered care for children with special health care needs*. Alexandria, VA: Association for the Care of Children's Health.

Short, K.H., & Johnson, C. (1997). Stress, maternal distress, and children's adjustment following immigration: The buffering role of social support. *Journal of Consulting and Clinical Psychology, 65*(3), 494–503.

Solomon, P., & Draine, J. (1995). Adoptive coping among family members of persons with serious mental illness. *Psychiatric Services, 44*(11), 1156–1160.

Thompson, R.J., Jr., Gill, K.M., Burbach, D.J., Keith, B.R., & Kinney, T.R. (1993). Psychological adjustment of mothers of children and adolescents with sickle cell disease: The role of stress, coping methods, and family functioning. *Journal of Pediatric Psychology, 18*(5), 549–559.

Thompson, R.J., Jr., Zeman, J.L., Fanurik, D., & Sirotkin-Roses, M. (1992). The role of parent stress and coping and family functioning in parent and child adjustment to Duchenne Muscular Dystrophy. *Journal of Clinical Psychology, 48*(1), 11–19.

Section III

THE INTERDISCIPLINARY PROCESS

CASE STUDIES

Chapter 11

An Infant at
Increased Risk

*David T. Scott, Douglas S. Cook, Nuhad D. Dinno,
Richard C. Folsom, Betty L. Lucas, Marcia W. Swanson,
Susan Wendel, and Joan C. Zerzan*

Hospital-based newborn follow-up clinics have evolved since the 1970s to assist parents and pediatricians in managing the health and development of infants with various "risk factors." These risk factors include an array of medical
complications: low birth weight (LBW), birth asphyxia, difficult deliveries, and
a variety of brain insults. Special attention may also be given to infants who
are at "double risk" because of social or familial factors that may operate to
potentiate their medical problems. Undesirable fetal exposures secondary to
maternal substance use, very low maternal age, and unstable family situations
are examples of circumstances that may put an infant at double risk.

The natural history of infants having very low birth weights prior to the
1960s was relatively unfavorable. Fortunately, rapid advances in perinatal
medical technologies, together with the evolution of newborn follow-up programs, have resulted in greatly improved outcomes for many diagnostic categories of infants at increased risk.

This chapter illustrates some, though by no means all, of the medical problems and social-contextual factors that come into play in managing the care of infants at increased risk. The chapter is designed to give the reader a glimpse of how such clinics can integrate information from a spectrum of disciplines to provide a program of services that is tailored to the needs of individual children. Background information has also been included to provide brief summaries of some of the complications of prematurity and some of the measurement problems involved in follow-up, as well as brief consideration of some of the other methodological issues that are encountered in this work.

RATIONALE FOR FOLLOW-UP CLINICS

The rationale for follow-up clinics has been based largely on two assumptions: 1) that infants who require admission to an intensive care unit will be at increased risk after discharge for neurodevelopmental sequelae and 2) that it is possible to provide services after discharge that might reduce that risk. Fortunately, newborn follow-up programs have now provided empirical data with which to evaluate these two assumptions.

History and Major Findings

Newborn follow-up clinics can trace their history back to early follow-up surveys in Europe in the first decades of the 20th century (Scott, 1983). These early follow-up efforts were typically research ventures that sought to determine what happened to infants who had survived a premature delivery or who had survived some other perinatal complication. The outcomes in these early studies were often subjectively assessed, and sample bias was usually a prominent factor that limited the usefulness of the early results.

The modern era of newborn follow-up probably begins with Drillien's landmark 1964 study in Scotland. Drillien attempted to follow a sample that was population based, and she took great care to avoid loss to follow-up. Her outcomes included some standardized developmental testing. At this time— just before the introduction of the first neonatal intensive care units (NICUs)— the prognosis for LBW infants was not particularly favorable. In a subgroup of infants with birth weights of 3 pounds or less who were followed into the primary grades at school, Drillien found that about a third had been placed in special schools for children with mental retardation and another third were in general schools but functioning below grade level. Only a third of these children were at grade level at the time of the assessment.

In the 1970s, there was renewed interest in newborn follow-up (e.g., Fitzhardinge, Kalman, Ashby, & Pape, 1978; Fitzhardinge & Ramsay, 1973). Much of this interest arose from the mounting evidence that technical advances in neonatology had enabled more and more LBW infants to survive. Moreover, infants were surviving at progressively lower birth weights as new technologies were introduced.

By the late 1970s, there had been a proliferation of newborn follow-up clinics to complement the proliferation of NICUs. The data that emerged from these follow-up programs varied widely, but literature reviews tended to find that within a given birth weight range, outcomes tended to become more favorable over time. However, this trend was offset, at least in part, by progressive reductions in the birth weights at which infants were surviving (e.g., Bennett, 1994; Scott & Tyson, 1999). There was still ample evidence that LBW infants were at increased risk (compared with those having normal birth weights) for a variety of neurodevelopmental complications (Bennett & Scott, 1997). The more common complications included developmental delays, chronic lung disease, retinopathy of prematurity (ROP), cerebral palsy, recurring infections, behavior problems, and learning disabilities.

Intervention Programs

During the 1970s, there was also a proliferation of interventions that were designed to facilitate favorable outcomes for infants with various disorders and risk factors. When the literature on these early intervention treatment strategies was reviewed in the early 1980s, many methodological limitations were noted. Some reviewers (e.g., Ferry, 1981) evaluated the evidence for the efficacy of these treatments and found it to be largely unconvincing.

In this context, a large clinical trial known as the Infant Health and Development Program (IHDP; 1990) was developed. The IHDP was a multisite, randomized clinical trial of one approach to early intervention in the population of infants born prematurely and at low birth weights. Across eight sites with demographically diverse samples, 985 infants were randomly assigned either to a follow-up–only condition or a condition that included the same follow-up protocol in addition to a comprehensive intervention program.

The children in the IHDP sample were evaluated at age 3, just before the end of the intervention program. In the Lighter Stratum (birth weights of 2,000 grams [g] or less), there were medium-size treatment effects in the cognitive domain (6.6 IQ points). For infants in the Heavier Stratum (birth weights between 2,001 and 2,500 g), the effects were considerably larger (13.2 IQ points).

Children who had participated in the randomized clinical trial were also invited to participate in two follow-up evaluations, one at age 5 (Brooks-Gunn et al., 1994) and another at age 8 (McCarton et al., 1997). Briefly, 2 years and 5 years after the end of the intervention program, there were some modest residual treatment effects in the Heavier Stratum but not in the Lighter Stratum. This finding appeared to suggest that this approach to early intervention—in the absence of ongoing services after age 3—may not be *sufficient* to produce benefits of the desired magnitude in later childhood. There are insufficient data to determine whether such services during the first 3 years might still be *necessary*.

In any case, the medium- to large-size treatment effects documented at age 3 (just as the intervention was ending) made it clear that such programs can alter outcomes for the better. This fact suggests that newborn follow-up clinics can play an important role in identifying children who should be referred for special services.

PRACTICAL CONSIDERATIONS

The high-risk infant follow-up (HRIF) clinic described next was originally developed to provide longitudinal neurodevelopmental surveillance of infants discharged from NICUs. Many NICU graduates have medical conditions that place them at risk for developmental delays, neuromotor conditions, sensory conditions, and other long-term complications. Some of the neonatal conditions that prompt a referral to the HRIF clinic include very low birth weight (e.g., birth weight of 1,500 g or less); birth asphyxia; genetic conditions; meningitis or other infections that may affect the central nervous system (CNS); CNS malformations; certain CNS vascular conditions (e.g., strokes, CNS hemorrhages); and significant fetal exposures (e.g., alcohol, other drugs) secondary to antenatal maternal substance use.

The structure of the HRIF clinic is somewhat different from the structure of interdisciplinary teams that take referrals from the community in general. Nearly all HRIF cases are followed longitudinally via a protocol of visits at specific ages. Because, by design, each child is seen on multiple occasions, most HRIF clinic visits are somewhat streamlined in relation to the comprehensive assessments conducted by the more conventional interdisciplinary diagnostic team. This streamlining takes various forms. First, in lieu of a preliminary conference, the preclinic planning is managed by the clinic coordinator, working in collaboration with the head of the nursing discipline; there are also informal contacts, as needed, with clinical staff in the other disciplines. Second, the clinical staff in the HRIF clinic tend to see more cases during each HRIF clinic day than they would see as part of a conventional interdisciplinary diagnostic team. Third, there are two case conferences during each HRIF day. At each conference, a series of cases is discussed, with 5–10 minutes available for a typical case. Fourth, parent conferences are scheduled in the HRIF clinic only on an elective basis. For children who are being followed just because they are at risk but seem to be doing well, there is often no need for a formal parent conference. Instead, each discipline gives immediate feedback both orally and via a brief-feedback form. (A more detailed packet of written reports follows later by mail.) When there are new findings or new diagnoses to report, however, parent conferences are scheduled. These conferences are usually staffed by the developmental pediatricians and, when scheduling permits, by staff from other disciplines. At the parent conferences, the parents' comments are invited; the results are given and interpreted; further comments and questions are sought; and, when indicated, further referrals are made.

The clinic coordinator meets briefly with parents just before their departure. At this exit meeting, the parents complete release-of-information forms and clinic evaluation forms, and the clinic coordinator has a chance to identify any other concerns or problems that need to be addressed. At this meeting, the clinic coordinator gives the parents one copy of the brief feedback form and retains a copy for the child's satellite file. As the brief feedback form includes the names, disciplines, telephone numbers, and comments of each staff member who saw the child, it is relatively easy for the parents to contact clinic staff subsequently if the parents have additional questions or experience some difficulty with a referral.

The detailed written reports are prepared by each discipline and mailed in a packet. Copies are sent to each individual listed on the release-of-information form. This typically includes the parents, the child's primary care provider, and any other health and education personnel involved in the child's care. Copies of these reports are also added to the child's hospital chart and satellite file.

FAMILY BACKGROUND OF AN INFANT AT INCREASED RISK

Pete was born to Susan, a 17-year-old unmarried high school student with a history of substance use. At the time of Pete's birth, Susan lived with her parents in an affluent Seattle suburb. The baby's grandparents both worked full time in a small high-technology company that they had co-founded (with two other partners) when Susan was in elementary school. Susan was an only child who attended the local public schools where she was a "B" student until midway through the ninth grade, when she began to get more and more "C"s. Early in ninth grade, she had begun to see Alex, a tenth-grade student who would later father Pete.

Alex's parents were divorced when Alex was 4 years old, and he had lived since that time with his mother, who worked as a receptionist in a busy group-practice dental office. Alex's mother had been in a 12-step program for alcoholism, but she had seldom been able to go more than a few months without relapsing.

Alex had begun to experiment with alcohol while in junior high school, and before long he began to use marijuana occasionally as well. By the time he was in high school, he had also tried several other drugs, including cocaine, and he introduced Susan to several of them. He did not feel that he was dependent on any drug that he had tried. About a year after she began to see Alex, however, Susan found that she was having a harder time managing her drug use. She discovered that she was pregnant during her junior year, shortly after she had turned 17. As soon as she found out about the pregnancy, she tried to stop using drugs and alcohol, but she found that she then became increasingly depressed. When this happened, she sometimes resorted to using either alcohol or cocaine again in an effort to make herself feel better.

Susan's relapses were exacerbated by Alex's behavior during her first trimester. Initially, he seemed pleased when she told him she was pregnant; after a few weeks, however, she began to notice that he didn't drop by her house and didn't telephone her as often as he had in the past. Susan began to worry that he was drifting away, and this left her feeling alternately anxious about the future or more depressed. Susan finally confided in a teacher at school, and the teacher worked with the school nurse to get help for Susan. Susan's parents initially reacted with denial regarding both Susan's drug use and her pregnancy, but they quickly realized that they must move quickly to implement the school nurse's recommendation that Susan be enrolled in an outpatient drug treatment program at a suburban hospital. Susan was in her second trimester when she began the program.

LABOR AND DELIVERY

Susan experienced a premature rupture of the amniotic membranes during the 29th week of her pregnancy. She was transferred to the university hospital and received intravenous antibiotics in order to prevent chorioamnionitis. A urine screen at the time of admission revealed no evidence of recent substance use. The obstetrical plan was to administer steroids and to leave Susan undelivered, as long as there was no fever or other sign of infection, in order to stimulate maturation of the fetal lungs and, thus, reduce the likelihood of respiratory distress syndrome (RDS). Yet labor began spontaneously about 26 hours after rupture of the membranes, and the infant was delivered vaginally via cephalic presentation (i.e., head first). At the time of birth, an area of old placental infarction was noted. Pete weighed 780 g, which was less than the 10th percentile for his gestational age. For this reason, he was classified as small for gestational age (SGA), probably because of mild placental insufficiency secondary to the area of placental infarction.

Some Common Complications of Prematurity

Being born prematurely meant that Pete was at risk for certain medical conditions. Various complications that can be linked to prematurity are now reviewed briefly.

Intraventricular Hemorrhage

Intraventricular hemorrhage (IVH) is bleeding into the fragile germinal-matrix tissues of the brain, with possible rupture of blood into the ventricles (i.e., brain chambers that ordinarily contain only cerebrospinal fluid). IVH is thought to be caused by unusual alterations in cerebral blood flow, possibly due to the premature infant's immature autoregulatory mechanisms. The risk for IVH may be increased if the fragile capillary structures of the germinal matrix have already been compromised by too little oxygen or by abnormal levels of blood flow (Ment, 1994).

Necrotizing Enterocolitis

Necrotizing enterocolitis (NEC) is an intestinal condition, the etiology of which is poorly understood. The symptoms include abdominal distention, blood (or its breakdown products) in the stool, vomiting, diarrhea, and retention of feedings in the stomach. Treatment involves antibiotics; intravenous feedings in lieu of oral feedings; suctioning of stomach contents when there is retention; and, in some cases, surgery to remove damaged sections of the intestine (Motil, 1994).

Respiratory Distress Syndrome

Infant RDS, also known as Hyaline Membrane Disease, results from the immaturity of the lungs of the infant born prematurely (Gross, 1994). The lungs of these infants can be relatively stiff, and the membranes across which gas exchange occurs are underdeveloped. Consequently, infants born prematurely sometimes require exogenous ventilatory support with methods such as supplemental oxygen, continuous positive airway pressure (CPAP), or some form of mechanical ventilation. The growing use of artificial-surfactant therapy in the 1990s has significantly improved the management of this condition.

Bronchopulmonary dysplasia (BPD), also known as chronic lung disease, is often diagnosed when an infant born prematurely fails to recover in a timely manner from RDS. A variety of causal factors have been implicated, including the possible toxic side effects of supplemental oxygen on immature lung tissue and increased air pressures entailed by artificial ventilation methods (Kennedy & Warshaw, 1994). Possible treatments are continued use of supplemental oxygen, if required; diuretic therapy; and bronchodilators.

Patent Ductus Arteriosus

During typical fetal development, more than half of the blood that would otherwise pass through the lungs is shunted from the pulmonary artery across to the descending aorta (Kopf & Dewar, 1994). At the time of birth, the lungs begin to function as the infant's primary organ of gas exchange, and, shortly thereafter, the ductus arteriosus begins to close. In some infants who are premature, however, this ductus remains open (patent ductus arteriosus [PDA]), and blood continues to be shunted past the lungs. This can result in congestive heart failure and other complications. Administration of indomethacin can sometimes close the ductus; when this fails, surgery to close the ductus is often required.

Hyperbilirubinemia

Among infants born prematurely, hyperbilirubinemia is a common condition in which there is an excessive level of bilirubin in the infant's blood serum (Cashore, 1994). When bilirubin pigment is deposited in skin, jaundice can result. Bilirubin is produced when red blood cells are broken down. During fetal development excess bilirubin is cleared from fetal circulation via the placenta. After birth, the infant's liver takes over most of this process. Bilirubin levels can become excessive if too much bilirubin is being produced, as in a hemolytic process, or if there is insufficient supply of the enzyme required for metabolizing bilirubin into forms that can be excreted. Unfortunately, high levels of circulating bilirubin can be toxic. When hyperbilirubinemia results in the deposition of bilirubin in brain cells, the result can be kernicterus, which may result in athetoid cerebral palsy; seizure disorders; hearing loss; and, in some cases, cognitive delays.

THE NEONATAL INTENSIVE CARE UNIT COURSE

Pete's Apgar scores were 6 and 8 at 1 and 5 minutes, respectively. He was suctioned in the delivery room and ventilated temporarily via a mask. On arrival in the NICU, he was initially ventilated with CPAP with an oxygen level of 35%. It became clear, however, that he was spending too much energy to fill his stiff, immature lungs with air; also, his blood gases were variable. For these reasons, he was intubated, placed on mechanical ventilation, and given a dose of surfactant. He remained on the ventilator for 6 days, with a peak fixed-inspiratory oxygen concentration of 45%.

On the second day of life, a cranial ultrasound examination was performed. No evidence was found for germinal-matrix hemorrhage (GMH) or for IVH. Pete was also started on parenteral nutrition to provide protein, fat, vitamins, and minerals and to support growth while he was slowly started on oral feedings. He worked up to oral feeding with a premature formula during the first 2 weeks, and he initially tolerated this.

During the second week, Pete's respiratory status improved, and he was taken off the respirator and returned to CPAP. He experienced some mild-to-moderate episodes of apnea and bradycardia, but these were managed successfully with caffeine. Yet by the end of the second week, there was increasing evidence that Pete was not tolerating his feedings. The formula was not being digested, and he had increased residuals (i.e., feedings retained in the stomach). He was started on antibiotics; when abdominal distention and tenderness were noted, his feedings were held back, and abdominal X-rays were obtained. The X-rays showed evidence of NEC, and a gastrointestinal (GI) specialist was consulted. When Pete's GI status did not improve after administration of antibiotics, a surgical resection of his distal ileum was performed. He required continued parenteral support over the next 2 weeks while enteral feedings were restarted and slowly advanced. He gradually tolerated continuous-drip feedings of a premature formula via nasogastric tube, and his rate of weight gain began to improve as well. Prior to discharge, Pete had another surgery to complete the repair of his GI tract.

NEONATAL AUDIOLOGY

Toward the end of the neonatal hospitalization, Pete was seen by the audiologist for hearing screening. Using the auditory brainstem response (ABR), the audiologist found clear responses to click stimuli at 30 decibels of hearing level (dB nHL) in each ear. This constituted a pass in the NICU's hearing-screening protocol; thus, there were no concerns regarding Pete's hearing at the time of NICU discharge. Responses were also obtained at 50 and 70 dB nHL, and the latency/intensity functions for each ear showed a normal slope. In addition, the interwave latencies (waves I–III, III–V, and I–V) of the ABR waveform were determined and also were shown to be within the normal range. This meant that the audiologist had no concerns regarding the neural transmission of auditory information to the level of the brainstem.

Neonatal Hearing Screening

Hearing is screened in infants from the NICU because this population is at risk for hearing loss. Infants graduating from the NICU are 20–30 times as likely to have significant, long-standing hearing loss as are infants from the general newborn nursery. For example, among infants from the NICU, 2–4 out of every 100 will have significant hearing loss, whereas 1–2 infants in 1,000 from the general newborn nursery will have a significant hearing loss. The use of a physiological procedure, such as the ABR, is necessary during early infancy because behavior responses to sound at this age are unreliable.

Three recording electrodes were attached to Pete's scalp: at the vertex (top of the head) and on each mastoid (behind the ears). Short, abrupt-onset clicks were presented through an insert earphone placed in Pete's ear canal. Samples from an electroencephalogram (EEG) were averaged in a computer until the background noise was reduced sufficiently to reveal the ABR. The ABR waveform is dominated by a positive-going peak labeled "wave V." Presence of wave V at low intensity levels is consistent with normal functioning of the cochlea and lower brainstem.

DISCHARGE PLANNING

At about 35 weeks' postconceptional age, NICU personnel had begun planning for Pete's NICU discharge. As part of this process, Pete was seen by the retina specialist from the ophthalmology department. No evidence of ROP was found. The cranial ultrasound was repeated. Again, no evidence for intracranial hemorrhage was found. However, there was some suggestion that the right cerebral ventricle was slightly larger than the left. In the nutritional domain, Pete was beginning to take more and more of his feedings via a bottle. Nonetheless, he continued to require small-volume, frequent feedings due to his GI surgery and immature feeding skills. Another aspect of the discharge planning involved a referral to the HRIF clinic. This referral was made by the physical therapist who had treated and followed Pete during his 8-week NICU course. The therapist had met Susan on a number of occasions when Susan was in the NICU to visit and to feed the baby. The first follow-up visit was scheduled for 4 months corrected age.

Choice of an Age Scale[1]

Early follow-up studies often calculated the age of infants from the date of their premature birth (Scott, 1983). Thus, children born prematurely were com-

---

[1]The material in this section is adapted from Scott, D.T., & Tyson, J. (1999). Follow-up of infants discharged from newborn intensive care. In J.A. McMillan, C.D. DeAngelis, R.D. Feigin, & J.B. Warshaw (Eds.), *Oski's pediatrics: Principles and practice* (3rd ed., pp. 212–213). Philadelphia: Lippincott, Williams & Wilkins © Lippincott, Williams & Wilkins; adapted by permission.

pared with those born at term who were the same postnatal age but a more advanced postconceptional age. Not surprisingly, the children who had been delivered at full term were almost always taller, heavier, and more advanced developmentally. It was unclear whether the delays among the children born prematurely were genuine sequelae of prematurity and its complications or only the consequences of their younger postconceptional ages. Subsequently, many studies have attempted to put premature children on the same biological footing as full-term controls by calculating age from the child's due date. The age calculated from the due date has been called the *postterm age* or, more commonly, the *corrected age*.

Although the use of the postterm age for premature children has gained ever-wider acceptance, the age range over which it should be used is still subject to some controversy. In some early studies in which the degree of prematurity was modest and the samples were small, the use of the postterm age did not seem to make a significant difference after a year or two, and the investigators thus changed from the corrected-age scale to the chronological age scale after that point. As more survivors were studied with greater and greater degrees of prematurity, however, the effects of using the corrected versus the chronological age could be seen at progressively later ages, at least into the primary grades at school. For this reason, some investigators now use the postterm age indefinitely. For children in whom it makes a difference, many clinicians also usually recommend that parents consider starting their children in kindergarten according to the age they would be had they been born at term.

One simple rationale for this practice is as follows: If it makes sense to use the child's postterm age (rather than the postnatal age) early on, why would it cease to make sense later? The use of the postterm age merely allows one to evaluate a child born prematurely with norms for children the same biological (postconceptional) age.

DISCHARGE DISPOSITION

Pete was discharged a little more than 8 weeks after his premature birth, at a postconceptional age of 37 weeks. He was discharged into his mother's care. However, given his mother's age and history of substance use, the case had been placed under the supervision of the state's Child Protective Services (CPS) agency. CPS had agreed to having Pete discharged into his mother's care largely because Susan planned to continue to live with her parents, and Susan's mother had taken a 6-week leave of absence from her job in order to spend some time with Susan and the baby. As an extra precaution, CPS made a referral for a public health nurse to make regular home visits to Pete and his mother.

By the time of discharge, Susan had demonstrated the ability to feed Pete, but he continued to feed with varying success; he needed frequent feedings and time to pace himself during feedings. Pete was sent home on a higher-energy formula to encourage growth, and his mother was instructed on how to prepare the formula. Pete was also referred to a GI clinic for follow-up, including nutrient supplementation.

INTERIM HISTORY BETWEEN
NICU DISCHARGE AND FIRST FOLLOW-UP

Pete did well during the first few days after discharge from the NICU. However, his mother began to notice that he was spitting up more and more of his formula. Also, at times he seemed hungry and took formula vigorously at first only to become irritable again midway through a feeding. When Susan took Pete in to her pediatrician's office, it was determined that Pete was not gaining weight as rapidly as expected. The pediatrician referred Pete to a pediatric gastroenterologist who ordered X-ray studies. Gastroesophageal (GE) reflux was diagnosed. This was treated with ranitidine, which reduces the secretion of stomach acid, and Pete's formula was thickened with cereal.

Prior to Pete's first HRIF visit, both the clinic coordinator and the physical therapist who had worked with him in the NICU talked with Susan by telephone. Based on these discussions, it was decided that Pete and his mother would be seen by four disciplines at the first visit: nutrition, occupational or physical therapy, social work, and pediatrics.

FOLLOW-UP VISIT AT 4 MONTHS CORRECTED AGE

The first HRIF visit was scheduled at 4 months and 2 days corrected age. Pete was brought to the clinic by his mother. Susan stated that she felt his development was "okay." Because Pete was nearly 7 months chronological age at this point, however, she wondered when he would start crawling. Susan's primary concern was Pete's feeding behavior: She reported that he continued to feed every 2–3 hours and was not yet sleeping through the night. She also expressed frustration with his fussiness and prolonged crying.

Nutrition

Pete was being fed 20-kilocalorie-per-ounce, iron-fortified formula thickened with cereal. Sometimes he took only about 16 ounces a day, but he usually drank more than that. His mother had to enlarge the nipple hole so that he was able to get the thickened formula through the nipple. The number of times Pete spat up during the day had decreased, but he continued to be fussy and "hard to feed." Feedings were taking about 30 minutes to an hour, depending on how long Susan persisted in trying to feed Pete.

Pete's intake of food worried Susan and her mother, as his length was at the 10th percentile and his weight was below the 5th percentile for his corrected age. Weight for height was at the 5th percentile. Susan's mother had been helping to take care of Pete when Susan attended school. About a month before the 4-month visit, the grandmother had begun to feed Pete solids while holding him on her lap. Susan's mother felt that this would help Pete gain weight; she also felt that, because he was older than 6 months chronologically, it was time for him to begin with solid foods. Pete often gagged on the solids, and it took at least 20 minutes to feed him. Susan had been told by her primary care pediatrician and by the nutritionist with the Women, Infants, and Children (WIC) program to wait on starting solids, but Susan's mother did not agree. Therefore, this had been an area of conflict between Susan and her mother.

During the 4-month visit, it was recommended that Pete's formula be concentrated to 24 kilocalories per ounce. Suggestions were made regarding a trial of feedings that were not thickened. Susan was told that Pete's feeding frequency was not atypical. Pete's feeding cues were reviewed with her, including his signals that he was done feeding. It was suggested that solids be limited at this time and that the occupational therapist provide additional guidance on supported positioning and the facilitation of spoon feeding.

Occupational/Physical Therapy

Pete was evaluated with the Bayley Scales of Infant Development–Second Edition (BSID-II; Bayley, 1993), and with the Movement Assessment of Infants (MAI; Chandler, Andrews, & Swanson, 1980). On the Mental Scale of the BSID-II, Pete demonstrated poor visual following of the test objects. He attended to objects and appeared to focus on them when they were stationary, but his tracking of slowly moving objects was inconsistent. He made some efforts to reach for objects. Nevertheless, these efforts mainly involved the proximal musculature of the upper extremities and were not, ordinarily, sufficiently well coordinated to result in his being able to grasp the object. He was sociable, he smiled at the examiner, and he vocalized vowel sounds. He responded to sounds with behavior changes (usually stilling), but he did not yet turn his head toward the source of the sounds.

Pete's Assessment Results

Pete's scores on the BSID-II were 89 for the Mental Scale and 86 for the Motor Scale. Because the BSID-II's Mental Development Index (MDI) and Psychomotor Development Index (PDI) were standardized to have a mean of 100 and an SD of 15, both of Pete's Bayley indexes would be considered to be within normal limits according to the Bayley Manual. Nonetheless, many clinicians might consider such scores to be in the low-normal range and, thus, an additional indication for continued follow-up. The Mental Index of 89 would be 23rd percentile, and the Motor Index of 86 would be 18th percentile.

On the MAI, Pete exhibited moderately increased muscle tone in the extremities with resistance to passive movement in the heel cords and shoulders. His spontaneous movements appeared stiff, especially in a prone position. In this position, he had difficulty pushing up on his arms and lifting his head. Primitive reflexes included the tonic labyrinthine reflex in a supine position with shoulder retraction and the neonatal positive-support reflex. Pete's head-righting reactions were immature, but he had good head control when pulled to sitting. His movements showed mild asymmetry with preferred use of and orientation toward his right side. This was somewhat worrisome, as Pete's last neonatal cranial ultrasound scan had suggested possible enlargement of the right cerebral ventricle, which might be associated with left-sided weakness or neglect.

In discussing Pete's inconsistent visual responses, Susan reported that she had forgotten to take Pete in for a follow-up examination by the pediatric ophthalmologist. Pete had been referred to the ophthalmologist because his primary care pediatrician had noticed what appeared to be an intermittent alternating esotropia (i.e., either the left eye or the right eye deviated toward the mid-line while the other eye was fixated straight ahead on a target), and the doctor was concerned about the development of a "lazy eye" if this was left untreated. Susan was advised to reschedule this appointment as soon as she could. She was also shown how to position Pete with his shoulders forward in order to diminish the tendency toward shoulder retraction. She was advised to encourage Pete to play in a prone position, using a towel roll to facilitate support on his forearms. A floor gym was recommended to develop reaching skills. Pete was scheduled to return in 4 months, at 8 months corrected age, for follow-up assessment.

Social Work

At this first social work interview in the follow-up clinic, Susan identified three major stresses in her daily life. She was worried that Pete wasn't taking enough food to grow well, was depressed because Alex was not helping with child care and only dropped by for a few minutes a week to see Pete (often at times when she was not at home), and felt angry that her mother seemed to take over Pete's care. At this visit, Susan had seen the nutritionist before meeting with the social worker, and she volunteered that she felt better having talked with the nutritionist but was worried that her mother would still insist on giving Pete solid foods. Susan thought it would be helpful for the nutritionist to call Pete's grandmother, and this was arranged after the social work interview.

After Susan was asked more questions about her depression, she identified sadness at Alex's "not really being there" for her or Pete; she also expressed irritation at her mother for not letting her be more "in charge" of Pete. Another source of depression involved her enrollment in an alternative school to complete her high school education. Her prior school friends were not there, and after a month she still felt isolated from the students at the alternative school. She voiced a strong desire to finish high school and said that she was going to do it, but she resented not being able to be with her friends. Further conversation revealed that it usually took Susan longer than a month to make friends and that there were already two or three girls with whom she had begun to interact with some frequency. It was suggested that she was making good progress at making new friends at a rate that felt comfortable for her, and Susan agreed. It was further suggested that she probably could anticipate feeling more connected to friends at school within another month or two.

Susan did not think that Alex would ever become really involved with Pete or in a "real relationship" with her. But she still was not ready to give up her hope that it would all work out somehow. Her fantasies had been that Alex would get a good job and that they would get an apartment of their own with Pete. When asked about this, Susan initially gave this about a 10% chance of happening. After a few seconds of silence, she then said, "Well, maybe 1%." Later in the interview, when asked about her drug treatment program, she said that it was "okay." Susan did not volunteer any other information; when asked if her drug problems had also been a part of her depression, she said that she did not want to talk about it. She did volunteer that she was not currently using alcohol or other drugs. When asked, Susan said that she was eating and sleeping well. She also appeared to be very focused on Pete and quite delighted when she held the child and interacted with him. Susan said that she was not usually depressed when she was taking care of him except for sometimes worrying whether he was eating enough.

Because Pete had been born prematurely and was at risk for developmental delays, Susan was eligible to use a family resource coordinator (FRC), funded by the health department, up to the time Pete turned 3 years old. It was suggested that an FRC might be helpful to Susan as a source of information about Pete's growth and development as well as other resources. It was explained that FRCs kept up on current resources in their community for babies and young children, usually worked over the telephone but could make home visits if needed, and were part of a free service. Susan was interested in this resource and was referred to an FRC in her health department district.

Pediatrics

Pete's hospital chart and shadow file were reviewed by the postdoctoral fellow in developmental pediatrics and discussed with the attending pediatrician. Prior to seeing Pete, the fellow also spoke briefly with the therapist who had seen Pete earlier in the visit; the concern about the mild asymmetry was communicated during this contact.

The fellow and the attending pediatrician introduced themselves to Pete's mother. They elicited a brief history at this time to confirm and clarify several points in Pete's medical chart. They also asked Susan about the concerns that she had brought with her to the clinic that day, and they inquired about the extent to which these concerns had already been addressed. The pediatricians concurred with the prior recommendations that Susan and her mother hold off on giving Pete solid foods for the time being.

The pediatricians then undertook Pete's physical examination and neurodevelopmental evaluation. They found that Pete's pupils were symmetrical, round, and reacted to light by constricting normally. Pete's eye movements were conjugate (coordinated) at times, but at other times the pediatricians noted an intermittent alternating esotropia. Moving on to an examination of the mouth, they found that the palate was somewhat high and slightly arched.

Examination of the ears with an otoscope revealed normal tympanic membranes. Auscultation of the chest revealed normal breath sounds bilaterally. The rest of Pete's physical examination was unremarkable.

The pediatricians' neurological examination revealed subtle asymmetries. Deep-tendon reflexes were a bit brisker on the left side at the knees and ankles. However, the asymmetry was felt to be too subtle to warrant the diagnosis of a hemisyndrome at this visit. The pediatricians reviewed with Susan the recommendations that had been made earlier in the day by the physical therapist.

Exit Process

At the end of the clinic visit, Susan met briefly with the clinic coordinator. Susan was asked to look over the feedback and evaluation form, and she was also encouraged to complete the form at her convenience, returning it either anonymously or with her name written in, according to her preference. The release-of-information form was also completed so that the reports could be sent to Susan and to Pete's primary care pediatrician.

Test Instruments Often Used in Follow-Up Clinics

It is important that those conducting evaluations choose the most appropriate tool for the child being tested. The professionals assessing Pete determined that the BSID-II and the MAI were useful tools for his evaluation. The next section provides additional background information about some of the assessment instruments commonly used in HRIF clinics.

Bayley Scales of Infant Development

Most newborn follow-up programs at medical centers or clinics have used the BSID (Bayley, 1969) and the BSID-II (Bayley, 1993). These tests are the products of decades of refinement and restandardization. Both editions of the Bayley Scales were standardized on large national samples constructed to be representative of the U.S. population. The 1969 test covered a nominal age range from 2 to 30 months; the 1993 version extended the age range up to 42 months.

Both editions of the Bayley Scales generate age equivalents and developmental indexes, both in the cognitive domain and in the motor domain. The age equivalents are the age for which a given level of performance would be typical. The Mental and Motor Indexes are standardized scores that are distributed in the same manner as IQ scores, with a population mean of 100 and standard deviations (SDs) of either 16 (1969 edition) or 15 (1993 edition). These indexes permit comparison of an infant with other infants the same age. When evaluating infants who were born preterm, most developmental clinicians use the infant's postterm or corrected age so that comparison will be with other infants the same biological or postconceptional age (see the preceding Choice of an Age Scale section in this chapter).

Interpreting the Bayley index requires caution. Pair-wise differences smaller than 7 or 8 points may well arise from measurement error. In a sample of children at increased risk, the correlation between the Bayley Mental Index and subsequent IQ scores (during the preschool years) is often about 0.5, so that only about a quarter of the variance in preschool IQ scores is associated with variance in the Bayley Mental Index.

During the 1990s, experience with the 1993 edition of the Bayley Scales raised questions about its suitability for use with children with atypical development (Washington, Scott, Johnson, Wendel, & Hay, 1998). The item-set format of the BSID-II can prove problematic in children with uneven development or with substantial developmental delays—both of which are encountered with increased frequency in newborn follow-up programs. For such children, at least, the 1969 Bayley is sometimes the more prudent choice.

Movement Assessment of Infants

The MAI evaluates motor development during a child's first year. It includes assessments of tone and reflexes, automatic reactions, and volitional movements. It can be helpful in identifying children who should be referred for physical or occupational therapy, and therapists often use the MAI to monitor the progress of children who are already in therapy. MAI results are not used to make long-range predictions about a child's motor development but, rather, to permit a more standardized evaluation of an infant's motor development in relation to the population of other infants the same age.

Stanford-Binet Intelligence Scale

The fourth edition of the Stanford-Binet Intelligence Scale (Stanford-Binet-IV; Thorndike, Hagen, & Sattler, 1986) is a revision and restandardization of the third edition of the Stanford-Binet Intelligence Scale, Form L-M (Terman & Merrill, 1973). Like its predecessor, the fourth edition nominally covers the age range from 2 years through adulthood. Unlike Form L-M, the fourth edition groups items into subtests, 15 in all. (This can be a disadvantage for preschool children with short attention spans.) These 15 subtests are used in an effort to assess cognitive ability in 4 areas: Verbal Reasoning, Abstract/Visual Reasoning, Quantitative Reasoning, and Short-Term Memory. Like the previous Form L-M of the Stanford-Binet, the Test Composite (proxy nomenclature for IQ score) has been standardized to have a mean of 100 and an SD of 16.

The Stanford-Binet-IV is often used in newborn follow-up clinics for younger preschool children. However, there are certain caveats to bear in mind when this instrument is used with that population. First, the fourth edition's efforts to assess developed ability in four diverse cognitive domains may well be a strength of this test when one is testing older children. Nonetheless, there is some evidence to suggest that early development is too undifferentiated to permit reliable assessments of different cognitive areas in children younger than about $3^{1}/_{2}$ years of age. Thus, such area scores should be interpreted with special caution, if at all, in young preschool children. In some cases, these area scores may prove to be only unreliable estimates of a unitary factor (e.g., IQ).

Second, there are some special basal constraints on the fourth edition of the Stanford-Binet. On tests such as the Wechsler scales (Wechsler, 1989,

1991, 1992), subtest raw scores of 0 are assigned very low scaled scores; usu-ally the scaled score is 1 when the raw score is 0. The fourth edition of the Stanford-Binet, however, has a different approach: When raw scores of 0 are obtained, any subtests on which 0 scores were obtained are dropped. The se-lective dropping of the subtests on which a child has the weakest performance sometimes has the paradoxical effect of increasing the child's test composite score (compared with the overall score that would have resulted had the child obtained a raw score of 1 [Delaney & Hopkins, 1987]). Great caution is rec-ommended under these circumstances (Scott, 1997). Prudence may suggest use of a different test instrument in nearly all 2-year-olds and in many 3-year-olds as well.

Differential Ability Scales

This assessment is a revision and restandardization of the earlier British Abil-ity Scales. The Differential Ability Scales (DAS; Elliott, 1990) include both a cognitive-ability battery and a school-achievement battery for school-aged children. The cognitive-ability battery comprises 17 subtests. Of these, six sub-tests were designed to be used with children ages 2 to 3 years old: The four core subtests are Block Building, Verbal Comprehension, Picture Similarities, and Naming Vocabulary; two additional diagnostic subtests are Recall of Digits and Recognition of Pictures. Because factor-analytic scrutiny suggested a lack of cognitive differentiation below $3^{1}/_{2}$ years of age, for children between 2 and $3^{1}/_{2}$ years old, the DAS generates only a single composite score, the General Conceptual Ability (GCA) score. For children between $3^{1}/_{2}$ and 6 years of age, six subtests are administered and two domain scores (Verbal Ability and Non-verbal Ability) are produced in addition to the GCA score. For school-age chil-dren, this instrument produces a GCA score and domain scores for Verbal Ability, Nonverbal Reasoning Ability, and Spatial Ability.

One approach is to use the DAS for 3-year-olds and for some 4-year-olds with developmental delays or limited tolerances for structured activities. The DAS's subtest format can be something of a disadvantage for young children with short attention spans, but the materials tend to be quite appealing for preschool children, which helps to maintain task commitment.

Wechsler Preschool and Primary Scale of Intelligence–Revised

The Wechsler Preschool and Primary Scale of Intelligence–Revised (WPPSI-R; Wechsler, 1989) is generally employed for children 4, 5, and 6 years of age. Structured much like its predecessors in the Wechsler family of tests, the WPPSI-R generates a Verbal IQ score, a Performance IQ score, and a Full-Scale IQ score; all three of these IQ scores have been standardized to have a mean of 100 and an SD of 15 in the general population. The Performance IQ score is based on five standard subtests (Object Assembly, Geometric Design, Block Design, Mazes, and Picture Completion) with one optional or replace-ment subtest (Animal Pegs). The Verbal IQ score is also based on five standard subtests (Information, Comprehension, Arithmetic, Vocabulary, and Similarities) with one optional or replacement subtest (Sentences). Interpretive software is available to assist with the analysis of subtest profiles.

The ability to generate Verbal and Performance IQ scores can be useful in follow-up clinics that provide services for children with sensory or motor findings. For example, it is often possible to get a reasonably accurate assessment of Verbal IQ in a child with visual findings secondary to retinopathy of prematurity. Children with hearing impairments, together with children for whom there may be language barriers, can sometimes still be assessed—though with great caution—with the performance subtests. Specialized tests, such as the Leiter International Performance Scale (Leiter, 1979) and the Leiter International Performance Scale–Revised (Roid & Miller, 1997), can also be employed for children with hearing impairments or children for whom language barriers might otherwise yield underestimates of cognitive ability (Scott et al., 1997). Although it has many advantages, a disadvantage of the WPPSI-R is its administration time. Children with short attention spans may find the WPPSI-R rather long and somewhat tiresome.

Wechsler Intelligence Scale for Children—Third Edition

The Wechsler Intelligence Scale for Children–Third Edition (WISC-III; Wechsler, 1991) is probably the premier cognitive-ability test instrument designed for use with school-age children. This test is often used during the last visits in follow-up protocols, primarily in children who are 7 years of age or older. Like the WPPSI-R, the WISC-III also generates a Verbal IQ score, a Performance IQ score, and a Full-Scale IQ score. The interpretation of WISC-III profiles is based on decades of experience with the WISC-III, the prior WISC-R, and the original WISC. Interpretive software also exists to aid in profile analysis for this test.

Once children are at least halfway through first grade, an achievement test is often added to the follow-up assessment. Recommended tests are either the Wechsler Individual Achievement Test (WIAT; Wechsler, 1992), or the Tests of Achievement from the Woodcock-Johnson PsychoEducational Battery–Revised (WJ-R; Woodcock & Johnson, 1990). The WIAT has the advantage that its standardization was linked to that of the WISC-III, thus facilitating the comparison of WISC-III scores with achievement scores. Nevertheless, there has probably been more experience with the Woodcock-Johnson tests in research on learning differences.

INTERIM HISTORY BETWEEN 4-MONTH AND 8-MONTH VISITS

Pete and his mother did not keep their initial appointment for the follow-up visit at 8 months corrected age. When Pete's grandmother was contacted at work, she reported that Susan had moved in with a girlfriend who was living in an apartment in a different suburb. The grandmother did not know whether

Susan was still enrolled in the drug treatment program. Pete's grandmother stated that Susan had never given her the telephone number of the friend with whom Susan was now living. Susan and the baby were subsequently located via CPS, and CPS became more actively involved when they discovered that Susan had dropped out of her drug treatment program and had moved out of her parents' house. After the CPS intervention, Susan reentered the drug treatment program. A second HRIF clinic appointment was then given to Susan by CPS; Susan explained that she had never received the reminder for the initial appointment because it had been sent to her parents' house.

FOLLOW-UP VISIT AT 8 MONTHS CORRECTED AGE
Susan and Pete kept the new appointment. Susan stated that Pete was doing well and that she no longer had any particular concerns regarding feeding. She did ask if Pete should have started crawling by that time.

Nutrition
Pete's weight for height was now at the 10th percentile, and Susan reported that he now rarely had reflux. She also reported that she had started giving him some bottles of whole milk over the past 2 weeks because she had run out of formula. (After she moved out of her parents' house, Susan had found it harder to pick up her WIC vouchers due to difficulties with transportation.) She had been offering Pete some solid foods, but he mostly played with them and continued to gag and choke occasionally with mixed textures. Susan had been offering fruit and cereal from a jar and trying to get him to take "second foods." Occasionally, she gave him crackers, but Pete often crumbled them instead of eating them.

Although Pete's growth had improved, it was noted that some of the recent foods were lower in energy content. Continuing formula until 12 months corrected age was recommended. Developmental feeding progression was discussed with Susan, and suggestions were made for more energy-dense solid foods. Appropriate and safe finger foods were discussed as well as using a cup to introduce drinking milk. It was recommended that, if Pete continued to have difficulty making the transition to solid food, a feeding evaluation should be sought. The HRIF clinic social worker and nutritionist helped identify a WIC program more accessible to Susan's new apartment, and Susan gave written permission for the HRIF nutritionist to contact the WIC nutritionist regarding WIC follow-up.

Occupational/Physical Therapy
Once again, during the occupational and physical therapy assessments the BSID-II and the MAI were administered. Pete initially showed little interest in the toys, but he gradually became more responsive. He showed fairly reliable visual following. Pete's head turning to sounds was inconsistent; his mother reported that he was on antibiotics for otitis media. His vocalizations were rela-

tively sparse for his corrected age; some vowel sounds and a couple of consonant-vowel syllables were heard but no double syllables such as "mama," "dada," or "baba." Pete was able to pick up cubes and grasp a ring, and he attempted to grasp a pellet. He transferred objects but did not combine objects together at the mid-line, and he showed a mild preference for the right hand by reaching with his right hand for objects that were somewhat to the left of mid-line. Pete's BSID-II MDI score was 93 (32nd percentile), and his PDI score was 84 (14th percentile).

On the MAI, Pete continued to show increased tone in his lower extremities with frank resistance to passive movement in the heel cords and hip adductors, but with full range of movement. His mother reported that at home he rolled from supine to prone positions, but in the clinic he rolled only from his back to his side. In a prone position, he was not able to move forward, but he did push up by extending his arms and was able to pivot to one side. He sat without support for brief periods but was not yet stable. At times, his lower back was rounded, and he sat with a narrow base of support, but at other times he arched backward suddenly and lost his balance. When held in a supported-standing position, Pete bore weight on his toes, but he was capable of coming down on his heels with some manipulation by the therapist. In the conversation between Susan and the therapist, the mother reported that Pete spent "a lot of time" in an infant walker, and, while in the walker, he made contact with the floor primarily with his toes.

Social Work
Susan had moved into an apartment with a new friend who worked as an aide at the alternative high school. Susan had turned 18 and obtained Aid to Families with Dependent Children (AFDC) for herself and Pete after the move, but she was having difficulty getting to the WIC clinic because she had no transportation. Alex was not involved with the mother or the child at this time, but it was unclear if that was his choice or if he simply did not know where Susan lived. Susan said that she had not told Alex or her mother where she lived because she wanted to have a clean start. Her roommate was said to share in the baby's care.

Money was a primary concern for Susan at this visit, and she said that the FRC had steered her to a clothing bank for Pete, as he was outgrowing many of his old clothes. Susan also had obtained some additional toys for Pete from a church that she had begun to attend. She felt very positive about the church and said that the pastor and several other people had helped her out. Her depression and sadness were said to have "pretty much disappeared" since she moved out of her parents' home. The only thing she resented was having to attend the drug treatment program, which she still insisted was not needed. She again said that she was not using alcohol or drugs but did think that she was probably still a little at risk for a relapse. It also was somewhat worrisome that her roommate supposedly had a drink "maybe once or twice a week" and kept beer in the refrigerator.

Susan was still attending the alternative school but did not have much energy to interact with other students at the school. She anticipated graduating in another 3 months and hoped to get a part-time job after that. It seemed that her roommate was providing the majority of her friendship contact, with the church being the other source of interaction and support. Locating a closer WIC site was accomplished with the help of the nutritionist, and this was the only resource need that Susan identified.

Elective Parent Conference

At a parent conference staffed by the pediatrician and the physical therapist, Pete's mother was commended for Pete's developmental progress, particularly for his improved hand functioning and diminished shoulder retraction. She was advised to give him a variety of objects with which to play, including tiny bits of age-appropriate food (e.g., Cheerios), as a way of cultivating his fine motor development. It was also recommended that she reduce or eliminate Pete's use of the infant walker. In addition to discussing the safety concerns associated with walkers, Pete's mother was told that play time on the floor would provide him with more opportunities to develop crawling skills.

Pete's tendency to bear weight on his toes was also discussed. His mother was told that this could be a temporary condition called *transient dystonia of prematurity* that is sometimes seen in infants born prematurely; alternatively, it could be a more static condition referred to as spastic diplegia (a type of cerebral palsy). A trial of physical therapy was recommended, and Susan agreed to having a physical therapist visit Pete in their apartment once a week. In consultation with the physical therapist, the HRIF pediatrician wrote a prescription for physical therapy. Finally, Pete was scheduled for a follow-up assessment at 12 months corrected age.

Cerebral Palsy versus Transient Dystonia

For a large majority of LBW children, parents can expect motor development within typical limits. Even so, LBW children are still at increased risk for certain forms of cerebral palsy (CP), especially spastic diplegia. Children with CP need physical therapy and other special management. Generally, it is believed that the earlier such treatments are initiated, the more effective they are likely to be. Follow-up programs for children discharged from NICUs have been developed in order to promote the early identification of CP and other neurodevelopmental disorders.

Unfortunately, the signs and symptoms that often indicate early CP tend to be subtle, and the specificity of these indicators is limited. Drillien and her colleague (Drillien, 1972; Drillien & Drummond, 1977) followed a series of LBW infants who showed early neurological abnormalities that were known to be associated with CP in later childhood. In some cases, these abnormalities later vanished; thus, it became clear that those children did not, in fact, have genuine CP (which is a chronic condition) but transient dystonia of prematurity. As a result, newborn follow-up programs are often confronted with a clinical dilemma. On the one hand, it may be harmful to withhold physical therapy from a child with, for example, increased extensor tone in the lower extremities. On the other hand, it may also be harmful to make a CP diagnosis in a child who, 6 months later, returns with a normal neurological examination. For this reason, LBW children who have findings such as increased extensor tone are often referred for physical therapy before a definite diagnosis is made. Even though some cases probably would resolve without treatment, the prudent course is often to provide physical therapy until subsequent findings clarify whether the child has CP or transient dystonia of the premature. In either circumstance, ongoing follow-up remains an important precaution. Among infants who are determined to have transient dystonia, a disproportionate number will later turn out to have other neurodevelopmental impairments (Nelson & Ellensberg, 1982).

FOLLOW-UP VISIT AT 12 MONTHS CORRECTED AGE

At this visit, the BSID-II was given again. Given the concerns noted at previous visits about shoulder retractions and increased extensor tone in the lower extremities, it was decided that the physical therapist would administer the Bayley Motor Scale and the psychologist would administer the Mental Scale.

Psychology

On the Mental Scale, Pete was by now making somewhat more varied vocalizations. He said "baba" and "mama" in the clinic, and he was reported to say several other double-syllable utterances (e.g., "nana," "gaga") at home. Nevertheless, he did not "jabber expressively" in the way that full-term 12-month-old children often do. He also did not imitate any words, which is occasionally seen at this corrected age.

At this visit, there was convincing evidence for object constancy. For example, when beads were put into a box and then rattled about, Pete stared down into the box in an obvious effort to see the beads once he was given the box. He did not have the fine dexterity necessary to remove the lid from the box, however. When given a tall cylinder with a pellet in it, he was not able to remove the pellet through some form of directed effort (e.g., turning the cylinder upside down). When the examiner placed a slotted lid on the box and then demonstrated how the beads could be put into the box through the hole in the lid, Pete did not imitate this activity. Rather, he was preoccupied with trying to put the small beads into his mouth, which could not be permitted for reasons of safety. At a somewhat younger level, he was able to place a 1-inch block into a cup after the examiner demonstrated. When given more blocks and asked to put them into the cup as well, Pete quickly became disorganized by the presence of so many objects on the table at once, and he began to rake the blocks off the table and onto the floor. Pete's BSID-II Mental Index was 86, which would be more in keeping with an 11-month-old. According to 12-month norms, a BSID-II Index of 86 is at the 18th percentile.

Occupational/Physical Therapy

On the Motor Scale, Pete achieved a score of 85. He sat independently, crawled reciprocally, and pulled to stand using the furniture in the room. Gross motor skills were functional but characterized by limited trunk rotation. He was just beginning to stand alone but was not yet taking independent steps. He could pick up a pellet with either hand (though somewhat more skillfully with the right hand), but he did not yet have a refined pincer grasp. Asymmetry was still evident in hand function with a persisting but mild right-sided hand preference. His muscle tone continued to be mildly increased in the lower extremities, but this was less remarkable in relation to previous evaluations. Although he usually stood on his toes when pulling up at furniture, he bore weight on his heels when standing alone. The overall impression was of immaturity in gross and fine motor skills, mild asymmetry, and resolving transient dystonia of prematurity.

Audiology

During Pete's 12 months corrected age visit to the HRIF clinic, he was seen by an audiologist for a hearing assessment. Using visual reinforcement audiometry (VRA), Pete's hearing was tested in each ear for the frequencies 500–4,000 hertz (Hz) and for speech. VRA is a test procedure in which the infant is conditioned to turn toward the sound source by introducing visual reinforcement following the head-turn response. Reinforcement in this approach consists of an animated, lighted toy situated to either side of mid-line. This head turn is an easily observed and reliable response. Once Pete learned that the sounds were linked to the reinforcer, the intensity level of the sound was reduced until the softest level that just produced a head turn was determined. In this manner, Pete's hearing threshold for a range of sounds was tested. Findings for Pete at 12 months corrected age showed his hearing to be in the normal range for each ear across the frequency range important for speech reception.

Pediatrics

During the pediatric assessment, Susan reported that her son had had several upper respiratory tract infections and also otitis media, for which he had received antibiotics. He had not been hospitalized for any of these episodes, however. Yet, Susan reported that Pete was being followed by a gastroenterologist at the local children's hospital for his GE reflux, which seemed to be improving with positioning and the medication. She reported that Pete was still taking a bottle and also some baby food. He seemed to tolerate the solids better. She reported that he was somewhat irritable so that she felt a need to carry him around at times to help him calm down.

Pete was babbling; he said "mama" and "dada." He also pointed to make his needs met. Susan stated that he was able to pull to stand and to take a few steps along furniture. He seemed to favor reaching with his right hand more than with his left. When standing against furniture, he had a tendency to stand on his toes. He had begun to crawl at 10 months corrected age. He was able to hold his own bottle and to drink from it, and he could also drink from a cup with assistance. Pete liked to look at pictures in a book. No significant sleep problems were reported.

On examination, his height was 75 centimeters (cm), at the 30th percentile; his weight was 8.91 kilograms, at the 10th percentile; and his head circumference was 46 cm, at the 25th percentile. Pete appeared small but reasonably proportionate for his age. He was in no cardiorespiratory distress. The anterior fontanel was closing. Both eardrums appeared dull, but there was no evidence of active infection. The rest of the physical examination—including the head and neck, chest, abdomen, genitalia, and extremities—was unremarkable.

The neurological examination revealed mild truncal hypotonia (low muscle tone), and when picked up, Pete had a tendency to hyperextend his lower extremities. The deep-tendon reflexes were rated 3+ (brisk) in the lower extremities and 2+ (normal) in the upper extremities but symmetric. Pete tended to reach most of the time with his right hand, and his pincer grasp was somewhat immature for a child his age. He was inconsistent in his responses to sounds when called although he seemed to be visually alert and social. As mentioned previously, he jabbered often. Pete also appeared to be somewhat active, more so than expected for his age.

In summary, the pediatrician's impression was that Pete presented with some evidence of CNS dysfunction; however, the child's development by report and by observation seemed close to age level. It was recommended that Pete return to his primary care physician for medical management of his chronic otitis. It was also suggested that the primary care physician consider a referral to an ear, nose, and throat specialist because of Pete's history of recurrent otitis media and the fact that dull tympanic membranes were found during this examination. Furthermore, it was recommended that Pete return for further hearing assessment as previously recommended. He was to continue his follow-up by the GI clinic, and a nutritionist through the GI clinic was to continue to monitor the child's nutrition intake. Pete was not seen by nutrition at this visit, but his weight for height continued at the 10th percentile. It was noted that Pete was still taking mostly second foods, and he was beginning to use whole milk instead of concentrated formula.

Social Work
A social work interview was not scheduled for this visit, as an interim telephone call to Susan had failed to identify any new issues or concerns about resources.

Susan had received her high school diploma and had also found a full-time job as a receptionist at a real estate office. She took a bus to and from her job, but she was hoping to get a car soon. Her roommate was said still to be helping with some child care, and Susan's mother had been delighted when asked to provide care 2 days a week. Susan was still in contact with the FRC and was becoming a member of the church that she had been attending. Her drug treatment program would be ending within the month, and Susan said that she still was not using alcohol or drugs. She sounded very happy about her new job and pleased with Pete's development. She was told that she could still see the social worker at future visits if she wished but that she wouldn't be routinely scheduled for a social work interview.

FOLLOW-UP VISIT AT 18 MONTHS CORRECTED AGE

On arrival at the clinic, it was noted that Susan seemed somewhat short-tempered with Pete. Most of her communications with him were directives regarding his behavior to which Pete seldom responded.

Psychology

The Mental and Motor Scales of the BSID-II were both administered by the psychologist at Pete's visit at 18 months corrected age. When the BSID-II Mental Scale was begun, it was clear that Pete was having trouble tolerating the structured activities contained in the 18-month BSID-II item set. He tended to become disorganized if there were more than one or two objects on the table at once. For example, when the pegboard and the six pegs were presented to Pete, on the third trial he picked up one peg and chewed on it briefly, and then he raked several other pegs off the table. There was a similar response to the BSID-II puzzles.

In fact, Pete passed only four of the items in the 18-month item set. He stacked one block onto another to make a tower of two cubes, but he quickly knocked the tower over instead of moving on to add a third cube as the examiner had demonstrated. He also imitated a crayon stroke, and Susan commented that she had spent a fair amount of time with Pete trying to get him to mark with a crayon on pieces of paper from a legal pad. He also used words to make his wants known on two occasions: When shown a red rubber ball, he vigorously said, "Bah!" (i.e., *ball*), and he also said, "Moe" for *more* on several occasions.

Because Pete had passed only four items in the 18-month item set, the BSID-II's basal criterion was not met, and the examiner therefore dropped back to the next lower item set. Pete passed all the additional items in the next lower item set, obtaining a raw score of 100. According to the 18-month norms, this raw score yielded a Mental Development Index of 75, which is at the 5th percentile. Among children born at term, this level of performance would be more typical at 15 months of age than at 18 months of age.

On the BSID-II Motor Scale, Pete met the basal criterion in the item set for 18 months by passing six items in that item set. In the Gross Motor domain, Pete was able to walk up the small BSID-II staircase while holding on to the wall for support, but he could not yet walk down the staircase in this manner. When given a pull-toy car on a string, Pete took both sideways and backward steps while watching the car move at the end of the string that he was pulling. He stood from a supine position after first rolling over to his side and then standing up without having to pull up on furniture. In the Fine Motor domain, when given a primary pencil and asked to draw a picture, Pete did use the pads of his fingertips to grasp the pencil. He also used his left hand to hold the paper in place while he scribbled with the right hand. Overall, Pete obtained a raw score of 71, which would be typical for 15-month-olds. According to the 18-month norms, a raw score of 71 receives a Motor Index of 83, which is 13th percentile.

During the BSID-II, there were a number of qualitative features that gave the examiner cause for concern. Pete's attention span was unusually short for a child of 18 months corrected age. He manifested diminished tolerance for minor frustrations (e.g., he sometimes became rather irritable at the transition from one toy to another), and these episodes of irritability tended to leave him somewhat disorganized even after the irritability had resolved. In addition, Pete's tolerance for structured activities was very limited, especially when the activities involved multiple small objects such as pegs or puzzle pieces. In the presence of many such items, Pete's behavior tended to become less mature and less organized. Susan commonly became impatient herself when Pete behaved in this manner, and her impatience seemed only to make her son's behavior even more disorganized.

Nutrition

Pete's rate of growth in weight had decreased since the 12-month visit. Weight for height had dropped to the 5th percentile. He had been taking bottles of 2% milk and had also been enjoying apple juice, which he took from a cup without a spout. Susan said that she gave him the juice throughout the day, especially when he became fussy. Pete was taking fewer baby foods now, but they were still a part of his diet. The other solids he was taking were soft foods with smooth textures (e.g., applesauce, oatmeal, pudding). Pete gagged or spat out many foods with lumps or coarse textures. Susan reported that she often ended up feeding her son because he was very slow feeding himself and made a mess when trying to use a spoon. A brief oral-motor evaluation revealed immature oral-motor patterns.

Pete's mother also reported that he frequently had a poor appetite and sometimes had bouts of diarrhea. At the end of the nutrition assessment, Susan was told that excessive juice intake can lead to diarrhea and can curb a child's appetite for other foods. Moreover, fruit juices are less energy-dense than other foods. It was recommended that Pete be given whole milk instead of 2% milk, and it was also noted that solid foods are, in general, more energy-dense. Susan and the nutritionist discussed the family meal pattern and worked out a schedule for Pete to have three meals and two or three planned snacks per day. Susan was encouraged to allow Pete to self-feed with a spoon and to use a cup more regularly, even though there would be messy consequences. Susan and Pete were then referred to a feeding team for more thorough evaluation and monitoring of Pete's feeding patterns.

Case Conference

Three areas of concern were identified during the case conference for Pete. First, there was concern about the tenor of the interactions between Pete and his mother. His mother had fallen into a pattern of talking to Pete primarily to give him behavioral directives. The friend with whom she had been sharing the apartment had expressed intermittent dissatisfaction with having a toddler in the small apartment, and Susan was feeling a need to "keep a lid on Pete's behavior." However, Susan did not seem to possess many techniques for cultivating more adaptive behavior in her toddler. Second, the apparent drop in Pete's BSID-II Mental Index was worrisome. Previous BSID-II scores had been in the 80s and low 90s—significantly higher than the current score of 75. The 18-month score was only 5th percentile and could be considered to be consistent with a borderline developmental delay. Fortunately, in many states, BSID-II scores of 77 and lower (i.e., $1^1/_2$ SDs or more below the mean) qualify young children for services via the state's early intervention network of birth-to-3 programs. Third, there was also concern about Pete's behavior findings. His short attention span, tendency to become disorganized if multiple objects were available at the same time, and diminished tolerance for minor frustrations and for structured activities were all worrisome, even though these findings are all seen with increased incidence in LBW infants.

Members of the case conference team were concerned that these three factors might act to potentiate each other. The professionals on the team worried that Susan's parenting style would only exacerbate Pete's behavior findings and that both of those factors could result in even lower Mental Indexes in the future. For these reasons, then, the consensus was that a referral to a birth-to-3 early intervention program should be recommended at the parent conference. Such a referral would, of course, require Susan's consent and participation.

Parent Conference

When this case conference recommendation was presented to Susan at the parent conference, she was pleased. She had become increasingly aware that she and Pete needed some help to negotiate their way through some of the challenges that they faced together. Pete's mother gave consent on the release-of-information form for the reports from the 18-month visit to go to the FRC serving the new area in which Susan resided. In addition, the FRC was contacted by telephone regarding this referral. During this telephone exchange, the FRC offered to work in conjunction with the CPS case manager to ensure that Pete received a comprehensive toddler program that included input from specialists in physical, occupational, and speech-language therapy, as well as the services of personnel with special training in early intervention. The birth-to-3 program also included a parent support group in which parenting techniques were presented and discussed. Finally, Susan was given an appointment for another visit at 24 months corrected age. She seemed relieved when she left the clinic building that she would be getting some additional help for Pete and for herself.

CONCLUSION

As initially noted, the IHDP demonstrated that it is possible to better the outcomes of LBW infants by providing high-quality services after they leave the hospital. Much research in this area remains to be done. Meanwhile, however, clinicians who work in the field of newborn follow-up must often rely on their clinical judgment to identify those infants who are at the greatest risk.

In the case of Pete, there was a spectrum of risk factors. Pete's mother was relatively young and had little prior parenting experience. Her situation was complicated further by her history of substance use and by her affective adjustment to becoming a single parent. Pete's early medical complications included mild intrauterine growth retardation, persisting GI difficulties, feeding problems, and worrisome neuromotor soft signs. His cognitive development began in the low-average to low-normal range but reached the borderline range by 18 months of age. Clearly, there were many reasons for his caregivers to be concerned. Fortunately, the results at 18 months postterm age made Pete eligible for a birth-to-3 program.

The long-term implications of the downward drift in Pete's Mental Indexes are not well defined. The fact that he was in a situation characterized by some social stress could possibly account, at least in part, for the gradual deterioration in scores. In that case, the referral for birth-to-3 services could produce a relatively rapid improvement that could be documented at the next follow-up visit at 24 months corrected age.

In the first 3 years of life in particular, standardized scores can fluctuate over a considerable range as a child's development passes through static plateaus and through bursts of rapid advance. It is for this reason that many follow-up programs for infants at the highest risk now follow these children into the early school years. A postterm age of 18 months would be much too soon to try to predict Pete's level of functioning in his early years at school. With ongoing specialty care from an interdisciplinary team, however, it is likely that the outcome will be substantially better than could be expected based on the natural history research that first launched the field of newborn follow-up.

REFERENCES

Bayley, N. (1969). *Bayley Scales of Infant Development.* San Antonio, TX: The Psychological Corp.

Bayley, N. (1993). *Bayley Scales of Infant Development–Second Edition.* San Antonio, TX: The Psychological Corp.

Bennett, F.C. (1994). Developmental outcome. In G.B. Avery, M.A. Fletcher, & M.G. MacDonald (Eds.), *Neonatology: Pathophysiology and management of the newborn* (4th ed., pp. 1367–1386). Philadelphia: Lippincott, Williams & Wilkins.

Bennett, F.C., & Scott, D.T. (1997). Long-term perspective on premature infant outcome, and contemporary intervention issues. *Seminars in Perinatology, 21,* 190–201.

Brooks-Gunn, J., McCarton, C.M., Casey, P.H., McCormick, M.D., Bauer, C.R., Bernbaum, J.C., Tysoin, J., Swanson, M., Bennett, F.C., Scott, D.T., Tonascia, J., & Meinert, C.L. (1994). Early intervention in low-birth-weight premature infants: Results through age 5 from the Infant Health and Development Program. *JAMA: Journal of the American Medical Association, 272,* 1257–1262.

Cashore, W.J. (1994). Neonatal hyperbilirubinemia. In F.A. Oski, C.D. DeAngelis, R.D. Feigin, J.A. McMillan, & J.B. Warshaw (Eds.), *Principles and practice of pediatrics* (pp. 446–455). Philadelphia: Lippincott, Williams and Wilkins.

Chandler, L.S., Andrews, M.S., & Swanson, M.W. (1980). *Movement Assessment of Infants: A Manual.* Rolling Bay, WA: Chandler, Andrews, & Swanson.

Delaney, E.A., & Hopkins, T.F. (1987). *Stanford-Binet Intelligence Scale (4th ed.): Examiner's Handbook* (pp. 68–69). Itasca, IL: The Riverside Publishing Co.

Drillien, C.M. (1964). *The growth and development of the prematurely born infant.* Edinburgh, United Kingdom: E. & S. Livingstone.

Drillien, C.M. (1972). Abnormal neurological signs in the first year of life in low-birthweight infants: Possible prognostic significance. *Developmental Medicine and Child Neurology, 14,* 575–584.

Drillien, C.M., & Drummond, M.B. (1977). *Neurodevelopmental problems in early childhood.* Oxford, United Kingdom: Blackwell Scientific Publications.

Elliott, C.D. (1990). *Differential Ability Scales.* San Antonio, TX: The Psychological Corp.

Ferry, P.C. (1981). On growing new neurons: Are early intervention programs effective? *Pediatrics, 67,* 38–41.

Fitzhardinge, P.M., Kalman, E., Ashby, S., & Pape, K.D. (1978). Present status of the infant of very low birth weight treated in a referral neonatal intensive care unit in 1974. In *Major mental handicap: Methods and costs of prevention. Ciba Foundation Symposium, n.s. 59.* Amsterdam: Elsevier/Excerpta Medica.

Fitzhardinge, P.M., & Ramsay, M. (1973). The improving outlook for the small, prematurely born infant. *Developmental Medicine and Child Neurology, 15,* 447–459.

Gross, I. (1994). Respiratory distress syndrome. In F.A. Oski, C.D. DeAngelis, R.D. Feigin, J.A. McMillan, & J.B. Warshaw (Eds.). *Principles and practice of pediatrics* (pp. 369–374). Philadelphia: Lippincott, Williams & Wilkins.

Infant Health and Development Program. (1990). Enhancing the outcomes of low-birth-weight, premature infants: A multisite, randomized trial. *JAMA: Journal of the American Medical Association, 263,* 3035–3042.

Kennedy, K.A., & Warshaw, J.B. (1994). Bronchopulmonary dysplasia. In F.A. Oski, C.D. DeAngelis, R.D. Feigin, J.A. McMillan, & J.B. Warshaw (Eds.), *Principles and practice of pediatrics* (pp. 388–391). Philadelphia: Lippincott, Williams & Wilkins.

Kopf, G.S., & Dewar, M.L. (1994). Cardiovascular surgery in the newborn. In F.A. Oski, C.D. DeAngelis, R.D. Feigin, J.A. McMillan, & J.B. Warshaw (Eds.), *Principles and practice of pediatrics* (pp. 565–573). Philadelphia: Lippincott, Williams & Wilkins.

Leiter, R.G. (1979). *Instruction Manual for the Leiter International Performance Scale.* Wood Dale, IL: Stoelting Co.

McCarton, C.M., Brooks-Gunn, J., Wallace, I.F., Bauer, C.R., Bennett, F.C., Bernbaum, J.C., Broyles, S., Casey, P.H., McCormick, M.C., Scott, D.T., Tyson, J., Tonascia, J., & Meinert, C.L. (1997). Results at age 8 years of early intervention for low-birth-weight premature infants: The Infant Health and Development Program. *JAMA: Journal of the American Medical Association, 277,* 126–132.

Ment, L.R. (1994). Intraventricular hemorrhage of the preterm infant. In F.A. Oski, C.D. DeAngelis, R.D. Feigin, J.A. McMillan, & J.B. Warshaw (Eds.), *Principles and practice of pediatrics* (pp. 347–352). Philadelphia: Lippincott, Williams & Wilkins.

Motil, K.J. (1994). Necrotizing enterocolitis. In F.A. Oski, C.D. DeAngelis, R.D. Feigin, J.A. McMillan, & J.B. Warshaw (Eds.), *Principles and practice of pediatrics* (pp. 436–443). Philadelphia: Lippincott, Williams & Wilkins.

Nelson, K., & Ellensberg, J. (1982). Children who "outgrew" cerebral palsy. *Pediatrics, 69,* 529–536.

Roid, G.H., & Miller, L.J. (1997). *Leiter International Performance Scale—Revised.* Wood Dale, IL: Stoelting Co.

Scott, D.T. (1983). Prospects for the premature: Past and present. In J.B. Warshaw & J.C. Hobbins (Eds.), *Principles and practice of care* (pp. 277–293). Menlo Park, CA: Addison-Wesley.

Scott, D.T. (1997). Rationale for selection of measures: Cognitive development. In R.T Gross, D. Spiker, & C.W. Haynes (Eds.), *Helping low birth weight, premature babies: The infant health and development program* (pp. 67–83). Stanford, CA: Stanford University Press.

Scott, D.T., Spiker, D., Kraemer, H.C., Bauer, C.R., Bryant, D.M., Constantine, N.A., & Tyson, J.E. (1997). Possible confounding issues concerning the primary child outcomes. In R.T. Gross, D. Spiker, & C.W. Haynes (Eds.), *Helping low birth weight, premature babies: The infant health and development program* (pp. 154–180). Stanford, CA: Stanford University Press.

Scott, D.T., & Tyson, J. (1999). Follow-up of infants discharged from newborn intensive care. In J.A. McMillan, C.D. DeAngelis, R.D. Feigin, & J.B. Warshaw (Eds.), *Oski's pediatrics: Principles and practice* (3rd ed., pp. 209–214). Philadelphia: Lippincott, Williams & Wilkins.

Terman, L.M., & Merrill, M.A. (1973). *Stanford-Binet Intelligence Scale* (3rd ed., Form L-M). Boston: Houghton Mifflin Co.

Thorndike, R.L., Hagen, E.P., & Sattler, J.M. (1986). *Stanford-Binet Intelligence Scale for Children* (4th ed.). Chicago: The Riverside Publishing Co.

Washington, K., Scott, D.T., Johnson, K.A., Wendel, S., & Hay, A.E. (1998). The Bayley Scales of Infant Development–II and children with developmental delays: A clinical perspective. *Developmental and Behavioral Pediatrics, 19,* 346–349.

Wechsler, D. (1989). *Wechsler Preschool and Primary Scale of Intelligence–Revised.* San Antonio, TX: The Psychological Corp.

Wechsler, D. (1991). *Wechsler Intelligence Scale for Children–Third Edition.* San Antonio, TX: The Psychological Corp.

Wechsler, D. (1992). *Wechsler Individual Achievement Test.* San Antonio, TX: The Psychological Corp.

Woodcock, R.W., & Johnson, M.B. (1990). *Manual for the Woodcock-Johnson–Revised Tests of Achievement.* Allen, TX: RCL Enterprises.

Chapter 12

A Child with Down Syndrome

*Anne Hay, Truman E. Coggins, Douglas S. Cook,
Nuhad D. Dinno, Richard C. Folsom, Vanja A. Holm,
Betty L. Lucas, and Susan Wendel*

This case study demonstrates the interdisciplinary team assessment process for a child with a well-known developmental condition, Down syndrome. It also illustrates the changes that must occur during a team assessment when the assessment questions initially presented to the team must be revised due to new information discovered in the course of the evaluation. Members of an interdisciplinary team have to realize that material collected before an assessment may be incomplete or that the family's, school's, or community professionals' primary issues of concern may not be those the team will eventually judge to be the most essential questions about a child's development. It is important to remember that the assessment is a dynamic process, and it must remain flexible as new information emerges.

PRELIMINARY CONFERENCE
The parents of Sam, a 4-year and 10-month-old child with Down syndrome, contacted the interdisciplinary team clinic staff by telephone to present con-

cerns regarding feeding. The parents' specific worries were about Sam's lack of chewing, refusal to finger feed, and high tactile sensitivity. Sam's parents also were concerned about the adequacy of their son's diet because he ate a very limited variety of foods. Furthermore, they worried that Sam was not making progress learning to talk or to use sign language as most children with Down syndrome eventually do.

The team decision at the preliminary conference was to combine a feeding clinic evaluation with a full team developmental assessment. The feeding clinic is one of the specialty subgroups included in many comprehensive interdisciplinary teams. The disciplines scheduled for the feeding clinic in this assessment were nursing, occupational therapy, and nutrition. A pediatrician, a psychologist, a speech-language pathologist, and an audiologist were to complete additional assessments as part of the larger interdisciplinary developmental assessment process. It was decided that one of the members of the feeding clinic would serve as the service coordinator. This person would be responsible for liaisons with the family and any school or other community professionals involved in the assessment process.

Additional information to be obtained was based on forms sent to the family. A feeding clinic parent questionnaire (see the Appendix at the end of this book) was sent to Sam's parents. It contained questions regarding Sam's current dietary intake and past problems and what his parents saw as the main feeding difficulties, as well as information about past interventions. A general parent questionnaire (see the Appendix) collected background material about family history and Sam's current status, early medical history, developmental milestones, and overall areas of concern. In addition, Sam's parents were asked to identify other medical, therapeutic, or school services they utilized in the community and to sign the appropriate release forms so that reports could be obtained. Because Sam was enrolled in a community developmental birth-to-3 program, questionnaires were sent to his teachers as well as to occupational, physical, and speech-language therapists to gather more detailed input regarding developmental progress and goals in those environments (see the Appendix).

PREASSESSMENT CONFERENCE

During the preassessment conference, all of the forms from Sam's family and community service providers were reviewed. It became apparent that feeding was only one of many important issues. Major concerns revolved around Sam's unusually slow developmental progress. Reports indicated that Sam was just beginning to engage in parallel play. He was also just beginning to be aware of his surroundings. Of special significance, both school personnel and his parents noted that Sam had no spoken language at all. In addition, he had not been able to learn sign language, and the school was just beginning a picture exchange communication system that had not yet become effective. All of these circumstances suggested that Sam was at a much lower developmental level than expected for a child his age with Down syndrome.

Based on this information, an alteration was made to the initial assessment plan: The team decided that it would be more appropriate for the psychologist to function as the service coordinator. Given the developmental concerns, this change would allow a more comprehensive array of assessments, providing the level of analysis required to evaluate Sam's behavior and development properly. In view of the complexity and uncertainty of the situation, all of the disciplines originally proposed were scheduled to participate in the assessment.

Following the preassessment conference, the team determined a preliminary schedule. This schedule was mailed to the family and was accompanied by a description of each of the disciplines participating in Sam's assessment. Consequently, the family could review and approve both items, or they could request additional information from other disciplines that were not on the schedule.

DISCIPLINARY ASSESSMENT PROCESS

The structure of Sam's assessment was discussed by the team. Possible adjustments to the typical evaluation were proposed in light of the unique learning and motivational challenges sometimes encountered when assessing children with Down syndrome. For example, longitudinal research on the learning problems of young children with Down syndrome has revealed important differences in learning style and motivation that are of special interest to clinicians (see Wishart, 1993). Specifically, children with Down syndrome tend to accept a low reward level when working on tasks and show evidence of developmental instability in that test items previously passed tend not to be well consolidated with other items intended to measure the same domains of development. Children with Down syndrome often do not actively pursue—or they may even avoid—learning opportunities (Wishart, 1993). This pattern, which seems to be particularly characteristic of children with Down syndrome, may well affect the outcomes of the assessment process. Consequently, not only should individual evaluators be attentive to this complex process, but the entire assessment schedule should be sensitive to these learning and motivational concerns (Wishart, 1993).

As the family was traveling across the state to reach the clinic and would only be able to make one trip, all assessments were scheduled on 3 consecutive days. Sam reportedly tired easily, so assessments were scheduled only for the morning. Professionals in two disciplines were scheduled to see Sam on a single day. Given that the family's initial concern was nutrition and related feeding issues, the feeding clinic evaluation was to be conducted first.

When the family arrived at the interdisciplinary assessment center for Sam's first evaluation, they were met by a staff member who reviewed the schedule of assessments. In order to help develop a successful parent–professional partnership, a detailed discussion with Sam's parents took place prior to beginning the assessment. In this meeting, the parents' concerns were explored, and they were introduced to the clinic assessment process.

DISCIPLINE ASSESSMENT SUMMARIES

The goal of interdisciplinary assessment is for the professionals to make team decisions and intervention plans. Nonetheless, these points are reached by members of each discipline conducting their own evaluations, in terms of their areas of expertise, of the child. An exception in this case is the feeding clinic evaluation, in which three disciplines conduct an arena assessment and report their findings and recommendations as a unit. An exploration of each discipline's findings during Sam's assessment follows.

Feeding Clinic: Nutrition, Occupational Therapy, and Nursing

A feeding clinic evaluates children whose nutrition, growth, feeding skills, or mealtime behaviors are a concern to parents or caregivers. As feeding problems in young children fall within the domain of several disciplines, the feeding clinic consists of a nutritionist, an occupational therapist, and an advanced practice nurse. The evaluation carried out in an arena format by the feeding clinic team members involves observations of the child eating with the family (videotaped with permission), a more structured oral-motor evaluation, and a team interview with the family. The family is involved in all aspects of the evaluation and subsequent planning.

The nutritionist uses current and past growth parameters, anthropometric data, food records, parental interview about early feeding history, and other food and feeding information. The occupational therapist uses structured feeding observations to assess oral-motor skills, self-feeding skills, and sensorimotor skills. These observations are also the context for demonstrating intervention techniques. The nurse uses structured parent–child interactions and related tools to determine patterns of parent–child interactions, feeding behaviors, and the adequacy of family support. A brief review of the child's overall health also is obtained.

History of Feeding Behaviors and Patterns

Sam's feeding history was received from his parents. Past significant feeding problems for Sam included a slow transition to textured foods, tactile sensitivity, and resistance to independent feeding. A videofluoroscopy swallowing study at 18 months of age showed normal functioning. The following interventions had already been utilized: an electric toothbrush and facial touching for tactile sensitivity and gradually removing parental assistance to encourage independent spoon feeding. Sam's parents had also used a number of creative interventions over the years and reported positive changes in the few months prior to assessment:

1. Sam fed himself during most meals. In the past he required greater assistance, but his parents encouraged Sam to become more independent. At the child care center, he did not usually receive help with feeding.

2. Sam's hunger and satiation cues had become more clear to his parents; at times, he would go to the refrigerator to show hunger or thirst.
3. Mealtimes had become a more social time for the entire family.

Diet and Nutritional Status

Sam's parents reported that their son typically ate three meals and two snacks per day, mostly at home and in child care. He would sit with other children at school snack time but did not usually eat. The 7-day food record showed his usual foods to be soft and moist (e.g., yogurt, pasta, mashed potatoes). At the time of assessment, Sam preferred mostly smooth textured food but had begun tolerating some lumps. He refused most fruits and vegetables, drank 2% milk, and ate nonfat yogurt. Sam had also taken a vitamin supplement in the past, but he refused all forms at the time of his evaluation. An analysis of the 7-day food record indicated an average daily intake of 1,142 calories (12.2 calories per centimeter [cm] of height). Nutrients that were low or inadequate in Sam's diet included vitamin C, zinc, and iron. Growth patterns were obtained as part of the pediatrics evaluation (see the section on pediatrics, to follow).

Oral-Motor Skills

For the feeding observation, Sam sat in a highchair, with the tray removed, pulled up to the table. This was typical of how he was fed at home. Sam displayed decreased tone (hypotonia) throughout his body, including the oral and facial muscles. He had good lip closure around the spoon and cup. He also used his lips to clean food off the spoon and maintained lip seal on the cup with no loss of liquid when drinking. Sam moved a bite of food laterally to the side of his mouth with his tongue. Sam's chewing pattern was immature, however: He moved his jaw up and down in an exaggerated munching pattern, his mouth slightly open. He lacked the more refined skill of rotary chewing movements with his lips closed.

Sam was most successful at self-feeding when he looked toward his bowl and was interested in eating. He held the spoon in a fisted and pronated grasp and scooped yogurt onto it using the side of the bowl to assist him. With more effort, Sam successfully scooped some pieces of cut-up fruit onto the spoon as well. He brought the food to his mouth, although he lacked the precision of wrist rotation to bring the food to his mouth without spilling food off of the spoon. He held a small open cup with one hand; at home, Sam's parents preferred to have their son use a covered cup to prevent spilling. During the feeding observation Sam would not use his fingers to pick up finger foods. His parents stated that at home he refused to pick up foods with a wet or sticky texture. Further exploring Sam's response to tactile sensations, his parents reported that Sam fussed when his face was wiped, frequently refused to have his teeth brushed, avoided getting his hands messy during play and eating, and sometimes avoided hugs or touching by other people. This suggested that Sam may have been hypersensitive to tactile sensations.

Feeding Interactions and Behaviors

Regarding communication during feeding, Sam displayed hunger cues such as mouth and hand movements, a cry, and an "um." Sam's parents responded to these cues by offering more food. They gave Sam verbal praise, and they identified by name the foods given to him. As the session progressed, Sam's verbal and nonverbal cues became less clear. It was difficult to distinguish whether he was still hungry, frustrated, or no longer interested in eating. Sam's parents continued to offer him food, but he ended the meal by getting down from the highchair and leaving the table. Sam's parents indicated that this was a fairly typical meal for Sam. During the feeding sessions, Sam's parents responded to his nonverbal cues and signs as they understood them. At times Sam looked in the direction of his parents when they spoke, but it was unclear if he made direct eye contact. Of note, Sam's unusual difficulties in social responses, severe communication problems, and lack of eye contact raised concern for possible co-occurring autism or autism spectrum disorder. The psychologist and the speech-language pathologist were alerted to this concern so that the issue of autism would be addressed in subsequent assessment sessions.

Feeding Clinic Findings and Tentative Recommendations

Based on observation, interview, and feedback from parent and community questionnaires, Sam displayed substantial impairments in oral-motor development and self-feeding skills when compared with other children his age. Oral and tactile sensitivity contributed to delays in acquisition of chewing as well as acceptance of handling finger foods. Fortunately, Sam had made some gains in tolerating a greater variety of foods and in using a spoon thanks to the consistent, coordinated efforts of his parents and school staff. At the time of observation, Sam was showing readiness cues to move on to more textures and finger feeding.

Sam's growth was typical for boys with Down syndrome (see the pediatrics section). His weight for height above the 95th percentile and other measurements indicated that he had ample fat stores, and excess weight gain should be avoided. He would still have reserves for any times he might eat less than usual. Nevertheless, Sam's caloric intake, based on the food record, did not seem excessive for his age and size. His parents had done an excellent job of providing low-fat foods and avoiding foods of limited nutritional value. However, because Sam refused many fruits and vegetables and his intake of meats and other animal proteins was low, vitamin C, iron, and zinc were inadequate in his diet. Yet, overall, Sam's parents had done well in feeding Sam while encouraging developmentally appropriate self-feeding behaviors. The process had been challenging, but they remained consistently supportive.

The feeding clinic team established tentative recommendations for the family, which are described in detail next.

Nutrition and Growth

Sam's parents should continue to offer a wide variety of foods at regular meals and snacks—including ones Sam has refused—as well as to encourage touching, tasting, or other exploration without pressuring him. In addition, they would be advised to keep using low-fat dairy products, limited fat in cooking, and other low-calorie efforts. A children's multiple vitamin containing iron and zinc would be suggested. An additional recommendation to Sam's parents would be to try crushing and dissolving the tablet in water or juice. Finally, periodic growth measurements should be taken by his primary care provider and charted on the growth charts for children with Down syndrome.

Oral-Motor and Self-Feeding

Sam's parents would be advised to continue his occupational therapy at school and to incorporate oral-motor and feeding activities in the school program and individualized education program (IEP). Encouraging finger feeding at each meal, by offering foods easily held by Sam, would also be suggested. Examples of such food include crackers of all types, fat pretzels, and strips of cheese. To promote Sam's chewing, he should practice with foods that require chewing, such as those listed previously as well as dried fruits. Sam should also be encouraged to dip foods (e.g., a pretzel in peanut butter) to promote hand-to-mouth functioning with familiar and accepted foods. In addition, Sam's parents would be asked to employ tactile play around his mouth prior to feeding to "wake up" the muscles and sensory receptors. Tapping or stroking the cheeks and mouth to music or while singing is one such activity. Other tactile play for decreasing sensitivity to hands would be suggested as well: using play dough, water play, sand play, and hand puppets. Furthermore, Sam should be taught the hand signs for "eat," "drink," and "all done" to allow communication and control during mealtimes. This recommendation should also be included in his IEP.

Mealtime Environment and Behavior Adaptations

The general goal was to make mealtime pleasant for both Sam and his parents and to encourage interaction and communication at this time. Specific recommendations were as follows: Sam's parents should continue to focus on making mealtimes social for everyone, including conversation about the meal as well as other subjects. It might be helpful to limit the number of questions asked of Sam and instead provide a number of playful interactions. In addition, positive feedback should continue to be offered to Sam during the mealtime for behaviors parents wish to encourage. For example, when finger feeding, it might be useful for his parents to praise Sam for simply holding the food in his hand. Finally, Sam's parents should continue to encourage their son's independence during mealtimes. For example, he should be allowed to wipe his face as needed. The family would also be advised to give Sam ample opportunities for developmentally appropriate independence in other activities (e.g., dressing, play) that might be pleasurable for him but would also support his generalized independence.

Developmental Pediatrics

Sam's family history disclosed no history of Down syndrome, other genetic disorders, mental retardation, or learning disabilities on either side of the family. Both parents and his older sister were in good health. Sam was born after a full-term gestation when his mother was 33 years old. Her pregnancy was essentially uncomplicated, and Sam weighed 7 pounds 14 ounces at birth. His length was borderline-short (18½ inches [in]), and his head circumference measurement indicated that he had slight microcephaly (32 cm or 12½ in). He had normal Apgar scores. Sam's condition of Down syndrome was recognized immediately after birth because of typical facial features and hypotonia. Genetic studies showed trisomy 21 and confirmed the clinical diagnosis of Down syndrome. While in the nursery, Sam had difficulties sucking and needed to be gavage fed. He remained in the hospital for 4 days.

Sam seemed to be doing well after he came home. However, his physician noted a heart murmur in early infancy, and Sam was referred for a pediatric cardiology evaluation. Extensive assessment of the child's heart showed that he had an "innocent" murmur with no evidence of congenital heart disease. At about 2 years of age, Sam's parents noted a "wandering eye," which was evaluated by a pediatric ophthalmologist who diagnosed alternating strabismus and recommended observation. The parents had no further concerns about vision. Sam frequently contracted upper respiratory tract infections and had two or three middle-ear infections every winter, so his parents worried about the child's hearing. X-rays of his neck have revealed no atlanto-occipital instability, and a review of organ systems was unremarkable. Sam's early development was somewhat delayed, as his parents had anticipated. He sat independently at 12 months of age, started to walk at 24 months, and said one word ("Mama") at 24 months. Yet further language development did not occur as expected. Sam's developmental delay was of great concern to the parents, as he seemed much more delayed than other children with Down syndrome.

Sam's overall physical characteristics at the time of assessment were noted. They were as follows:

- Height: 93.5 cm (between the 25th and 50th percentiles on the Down syndrome chart)
- Weight: 16.9 kilograms (between the 75th and 90th percentiles on the Down syndrome chart)
- Weight for height: (above the 95th percentile National Center for Health Statistics [NCHS] growth charts)
- Head circumference: 48.0 cm (below the 2nd percentile NCHS chart)
- Upper arm circumference: 18.9 cm (between the 90th and 95th percentiles)
- Triceps fatfold: 10.0 millimeters (between the 50th and 75th percentiles)

Several of Sam's physical characteristics were consistent with the diagnosis of Down syndrome. His occiput was flat and his neck was short. His ears were small (less than the 3rd percentile); tympanic membranes were not well seen because of small ear canals. His eyes showed an upward slant and epicanthal folds, and his irises were blue with white speckles (Brushfield spots). Strabismus was suspected on the cover test, but no evidence of cataracts was observed. He also had a flattened facial profile; a depressed nasal bridge; and a large, fissured tongue. His hands were short (less than the 3rd percentile) with a simian crease on the right hand, but not on the left. In addition, his fifth fingers were short and incurved on both sides with single phalangeal creases. His feet were also shorter than the 3rd percentile with a wide space between the first and second toes with a marked transverse plantar crease. The heart murmur was no longer detected. The genitals were unremarkable for a prepubertal male. Sam had hypotonia throughout and his gait was wide based, but there were no atypical neurological findings. He was physically active but had limited social interaction with the environment and had poor eye contact.

Serous otitis media (sterile middle-ear fluid) and strabismus needed to be ruled out as factors contributing to Sam's apparently pronounced developmental delays and lack of social interaction. The team recommended that the parents take Sam to an otolaryngologist for further evaluation of the otitis media and to an ophthalmologist for further evaluation of the strabismus.

Psychology

The information provided by Sam's parents and his developmental preschool included the facts that Sam was just beginning parallel play and to become aware of his surroundings. The fact that he did not yet talk or communicate suggested that Sam was functioning at a lower developmental level than is typical of children with Down syndrome, and it also called into question Sam's social responsiveness and reactions to his world. Children with Down syndrome commonly show delays in social interaction and communication skills and can show a wide range of cognitive functioning. However, most children with Down syndrome do develop both social interaction skills and expressive language or some type of expressive communication skills by Sam's age (Beeghly, Weiss-Perry, & Cicchetti, 1990; Berger, 1990; Serafica, 1990). The psychologist also noted the feeding clinic personnel's concerns that Sam showed characteristics that suggested autism. Therefore, the task of the psychologist was to ascertain the level of Sam's cognitive and adaptive development. The psychologist also planned to attempt to determine if the unusual characteristics noted by the feeding team were autistic-like behaviors not uncommon in children with severe developmental delays or whether Sam had autism co-occurring with Down syndrome (Howlin, Wing, & Gould, 1997). This exchange of information reflected the assessment's dynamic nature, in which flexibility and communication with other team members was essential even during a time-limited assessment process.

The preliminary plan was for the psychologist to assess Sam's developmental status and adaptive functioning formally and appropriately. In addition, the evaluation focused on Sam's reaction to social stimuli through observing his play, interviewing his parents, and using standardized questionnaires. The assessment tools planned to evaluate his general development were the Bayley Scales of Infant Development–Second Edition (BSID-II; Bayley, 1993) and the Vineland Adaptive Behavior Scales (VABS) interview form (Sparrow, Balla, & Cicchetti, 1984). The BSID-II is normed for children from birth to 42 months of age, and given Sam's developmental level, he would fall well within the BSID-II range. The BSID-II Mental Scale only was planned, as Sam's motor skills had already been evaluated by the occupational therapist.

In addition, the issue of autism was to be addressed by observations of Sam's behavior during free play and by discussion of Sam's developmental history with his parents. Gathering a history relevant to autism includes asking questions about the child's development of communication skills, current and past social interactions, play patterns, sensory responsiveness, and the ability to share gaze and reference with others. The psychologist also planned to use the Childhood Autism Rating Scale (CARS; Schopler, Reichler, & Renner, 1988) questionnaire, which employs interaction with and observation of the child during the assessment. The *Diagnostic and Statistical Manual of Mental Disorders, Fourth Edition* (DSM-IV; American Psychiatric Association, 1994), criteria for the diagnosis of autism were also considered when evaluating Sam.

Behavior Observations

Sam was accompanied to the psychology testing room by his father, and they were later joined by Sam's mother. Sam did not respond to the examiner's greeting. He resisted social contact, initially leaving the lobby and later sitting down in the testing room. Sam showed his displeasure by screaming and turning his back, although Sam's father was able to calm him by letting Sam cuddle with his favorite stuffed toy. When Sam became calm, he was willing to explore some of the testing toys. However, he interacted with the toys in an unusual way, such as dropping all round objects to watch them clatter and spin. He briefly handled other toys, then threw them aside. Sam directed his attention to his parents for brief periods of time but did not respond to the evaluator at all. When he became frustrated, Sam slapped his head and screamed angrily. He gave a variable effort on the evaluation, which was judged to reflect his functional level but perhaps not his best performance.

Test Results

On the BSID-II Mental Scale, Sam achieved an approximate developmental level of 6–9 months, which was significantly lower than his chronological age of 4 years and 10 months. Sam was willing to attempt only a portion of the tasks in any item set, so this evaluation may have underestimated his abilities in familiar or more comfortable surroundings. In addition, the approximate developmental level obtained from the BSID-II assessment may have been somewhat lower because Sam was not willing to attempt more tasks. Thus, concern arose with respect to the ecological validity of his test results. Nevertheless, these results appeared to confirm Sam's limited cognitive development. As suspected, based on his parents' and the school's reports, Sam's development was more delayed than expected for a child with Down syndrome. On the VABS, based on his parents' responses to interview questions, Sam's adaptive functioning in all areas was also very significantly delayed (Communication: 11 months; Daily Living Skills: 16 months; Socialization: 14 months). Behaviors of note at home included Sam's tendency to spend his time awake roaming around the house, experimenting with objects that made noise, and exploring objects with his mouth. He was interested in the computer and was unexpectedly accurate using the computer's mouse. His play was not social, although he sometimes engaged in parallel play beside children at preschool.

With respect to possible co-occurring autism, the psychologist used the CARS questionnaire, which includes judgments made while observing and interacting with the child as well as a parent report. Sam showed a number of characteristics typical of children with autism, including limitations in communication and social responsiveness that were more severe than would be expected even for a child with significant developmental delays. Other worrisome characteristics were unusual body use, such as finger posturing and slapping himself when angry; unusual object use, such as spinning objects and banging them to make noise; extreme resistance to changes in activities and routines; and unusual reactions to some textures, such as carpet. It was also likely that Sam's aversion to food textures and to finger feeding was related to autism. Furthermore, Sam was easily upset in social groups, such as family gatherings. Based on his score on the CARS questionnaire, observations of his behavior, and his parents' descriptions of their son's history and current functioning, Sam's characteristics were consistent with a diagnosis of mild-to-moderate autism. Sam's functioning also fit a categorical diagnosis of autism based on the criteria in the DSM-IV. Although children who have a significant cognitive delay sometimes show autistic-like behaviors (e.g., finger posturing), the number and cohesiveness of Sam's characteristics consistent with autism indicated that a diagnosis of co-occurring autism would be appropriate. This diagnosis would help Sam's family and school district develop an appropriate educational program for him.

Down Syndrome and Autism
Autism in children with Down syndrome is relatively rare, but it has been documented and estimated to occur at a rate of 4 to 5 per 100 children with Down syndrome. This small subgroup of children with Down syndrome tends to present with behavior problems and notable difficulty with social and communication skills (Ghaziuddin, Tsai, & Ghaziuddin, 1992; Howlin et al., 1997).

Typically, children with Down syndrome show comparatively strong social skills and are interested in other people and their surroundings. Their behavior is generally commensurate with their developmental level, and families of children with Down syndrome report relatively few behavioral or social concerns. In addition, children with Down syndrome usually show communication difficulties in areas of syntax and articulation rather than in pragmatic or social aspects (Kumin, 1994). For children in whom Down syndrome and autism co-occur, difficulties with communication are more extensive, including the limitations in developing joint attention and nonverbal communication skills seen in children with autism (Mundy, 1995). When evaluating a preverbal child such as Sam, one would look for attempts to establish joint attention to objects, such as coordinating his gaze with his parents' gaze. One would also look at whether the child was actively initiating nonverbal communication (e.g., pointing) for social purposes.

Psychology Summary and Tentative Recommendations
Based on this assessment, the psychologist's tentative conclusion was that Sam showed mild-to-moderate autism, as well as development of cognitive and adaptive skills below the norm for children with Down syndrome at his age. Pending confirmation of the diagnosis of autism from other team members, a number of specific recommendations that take into consideration these co-occurring diagnoses would be presented to the family. In particular, Sam would benefit from teaching techniques and curricula that have been developed for children with autism. These programs include the practice of building new skills using routines and scripts, increasing imitation and joint attention skills, increasing functional communication skills, and helping the child adapt to transitions.

Speech-Language Pathology
Sam willingly entered the speech-language pathology testing suite with his father. Once inside, the child put his hands over his face and did not respond to his father's repeated invitations to play. When the clinicians entered the room, Sam remained largely noncompliant or engaged in competitive behaviors. For example, he continually turned away from the clinicians, climbed on tables and chairs, and often yelled.

Sam was not particularly responsive to the clinicians when they attempted assessment by inviting him to play with toys. Physical prompts and verbal cues were not effective in getting Sam to interact socially. The clinicians therefore attempted to assess Sam's understanding of familiar words without contextual cues. He did not, however, give any overt evidence of understanding the lexical items tested. The clinicians then attempted to engage Sam in several communicative–social-action games (e.g., Pat-a-cake, Peekaboo). Regardless of the amount of cuing provided by the clinicians, Sam did not participate in these structured social interactions.

Parental reports are invaluable sources of information about a child's day-to-day progress in the early stages of language development. Therefore,

Sam's father was requested to complete the Words and Gestures portion of the MacArthur Communicative Development Inventories (CDI; Fensen et al., 1993). Results revealed that Sam's understanding of familiar phrases was near the 13-month level of functioning while his understanding of words was near the 10- to 11-month level. In addition, data from clinical observation and the CDI indicated Sam was just beginning to use communicative gestures, which is typically observed near the 10- to 11-month level. Furthermore, the CDI demonstrated that Sam did not imitate others or use words to communicate. Also of note was that Sam did not spontaneously produce or imitate words during low-structured interactions with his father. Although the clinicians were able to prompt Sam to imitate /i/ and /a/ on one occasion, structured elicitation tasks were largely ineffective. Sam was, however, beginning to engage in some vocal turn-taking.

Speech-Language Summary and Tentative Recommendations
Sam's comprehension, production, and social use of language were significantly delayed. The results obtained through nonstandardized assessments and parent report indicated an overall level of functioning of approximately 12 months. At the time of assessment, Sam's linguistic and communicative skills generally appeared to be commensurate with the nonverbal schemes he used for playing with objects. The fact that the clinicians' structured prompts and verbal cues had virtually no effect on Sam's linguistic performance suggested limited potential for immediate change in his expressive language. Finally, the evidence collected during the assessment was consistent with information reported by Sam's parents and school personnel, and it indicated possible autism.

Before this assessment, Sam had been receiving support services from the speech-language pathologist at his school. The Picture Exchange Communication System (PECS; Frost & Bondy, 1994) had been implemented, but its success was not yet clear. Based on the findings from this assessment, the PECS program remained an appropriate communicative system for Sam. Moreover, the interdisciplinary team believed that Sam would benefit from a treatment program designed to shape current vocalizations and communicative intentions into more salient and conventional acts. Sam's protests could be molded into more functional communication, and he could be enticed (using food or drink as a reward) to produce an intentional request.

Audiology
The most reliable procedure for testing hearing levels is the conditioned head-turn response (Wilson & Thompson, 1984). The use of a head turn toward a sound source has been used as a means of auditory assessment since the early 1980s. Visual reinforcement audiometry (VRA) has become a generic term to describe this approach to evaluate young children's hearing.

Previous research has shown that VRA can be used effectively to test the hearing of infants with typical development who are 6 months of age and older. Infants with Down syndrome, however, do not learn this task at the same age. Whereas infants with typical development who are 5 months of age initially localize to sound, only a small percentage of infants with Down syndrome are able to do so. Furthermore, analysis of the performance of infants with Down syndrome on the basis of developmental age shows that those with Down syndrome do not successfully learn the conditioned head-turn response until 10–12 months of developmental age. The difference in age between children with typical development and children with Down syndrome in terms of acquiring the conditioned head-turn response cannot be explained on the basis of underlying auditory systems. More likely, delays in cognitive development as well as differences in problem-solving behavior and skill maintenance undermine acquisition of this behavior (Wishart, 1991, 1993).

Previous attempts to assess Sam's hearing were unsuccessful. The child's hearing was evaluated initially using VRA, but Sam was unable to achieve a level of conditioning required to carry out reliable hearing assessment. An attempt was then made to test Sam's hearing using behavioral observation audiometry (BOA). In BOA, sounds are presented and any reaction by the child is used to assess response to sound. Sam demonstrated no observable responses to any of the auditory stimuli presented during VRA or to noisemakers presented during BOA. This lack of responsiveness may have been due to the autistic characteristics and significant developmental delay noted in the other discipline evaluations.

Because neither conditioned nor unconditioned behavior responses to sound were observed, yet Sam reportedly responded to sound at home, physiological assessment of hearing was carried out. The auditory brainstem response (ABR)—a surface-recorded, electrophysiological response—can provide an estimate of hearing sensitivity in children who cannot otherwise actively participate in hearing assessment (see Chapter 2). Click-evoked ABRs were obtained from Sam and the intensity of the stimulus was manipulated to determine the lowest level at which a detectable response was elicited. Upon completion of the test, all recordings were analyzed for both presence of a response and the latency of the waves within each response. The click-evoked ABR provides an indication of hearing sensitivity for the frequency range of approximately 2,000–8,000 hertz. Using this method for Sam's assessment, clear ABRs were recorded down to an intensity level of 10 decibels of hearing loss for both the right and left ears. Latencies were within the expected range for children of his age with Down syndrome. These findings were consistent with typical hearing sensitivity in each ear.

Audiology Summary and Tentative Recommendations
Given these findings of normal hearing sensitivity, hearing loss did not appear to contribute to Sam's developmental delays. Nevertheless, it was recommended that Sam's hearing be rechecked (including utilizing tympanometry) at 6-month intervals to monitor possible change resulting from either conductive

or sensory disorder, which is more frequent in children with Down syndrome than in children with typical development, or other hearing impairments.

INTEGRATION OF DISCIPLINARY INFORMATION AND RECOMMENDATIONS

The interdisciplinary team members assembled briefly before meeting with Sam's parents and Sam's teacher at his preschool (who was included because recommendations for education were a primary issue). The team members discussed their findings, and conclusions were drawn based on the results of all the professionals involved. Sam's parents were already aware of the atypical nature of their son's developmental delays, but the finding of autism would be new to them. Information provided by all disciplines—including the feeding team (nursing, nutrition, and occupational therapy), pediatrics, psychology, speech-language pathology, and audiology—was important to establish a diagnosis of autism. All of the disciplines concurred with the finding of autism.

Sam's parents and preschool teacher then joined the discipline members for the conference. The general findings of each discipline were presented to them, and Sam's strengths were emphasized whenever possible and integrated into the recommendations. The team members also focused on those aspects of Sam's development that were unique to his case and on the specific concerns of his parents. For example, Sam's sensitivity to food textures and other sensory input was noted, as were his lack of both social responsiveness and communication skills (beyond the delays expected for a child with Down syndrome), limited play skills, and unusual behaviors. It was explained that these characteristics suggested that Sam had an autism spectrum disorder in addition to the delays and characteristics associated with Down syndrome. The co-occurrence of autism with Down syndrome is rare but documented in the literature (e.g., Ghaziuddin et al., 1992; Howlin et al., 1997). In Sam's case, autism and developmental delay appeared to interact with each other, resulting in a very low level of functional skills. Some of the behaviors associated with autism but not Down syndrome (e.g., differences in reactions to sensory stimuli, resistance to changes in routine) were likely contributing to Sam's difficulty with feeding. Sam's parents and his teacher discussed the issue of autism with the team. The teacher said that his behavior resembled that of other children with autism she had in her class. Sam's parents agreed that it explained some of their concerns about Sam's development.

The team, Sam's parents, and the teacher then discussed recommendations that might be helpful at school and at home. Team suggestions focused on consideration of present and future services and supports. The feeding recommendations were discussed first, as feeding was the issue of concern that prompted this evaluation. The group also agreed that Sam should continue attending his developmental preschool. At the time of assessment, it was decided that although Sam would probably function best in a self-contained classroom, some inclusion with peers having typical development would encourage Sam's social development. His educational program should focus on communication, encouraging social skills, and improving life skills. Sam's teacher was familiar with the various resources available for the teaching of children with autism (e.g., the TEACCH System, as outlined in Schopler, Mesibov, & Hearsey, 1995). A list of reading resources on this subject was given to Sam's parents and his teacher. The team also noted that occupational and speech-language therapy would be needed in the foreseeable future. Furthermore, planning for the special education services that Sam would require throughout his school years was recommended.

Sam's parents were also given information about autism and appropriate parent support groups. They were referred to the Autism Society of America, a national organization that provides resources and support. In addition, they were given handouts that answered specific questions about autism and described some useful behavior management techniques (Dawson & Osterling, 1997; Freeman, 1997). Sam's parents already belonged to a Down syndrome parents' support group and did not appear to require more information about Down syndrome.

Finally, the group agreed that the feeding clinic recommendations outlined previously should be given to Sam's preschool occupational therapist. New aspects of his therapy should involve working on sensory sensitivity and helping him adapt to changes in his feeding routine. The interdisciplinary team speech-language pathologist agreed to share the recommendations and information about the PECS system directly with Sam's school speech-language therapist. A reevaluation of Sam's hearing was also recommended for the next clinic evaluation. A comprehensive reassessment of Sam's development in approximately 1 year was suggested to evaluate his progress after the implementation of new educational and feeding strategies. The team expressed optimism that Sam's skills and general responsiveness would improve with the additional intervention.

REFERENCES

American Psychiatric Association. (1994). *Diagnostic and statistical manual of mental disorders* (4th ed.). Washington, DC: Author.

Bayley, N. (1993). *Bayley Scales of Infant Development–Second Edition*. San Antonio, TX: The Psychological Corp.

Beeghly, M., Weiss-Perry, B., & Cicchetti, D. (1990). Beyond sensorimotor functioning: Early communicative development of children with Down syndrome. In D. Cicchetti & M. Beeghly (Eds.), *Children with Down syndrome: A developmental perspective* (pp. 329–368). Cambridge, United Kingdom: Cambridge University Press.

Berger, J. (1990). Interactions between parents and their infants with Down syndrome. In D. Cicchetti & M. Beeghly (Eds.), *Children with Down syndrome: A developmental perspective* (pp. 101–146). Cambridge, United Kingdom: Cambridge University Press.

Dawson, G., & Osterling, J. (1997). Early intervention in autism. In M. J. Guralnick (Ed.), *The effectiveness of early intervention* (pp. 307–326). Baltimore: Paul H. Brookes Publishing Co.

Fensen, L., Dale, P., Reznick, J.S., Thal, D., Bates, E., Hartung, J., Pethcik, S., & Reilly, J. (1993). *MacArthur Communicative Development Inventories (CDI)*. San Diego, CA: Singular Publishing Group.

Freeman, B.J. (1997). Guidelines for evaluating intervention programs for children with autism. *Journal of Autism and Developmental Disorders, 27,* 641–651.

Frost, L., & Bondy, A. (1994). *The Picture Exchange Communication System (PECS) Training Manual.* Cherry, NJ: PECS.

Ghaziuddin, M., Tsai, L., & Ghaziuddin, N. (1992). Autism in Down syndrome: Presentation and diagnosis. *Journal of Intellectual Disability, 36,* 449–456.

Howlin, P., Wing, L., & Gould, J. (1997). The recognition of autism in children with Down syndrome: Implications for intervention and some speculations about pathology. In M. Hertzig & E. Farber (Eds.), *Annual progress in child psychiatry and child development–1996* (pp. 406–414). Levittown, PA: Brunner/Mazel Publishing.

Kumin, L. (1994). Intelligibility of speech in children with Down syndrome in natural settings: Parents' perspective. *Perceptual and Motor Skills, 78,* 307–313.

Mundy, P. (1995). Joint attention and social-emotional approach behavior in children with autism [Special issue: Emotions in developmental psychopathology]. *Development and Psychopathology, 7,* 63–82.

Schopler, E., Mesibov, G., & Hearsey, K. (1995). Structured teaching in the TEACCH System. In E. Schopler & G. Mesibov (Eds.), *Learning and cognition in autism* (pp. 243–268). New York: Plenum Publishing Corp.

Schopler, E., Reichler, R.J., & Renner, B. (1988). *The Childhood Autism Rating Scale (CARS).* Los Angeles: Western Psychological Services.

Serafica, F. (1990). Peer relations of children with Down syndrome. In D. Cicchetti & M. Beeghly (Eds.), *Children with Down syndrome: A developmental perspective* (pp. 369–398). Cambridge, United Kingdom: Cambridge University Press.

Sparrow, S., Balla, D., & Cicchetti, D. (1984). *Vineland Adaptive Behavior Scales (VABS).* Circle Pines, MN: American Guidance Service.

Wilson, W.R., & Thompson, G. (1984). Behavioral audiometry. In J. Jerger (Ed.), *Pediatric audiology* (pp. 1–44). San Diego, CA: College-Hill Press.

Wishart, J. (1991). Take the initiative in learning: A developmental investigation of infants with Down syndrome. *International Journal of Disability, Development and Education, 38,* 27–44.

Wishart, J. (1993). The development of learning difficulties in children with Down's syndrome. *Journal of Intellectual Disability Research, 34,* 389–403.

Chapter 13

An Infant
with Phenylketonuria

*Cristine M. Trahms, Anne Leavitt,
Janie Heffernan, and Janet Garretson*

Phenylketonuria (PKU) is an impairment in the enzyme phenylalanine hydroxylase (PAH), which causes phenylalanine and some of its metabolites to
accumulate in the blood and other body tissues. The buildup of these compounds leads to toxicity that results in mental retardation and related neurodevelopmental problems. In terms of genetics, phenylketonuria is the absence
or inactivity of PAH and is an autosomal recessive disorder. Autosomal recessive disorders are expressed only in the individuals who have inherited an affected gene from each parent. If both parents are carriers of the affected gene,
the risk of passing the affected gene to their children is one in four with each
pregnancy. The overall incidence of phenylketonuria is about 1 in 16,000 live
births in most populations. It is believed that the genetic alterations that cause
phenylketonuria are more common in people of northern European descent.

It was once thought that PAH was inactive or deficient in all children
with elevated phenylalanine levels. However, it was determined in 1985 that

1%–3% of these children have a normal PAH gene, and the elevated blood phenylalanine levels are due to an impairment in a co-factor of PAH (tetrahydrobiopterin, BH_4). These children do not respond to the phenylalanine restricted diet and require the administration of other compounds to normalize the affected neurotransmitters. Prenatal diagnosis for phenylketonuria is available for families with at least one affected child.

Before newborn screening programs were established, phenylketonuria was first suspected when a child presented with mental retardation or neurological symptoms such as seizures, ataxia, or behavior disorders. Newborn screening of infants, plus early and rigorous treatment, has changed this once devastating disorder into a manageable condition, and mental retardation can be prevented. However, the critical timing of initiation of treatment and the continuous need for dietary intervention and controlling blood phenylalanine levels to prevent neurological damage present challenges for the child, the family, and the interdisciplinary support team.

TREATMENT OF PHENYLKETONURIA

The goal for managing phenylketonuria is to achieve and maintain blood phenylalanine concentrations between 2 and 6 milligrams per deciliter (mg/dl) as quickly as possible. Dietary management must begin as soon as possible in the neonatal period to prevent interference with typical growth and development of the brain and nervous system (Medical Research Council Working Party on Phenylketonuria, 1993). It is expected that blood phenylalanine concentrations can be decreased to a safe range within 3–4 days of starting treatment. Due to the fact that infants and young children grow rapidly, blood phenylalanine concentrations must be measured frequently. When phenylketonuria is first detected, blood samples are taken every other day. This need for testing subsides to once per month by the time a child is 6 months of age, as blood phenylalanine concentrations, tolerance for phenylalanine, and growth stabilize.

Nutritional Considerations

As phenylalanine is necessary for typical growth, development, and protein metabolism, changes in an infant's formula prescription are frequent to ensure the provision of adequate nourishment. In addition, because tyrosine is an amino acid that is produced as a result of the breakdown of phenylalanine, it must be supplemented to obtain proper metabolic functioning. Thus, nutritional treatment of phenylketonuria consists of a low-phenylalanine, tyrosine-supplemented diet plus the recommended intake of calories of energy and all other nutrients to promote typical growth and neurological development.

Phenylalanine and tyrosine levels are usually 1–2 mg/dl in the blood of unaffected people. Some clinical management teams consider phenylalanine levels of 2–10 mg/dl appropriate for individuals having phenylketonuria. However, it is believed that safe blood phenylalanine concentrations, which promote typical cognitive and physical development, are in the range of 2–6 mg/dl, with tyrosine levels of 1–2 mg/dl (Diamond, 1994; Report of the Medical Research Council Working Party on Phenylketonuria, 1993).

Safe blood phenylalanine concentrations cannot be achieved without the use of a phenylalanine-free, tyrosine-supplemented medical formula to provide 80%–90% of daily nourishment. It is expected that blood phenylalanine concentrations will rapidly decrease and then stabilize after the initiation of treatment. No food other than formula is offered for the first 6 months so that families have an opportunity to adjust to the diagnosis before they are involved in the manipulation of foods. All protein foods (e.g., meat, chicken, fish, dairy products, legumes) are eliminated from the food pattern. Fruits, vegetables not from the legume family, low-protein pasta, breads, and cereals provide energy. This dietary treatment demands time and commitment from parents and other caregivers and requires learning, assimilating, and putting into practice a great deal of new information by all involved (Trahms, 1996).

Phenylketonuria treatment is lifelong; therefore, there is no time at which treatment can safely be discontinued. Education of families and primary care providers (PCPs) is important. Achieving the narrow band of biochemical control requires the support of the family by the PKU clinic team and all community providers, who must have an adequate knowledge base so the families are not confused by conflicting information.

OUTCOME OF PHENYLKETONURIA TREATMENT

Untreated, phenylketonuria results in an IQ score of less than 50. There are several factors related to IQ score in cases in which phenylketonuria is treated. These are the infant's age at diagnosis, the age at which the infant achieved safe blood phenylalanine concentrations due to nutrition therapy, and biochemical control over time. The age at diagnosis and start of the nutrition therapy depend on the effectiveness of a hospital's newborn screening program and the availability of an organized treatment program, as infants with phenylketonuria do not manifest any impairments until they are several months of age (Committee on Genetics, 1996).

IQ scores fall linearly and progressively with each week treatment is delayed and with each continued elevation of phenylalanine concentration during treatment. The National PKU Collaborative Study (Williamson, Koch, Azen, & Chang, 1981) identified several predictive factors for IQ score attainment. First of all, the study data supported a relationship between the age of an infant at diagnosis and eventual IQ scores as well as one between long-term blood phenylalanine concentrations and eventual IQ scores (Koch & Wenz, 1987). In addition, the study suggested that blood phenylalanine concentrations in the range of 2–10 mg/dl supported development of typical global IQ score attainment (Azen et al., 1991; Waisbren, Mahon, Schnell, & Levy, 1987). Furthermore, it was suggested in the 1990s that lower blood phenylalanine concentrations, between 2 and 6 mg/dl, foster improved prefrontal lobe functioning (Diamond, 1994; Smith, Beasley, & Ades, 1990). However, although children with well-managed cases of phenylketonuria may not develop mental retardation, they may have subtle learning delays that can interfere with academic performance. There continues to be the need to evaluate treatment in an effort to optimize growth and cognitive development.

People who have discontinued nutrition treatment or who have elevated blood phenylalanine concentrations due to nonadherence to treatment guidelines have manifested neuropsychiatric disturbances, agoraphobia, and memory impairments. Magnetic resonance imaging scans have shown changes in the brain's white matter and effects in the frontal cortex (Legido et al., 1993; Seashore, Friedman, Novella, & Bapat, 1985).

PROTOCOL FOR NEWBORN SCREENING AND CONFIRMATION OF DIAGNOSIS OF PHENYLKETONURIA

Newborn screening for phenylketonuria is available throughout the United States; however, each state has its own legislative guidelines. For example, in some states, it is required that infants have a Guthrie test—a heelstick blood sample drawn for qualitative newborn screening—in the newborn period. Presumptive positive tests are those with blood phenylalanine concentrations greater than 3 mg/dl in infants at birth or at 1 day of age. A follow-up test is immediately requested for these infants. In addition, a second test is requested for all infants at the first well-baby checkup, usually at 7–10 days of age.

If the second Guthrie bacterial inhibition assay test results are above 3 mg/dl, the infant is referred for quantitative blood tests and confirmation of the diagnosis of phenylketonuria. Confirmation of phenylketonuria requires at least two blood phenylalanine concentrations greater than 6 mg/dl and a tyrosine concentration less than 2 mg/dl. The goal is to identify and initiate treatment for affected infants as quickly as possible. It is generally accepted that treatment should be initiated before the infant is 14 days of age.

PKU TEAM

A PKU team is committed to two strategies for effective treatment: immediate confirmation of diagnosis and initiation of the low-phenylalanine diet as well as long-term education and support for children with phenylketonuria and their families (Trahms, 1986). A PKU clinic team is structured to meet these two objectives. All infants, children, adolescents, and adults with phenylketonuria are followed longitudinally with frequent, regularly scheduled clinic visits for nutritional assessment, neurological evaluation, parent support groups, and activities to develop self-management. There is a protocol for formal neuropsychological assessment at specific ages. Because each family is seen many times after the initial diagnostic visit, PKU clinic visits may be somewhat streamlined and team members might share roles depending on the needs of the family.

The preliminary conference is often conducted on an urgent basis because of the need for confirmation of diagnosis and initiation of treatment. The PKU team is a specialized, interdisciplinary team consisting of members from various disciplines: medicine (genetics, pediatrics), nutrition, social work, psychology, nursing, and genetic counseling. The team members work together to confirm the diagnosis, to initiate appropriate treatment, and to help and educate families and children as they work to manage this potentially devastating disorder. To activate effective treatment and to build a reliable support for the family, team members need to be firmly grounded in the expertise of their disciplines, to be experienced in the treatment of metabolic disorders, and to have a firm belief in the effectiveness of the interdisciplinary team process as well as family-centered care. It is the recommendation of the American Academy of Pediatrics that "a facility that specializes in the management of inborn errors of metabolism" be involved with the care of these children (Committee on Genetics, 1996, p. 489). Regional Genetics Centers are valuable resources in this regard because the staff have experience in the diagnosis and long-term treatment of metabolic disorders. Children with phenylketonuria require intense and consistent management of biochemical parameters and developmentally specific nutrition management and education. This goal is best achieved by a team consisting of families and professionals committed to phenylketonuria treatment.

This team effort is explored in the following case study. Included are discussions regarding a newborn screening program, the coordination process within a PKU team, the critical timing for diagnosis, the initiation of treatment, and the management of phenylketonuria. In addition, the case study describes the interaction with community providers—such as PCPs, public health nurses (PHNs), and Child Protective Services (CPS) workers—to support families as they work to manage phenylketonuria. Finally, a system of support services for families whose children have phenylketonuria is detailed.

CASE STUDY INVOLVING AN
INTERDISCIPLINARY TEAM ASSESSMENT

The state newborn screening program reported a presumptive positive diagnosis of phenylketonuria for a newborn named Sally. The sample for Guthrie bacterial inhibition assay, drawn at 1 day of age and evaluated when the infant was 1 week old, indicated a phenylalanine level of 8 mg/dl. The newborn screening coordinator contacted the PKU team and Sally's PCP to report the initial presumptive positive blood level.

The PCP, a family practice physician, discussed the newborn screening report with the family. As the family lived a significant distance from the laboratory, it was decided that rather than following the usual procedure to repeat the Guthrie test, blood for a quantitative sample would be drawn and sent to the central laboratory at a children's hospital. The results of the quantitative sample were received 2 days later, when Sally was 9 days old. The blood phenylalanine concentration was 29.4 mg/dl, and the tyrosine concentration was 0.9 mg/dl. These laboratory results confirmed the diagnosis of phenylketonuria. Blood and urine samples were also collected for standard biopterin and dehydropteridine reductase screening to rule out the possibility of the potentially fatal secondary disorders of phenylalanine metabolism.

Preliminary and Preassessment Conference
All information available from the newborn screening program referral was reviewed by the PKU team at an intake conference prior to meeting with the family. This information consisted primarily of the birth report and laboratory values (see the PKU clinic intake form in the Appendix at the end of this book). Because of the urgency of intervention, the family was given an immediate referral and an appointment for the next day with the PKU team for initiation of treatment and an introduction to phenylketonuria and its management.

Initial Meeting with the Family
The initial family assessment and commencement of the treatment process was conducted by the pediatrician, the nutritionist, and the social worker. The goal of these professionals would be to work together to minimize assessment time and to coordinate contacts with the family and Sally's PCP. The nutritionist was chosen as the initial service coordinator because of the urgency of nutrition management. However, all team members knew that this designation could change depending on the strengths, needs, and concerns of the family.

Sally's parents were anxious at the initial meeting because their child was not "perfect." In addition, they were confused: They had been urged to have Sally's blood drawn again, and the answers to their questions and worries were not yet available. The team functions at this point were to confirm the diagnosis, to explain phenylketonuria to Sally's parents, to reassure them of the positive long-term prognosis with early diagnosis and treatment, and to begin building the bonds for a long-term partnership with this family. It was also made known that teaching protocol might take several sessions, depending on the family's needs and their ability to begin adjusting to the diagnosis. The initial team members described their roles and the services they could offer to the family. Sally's parents were also given a "PKU Pal," a notebook containing all of the information described in the early clinic visits.

Discipline Summaries
After this introductory meeting, individual assessments were conducted according to each team member's discipline. The findings of the pediatric, nutrition, and social work assessments are summarized in the next three sections.

Pediatrics
At the initial clinic appointment, the diagnostic process was completed by collecting blood and urine samples for co-factor variant screening, which eliminated the possibility of the biopterin defect in phenylalanine metabolism for

Sally. Her blood phenylalanine concentrations at this visit were phenylalanine at 37 mg/dl and tyrosine at 0.9 mg/dl.

The physical exam showed that Sally was a typical 9-day-old infant who was born after a typical full-term pregnancy and an uncomplicated labor and delivery. Her birth weight was 3.4 kilograms (kg), which was in the 50th percentile according to National Center for Health Statistics (NCHS, 1976) growth charts. Sally's birth length was 48 centimeters (cm), at the NCHS growth charts' 25th percentile. Finally, her birth head circumference was 34.5 cm, placing her in the 50th percentile of NCHS growth charts.

At the time of assessment, the infant's weight was 3.6 kg (50th percentile), her length was 48 cm (25th percentile), her weight for length was at the 50th percentile, and her head circumference was 35 cm (50th percentile). She had normal muscle tone and deep tendon reflexes, good sucking ability, and no odor of phenylacetic acid. Examination of her cardiac status, auscultation of lungs, and palpation of abdomen as well as an evaluation of extremities were all normal.

A telephone contact was made with the PCP to discuss plans for immediate follow-up and to schedule weight checks and blood draws. Conversations with parents and PCP resulted in a contract for such visits to the PCP every second day until blood phenylalanine levels were decreased and stabilized in a safe range. In addition, the family was referred to a genetic counselor for discussion of the recurrence risk of phenylketonuria in subsequent pregnancies.

Nutrition

The nutritional assessment indicated that Sally was feeding well, taking 20–22 ounces (oz) of standard infant formula in 24 hours. Her parents reported appropriate formula preparation. Furthermore, they responded appropriately to cues from Sally for cuddling and attention. As a result, Sally was growing well, having gained 200 grams (g) since birth.

Treatment via diet was started immediately. A phenylalanine-restricted formula was prescribed to meet the nutrition goals for treating phenylketonuria. The initial formula prescription was organized to provide adequate energy and protein but to eliminate all phenylalanine for 48–72 hours. This served to reduce blood phenylalanine concentrations from toxic levels to the safe range more quickly. However, this process necessitated careful monitoring of blood phenylalanine concentrations to avoid a phenylalanine deficiency; phenylalanine deficiency can be as devastating as phenylalanine excess for the young infant. Therefore, the primary formula prescription was set to provide enough phenylalanine to meet requirements for Sally's physical growth and brain development; to meet her protein, energy, and fluid needs; and not to exceed her renal concentrating capability. (In general, these parameters are 60 mg phenylalanine/kg, 2.5 g protein/kg, 110 kilocalories (kcal) energy/kg, and 20 kcal/fluid oz of formula.)

Sally's parents were instructed on formula preparation for phenylketonuria management. They were also given written instructions for both the initial and primary formula preparations, enough phenylalanine-restricted formula for 2 weeks, a scale to use to weigh formula powder accurately, and a notebook in which to record Sally's daily formula intake. In addition, the booklet *New Parents' Guide to PKU* (Trahms & Luce, 1990) was provided for the family.

Social Work

Sally's parents were a young married couple whose parents opposed their relationship; thus, they eloped when the pregnancy was identified. Both had completed substance abuse rehabilitation programs. The father did not finish high school and was unemployed; the mother, who finished high school, provided child care for her aunt's children. As a result of these circumstances, finances and transportation were significant problems for this couple. They also did not have a telephone. Based on this assessment, the family was immediately placed in a high-risk category for future interventions.

Information was gathered for the family regarding the following resources and services: the local department of health services for possible financial assistance; transportation assistance; medical coupons; the Special Supplemental Nutrition Program for Women, Infants, and Children (WIC) program vouchers; and the department of health for a regular supply of phenylalanine-restricted formula for Sally. Because the family did not have a telephone, the aunt's telephone was established as the means for contacting the family.

Integration of Disciplinary Information and Recommendations

A PKU team generally meets weekly to discuss the current statuses of children with phenylketonuria, their progress, and the needs of their families. In this situation, the team met to determine the primary concerns in Sally's case, agree on an approach to the family, and organize as much support as possible for them. It was recognized by the team that, in spite of the imperative need to initiate treatment, the family may not have been ready to act on all aspects of care. It was the PKU team's responsibility to build connections with community providers for Sally's ongoing care as well as to help the family remove as many barriers to care as possible. Thus, the PKU team sought to establish such links for Sally and her family because of their limited communication and transportation resources. As the couple was inexperienced at parenting and appeared to have a limited family support system, resources in the community to support family life were sought for them. In addition, the need to bring blood phenylalanine concentrations into a safe range was critical for Sally's welfare, so local support services were sought in cooperation with the PCP.

The PCP was designated the primary community contact because of the need for monitoring Sally's physical progress and for blood draws. Because blood samples would be needed every second day until levels were in a safe range, a system was put in place to transport blood samples quickly to a children's hospital. This would relieve the family of having to make frequent trips to the PKU clinic while still meeting the progress monitoring needs. The PKU clinic nutritionist would report blood draw results to the PCP and to the family. The PCP would report physical findings to the PKU team. In this way, Sally's phenylketonuria treatment could be coordinated. Finally, the PKU clinic social worker would continue to organize efforts for providing appropriate resources for this family. A letter detailing the recommendations from this visit was dictated and mailed to the PCP, along with current articles and phenylketonuria treatment guidelines (see the Appendix at the end of this book for PKU management guidelines).

Follow-Up Communications

As previously stated, a PKU clinic team must make every effort to establish communication systems with families and care providers of children with phenylketonuria because treatment is urgent and rigorous and requires extensive family, clinical, and community resources. Management of phenylketonuria is not easy for a well-organized family with adequate resources; it is especially difficult for a family at high risk, having few resources and support systems. Therefore, follow-up in all cases is essential.

Within 1 week of Sally's initial visit, the PCP and the PKU team became concerned about the family's progress due to lack of follow-through by the parents. Specifically, this was the result of the following problems: 1) the family was not available as agreed for telephone contact, 2) the family did not keep appointments with the PCP for blood draws and weight checks, and 3) the family did not attend appointments regarding financial assistance and medical transportation. The PKU clinic social worker tried to contact the family. There was no answer and no message-taking device at the message telephone. Consequently, the PKU team initiated discussions with the PCP about a CPS referral to facilitate family support by providing medical transportation and a telephone by which to receive calls. Furthermore, a letter was sent to Sally's parents outlining the concerns about their daughter's blood phenylalanine concentrations and the need for monitoring. The letter again provided telephone numbers and addresses of available resources.

One week later the family had an appointment with the PCP, who later shared her concerns with the PKU team. Sally had not gained weight, and the parents reported having difficulty encouraging her to feed. Sally appeared to be irritable, had decreased muscle tone, and was taking only 10 oz of the prescribed 22 oz of formula per day. Blood was drawn for phenylalanine and tyrosine determinations. A dangerously elevated blood phenylalanine concentration of 19.5 mg/dl was reported from the laboratory and the PKU team to the PCP. A plan, negotiated by the nutritionist and the PCP (who contacted the family), was developed to increase the concentration of the formula to 24 kcal/oz to maximize energy intake in a tolerable volume, to make a PHN referral to assess the feeding situation and the parents' responses to Sally's hunger cues, and to continue coordinating with the PCP and the PHN with respect to checks for weight gain and monitoring for blood phenylalanine levels.

The nutritionist was not able to connect with the family to assess Sally's intake of formula, and the PCP was notified of this situation. A second attempt to reach the family was unsuccessful. This was a critical problem because the PKU team felt reassessment of Sally's status was critical and a change in formula was needed. The PCP agreed. The social worker was redesignated as the service coordinator because it was his discipline's specialty to determine and resolve family barriers. The social worker was also willing to continue working with community providers to establish a system of appropriate services and monitoring.

Telephone contact was finally established with the family 2 days later. The father adamantly asserted that they did not want the PHN to visit them and that they felt harassed by the health care system. The PKU team's concerns about problems with communication were stated, and Sally's father reluctantly agreed to provide a time and place for regular telephone contact. The PKU team and the PCP's concerns about the blood phenylalanine concentrations and the growth of the infant were shared as well. The father asserted that he had not been given any information about the danger of high blood phenylalanine concentrations and did not know that there was a need to worry about his daughter's growth. He stated that now that he was aware of these concerns, he would agree to a PKU clinic visit in 1 week.

The family failed to keep the appointment. In a follow-up telephone conversation with Sally's father, he refused an appointment with the PCP and a PHN visit. CPS was contacted and, based on a report of medical neglect, they provided transportation and mandated a visit to the PKU clinic for reevaluation of the infant.

Reevaluation

The information noted in the medical record from telephone conversations with the PCP and Sally's family was reviewed by the PKU team prior to meeting with her parents. The main issues were identified as 1) the critical need to bring Sally's blood phenylalanine concentrations into the safe range for management and prevention of mental retardation, 2) Sally's failure to grow and the possible relationship of this poor growth to inadequate parental response to hunger cues and preparation of formula, 3) the parents' level of understanding of Sally's disorder and its management, 4) the difficulties her parents had with responding to the concerns of health care providers about their child, and 5) the need to continue gathering resources for the benefit of Sally and her parents. All of these matters were discussed in the context of needing to build a trusting relationship with the family.

Child Protective Services Referral

CPS referrals are usually discussed with the child's PCP. A PKU clinic team may refer a child with phenylketonuria to CPS for several reasons. Examples include the following:

1. Families of children with phenylketonuria who demonstrate poor meta-bolic control or who are not willing to meet with the PKU clinic team are putting their children in danger. An unwillingness to bring children to the clinic, to work with a local PHN, or to have blood phenylalanine levels measured regularly are all manifestations of such unwillingness.
2. Children who demonstrate a condition secondary to phenylketonuria, such as failure to grow, or appear to be mistreated or abused may also be referred. The conditions of neglect or a secondary illness can influence ef-fective management of phenylketonuria.
3. Families that do not have access to adequate resources based on financial eligibility may also cause a report to CPS. In these cases, a discussion is held with the family to help them attain such resources, which might in-clude family counseling, respite care, parenting classes, or transportation.

Before a referral to CPS is made, the PKU team makes every effort to work with the family to meet the child's needs and to institute effective preven-tive treatment. In these situations, PKU team discussions center on the barriers to compliance from the family's point of view, a decision regarding when fail-ure to foster weight gain and noncompliance with phenylketonuria treatment become medical neglect, and a determination if additional services would sup-port the family as they struggle to manage this rigorous medical therapy.

CONCLUSION

In general, families do not have as much difficulty as Sally's did in adjusting to the diagnosis and required treatment of phenylketonuria. However, because newborn infants show no outward signs of this disorder, the diagnosis of phe-nylketonuria always surprises families. They further respond to the diagnosis in different ways. The denial and fear shown by Sally's parents is an unusually strong response. Most families are sad and fearful but respond positively to in-formation and support. All families need time and encouragement as they ad-just to having a new child in the family and at the same time adjust to the di-agnosis of phenylketonuria.

Some families prefer learning new information by reading; others prefer discussion. Some families want all available information; others want the tools to make changes and detailed information later. The effective PKU clinic team tries to accommodate different learning and coping styles as they work with families. Families are assured that learning about phenylketonuria is a gradual process and that the PKU team will support them at each step.

Families are usually able to comply with the early treatment requirements of frequent blood draws and contact with the PKU team. Often grandparents or other extended family members who are involved in the child's care attend PKU clinic appointments, both for their own education as well as to support the immediate family.

It is expected that children with phenylketonuria who are diagnosed as a result of newborn screening and who maintain stable blood phenylalanine concentrations will have typical intellectual and physical development. Although the requirements for treatment are rigorous, there is cause for optimism because the devastating neurological damage from phenylketonuria can be avoided. Families are provided support and information as they work with their children to develop self-management skills and independence in taking care of their own disorder.

REFERENCES

Azen, C.G., Koch, R., Friedman, E.G., Berlow, S., Coldwell, J., Krause, W., Matalon, R., McCabe, E., O'Flynn, M., Peterson, R., Rouse, B., Scott, C.R., Sigman, B., Valle, D., & Warner, R. (1991). Intellectual development in 12-year-old children treated for phenylketonuria. *American Journal of Diseases of Childhood, 145*, 35–39.
Committee on Genetics. (1996). Newborn screening fact sheets. *Pediatrics, 98*, 473–498.
Diamond, A. (1994). Phenylalanine levels of 6–10 mg/dL may not be as benign as once thought. *Acta Paediatrica Supplement, 407*, 89–91.
Koch, R., & Wenz, E. (1987). Phenylketonuria. *Annual Review of Nutrition, 7*, 117–135.
Legido, A., Tonyes, L., Carter, D., Schoemaker, A., DiGeorge, A., & Grover, W.D. (1993). Treatment variables and intellectual outcome in children with classic phenylketonuria. *Clinical Pediatrics, 32*, 417–435.
Medical Research Council Working Party on Phenylketonuria. (1993). Phenylketonuria due to phenylalanine hydroxylase deficiency: An unfolding story. *British Medical Journal, 306*, 115–119.
National Center for Health Statistics. (1976). NCHS Growth Charts. *Monthly Vital Statistics Report, 25*(3) (Suppl. [HRA]), 76–1120.
Report of the Medical Research Council Working Party on Phenylketonuria. (1993). Recommendations on the dietary management of phenylketonuria. *Archives of Diseases in Childhood, 68*, 426–427.
Seashore, M.R., Friedman, E., Novella, R.A., & Bapat, V. (1985). Loss of intellectual functioning in children with phenylketonuria after relaxation of dietary phenylalanine restriction. *Pediatrics, 75*, 226–232.
Smith, I., Beasley, M.G., & Ades, A.E. (1990). Intelligence and quality of dietary treatment in phenylketonuria. *Archives of Diseases in Childhood, 65*, 472–478.
Trahms, C.M. (1986). Long-term nutrition intervention model: The treatment of phenylketonuria. *Topics in Clinical Nutrition, 1*, 62–72.
Trahms, C.M. (1996). Nutritional care in metabolic disorders. In L.K. Mahan. & S. Escott-Stump (Eds.), *Krause's food, nutrition, and diet therapy* (9th ed.). Philadelphia: W.B. Saunders Company.
Trahms, C.M., & Luce, P. (1990). *New parents' guide to PKU.* Seattle: University of Washington Press.
Waisbren, S.E., Mahon, B.E., Schnell, R.R., & Levy, H.L. (1987). Predictors of intelligence quotient and intelligence quotient change in persons treated for phenylketonuria in early life. *Pediatrics, 79*, 351–355.
Williamson, M.L., Koch, R., Azen, C., & Chang, C. (1981). Correlates of intelligence test results in treated phenylketonuric children. *Pediatrics, 68*, 161–167.

Chapter 14

A Child with an
Autism Spectrum Disorder

*Julie A. Osterling, Carla A. Brooks,
Alan S. Unis, and Renee Watling*

Since the late 1980s, considerable progress has occurred in the field of early identification and treatment of young children with autism. In the area of early intervention, outcomes of children with autism who receive intervention are more positive than once achieved. For instance, a review by Dawson and Osterling (1997) found that approximately 50% of children enrolled in autism-specific preschool programs were included in general education classes by the first grade, and children made IQ score gains, on average, of 20 points. In addition, the field's literature also suggests that children with autism who receive intervention by 2–3 years of age tend to have better outcomes than those who receive intervention later in their preschool years (Fenske, Zalenski, Krantz, & McClannahan,1985; Simeonsson, Olley, & Rosenthal, 1987).

As of 2000, there is an active discussion regarding the type and intensity of effective interventions for young children with autism. Although the controversy can be confusing for families that are desperately trying to secure appropriate intervention for their children, the discussion has dramatically increased the interest and resources devoted to the development and evaluation of treatments for young children with autism. Thus, it is likely that improvements in the efficacy of interventions for children with autism will continue.

In the area of diagnosing autism, there have been a number of important developments. Research in early identification has shown that a significant number of infants or toddlers with autism can be identified retrospectively via home videotapes when compared to typically developing infants (Mars, Mauk, & Dowrick, 1998; Osterling & Dawson, 1994) or infants with global developmental delays (Baranek, in press). Baron-Cohen and colleagues (Baron-Cohen, Allen, & Gillberg, 1992; Baron-Cohen et al., 1996) have demonstrated that reliable diagnosis at 18 months of age is very possible. Although it is still unusual for community professionals to diagnose autism in 18-month-olds, professionals are being asked to make a diagnosis of autism at younger and younger ages.

A number of issues arise in evaluating autism in children younger than 3 years of age. First, some *Diagnostic and Statistical Manual of Mental Disorders, Fourth Edition* (DSM-IV; American Psychiatric Association, 1994), categories require refinement in their application to children younger than 3 years of age. Charman (2000) provided a detailed description of the developmental course of many social and communication behaviors in children with autism during the second to fourth years of life and discussed the implications for diagnosis in children younger than 3 years of age. In a review of the early identification literature, Stone (1998) reported that the third category of DSM-IV behaviors (i.e., restricted, repetitive, and stereotyped activities and behaviors) does not appear as consistently in very young children with autism, particularly adherence to routines or rituals (Stone et al., in press). There also are some diagnostic criteria that are often not applicable to very young children. These include impairments in peer relationships and in conversation and the use of stereotyped language. It is important to note that impairments in nonverbal social behaviors and in reciprocal social interaction are robust diagnostic criteria for young children with autism (Stone et al., in press).

A second issue in the early diagnosis of very young children with autism involves diagnostic stability. A number of studies (Baron-Cohen et al., 1992, 1996; Lord, 1995; Stone et al., in press) suggest that the diagnosis of an autism spectrum disorder is quite invariable even in children at 18 and 20 months of age. However, no prospective studies of younger toddlers and infants have been conducted, so the stability at younger ages is unclear. Consequently, the firmness of a particular diagnosis is not as strong, particularly for a diagnosis of pervasive developmental disorder (PDD). Given the difficulty of applying some diagnostic criteria to this age range, the lack of diagnostic stability is understandable.

Finally, a third issue in the diagnosis of very young children with autism is the difficulty in using standardized measures with the majority of toddlers with autism. Many of these young children tend to become easily confused and anxious in new environments, and their abilities can vary greatly among different settings. Because of their struggles making the transition from one environment to another, their high need for control at times, and their tendency not to be motivated by social interaction or rapport, young children with autism may not be able to comply with standardized testing. Any direct standardized assessments of a child's skills that provide accurate pictures of the child's general abilities are often challenging, if not impossible, to conduct. Therefore, the case study in this chapter illustrates the usefulness of assessing a child's skills across different levels of structure, such as free play, a semistructured interview, and standardized assessments.

In addition to discussing the clinical issues involved in the assessment of young children with autism, this case study also shows how an evaluation can take place within an interdisciplinary environment. The holistic atmosphere of an interdisciplinary center is optimal for evaluating a young child with autism. Autism disturbs social, cognitive, communicative, neurological, motor, and sensory development. Especially in very young children, these systems are often inextricably entwined; each system is only understood within the context of the whole and in its relation to other systems. For example, a child's social capacity is determined by his or her ability to attend to and process social and communicative information. If a child is easily overstimulated by auditory or tactile information, he or she will likely withdraw from social contact and may not be able to speak. If a child's attention capabilities are disrupted, he or she may not be able to identify the salient social information in her environment. In this way, the onus is on interdisciplinary centers to conduct the comprehensive evaluation that is needed to obtain a complete and integrated picture of the child's development.

Another purpose of the case study presented in this chapter is to illustrate issues that are relevant to evaluating toddlers with possible autism. Again, most interdisciplinary centers routinely diagnose autism in preschool-age children, but they are being called to make their diagnostic protocols more appropriate for toddlers. It is hoped that this case study contributes toward this goal.

In order to provide the reader with a clear picture of how Josh's evaluation was conducted and interpreted, the interdisciplinary team's overall assessment process is described, beginning with the preliminary case conference. Then each team member's assessment procedures and findings are given, in addition to commentary on the structure and results of the evaluation.

PRELIMINARY CASE CONFERENCE

This case history involves an interdisciplinary evaluation of a 20-month-old boy known as Josh. Josh was referred to the interdisciplinary team by his primary physician due to parental concerns regarding Josh's ability to communicate and difficulty gaining his attention. Josh was not receiving any intervention services at the time of assessment. His parents noted a great deal of variability in

Josh's ability to use gestures and words and to respond to others. At 18 months of age, Josh was sent for an audiology evaluation due to his difficulty responding to others, and results indicated hearing was within normal limits. Josh's physician and family requested an interdisciplinary evaluation at this time to assess Josh's development and to obtain a thorough medical evaluation to examine the possible biological basis for Josh's presenting concerns.

In a telephone conversation, Josh's mother reported that her son was the fourth child in his family. His oldest sibling was 12 years old and had autism and mental retardation. Josh's parents were very knowledgeable regarding autism and involved in their older son's intervention programs. Josh's mother said she was watching her younger children's early development carefully because of concerns about having another child with autism. She stated that Josh was able to engage in many age-appropriate activities; at times, he used words and gestures, responded to his name, and pointed. However, she observed Josh had some autistic-like characteristics, such as becoming overly focused on tasks, being nonresponsive to others' attempts to get his attention, and tending toward solitary activities. She also believed Josh had sensitivities to sound and tactile stimulation, but he ate a variety of foods. Overall, his mother requested information for helping Josh develop language skills and for managing his tantrums.

Based on the preliminary information, the team decided that evaluation should include professionals from the fields of speech-language pathology, psychology, psychiatry, and occupational and physical therapy, with the psychologist as the service coordinator. The purpose of the assessment was to provide diagnostic impressions and to evaluate the findings so that recommendations could be made for treatment. In addition, because this child was so young, the team decided that speech-language pathology, occupational therapy, and psychology clinicians would observe Josh and his parents during play before a specific assessment plan was developed. No preassessment conference was needed, as no new information was provided prior to the assessment.

DISCIPLINARY ASSESSMENT PROCESS

Josh was seen on 2 consecutive days of evaluation beginning at 8:30 A.M., with each team member assessing Josh for 2 hours. The team decided that Josh first needed to be observed in a familiar and minimally stressful context to ascertain his usual level of functioning, so they began with a play-based assessment. Ideally, this observation would allow time for Josh to become maximally comfortable. However, based on the constraints of scheduling, this observation lasted for approximately 20 minutes.

Interdisciplinary Play-Based Assessment

It was decided that the speech-language pathologist, the occupational therapist, and the psychologist would combine their play-based assessments because, in the early stages of development, social, adaptive, and communication skills are very difficult to separate into specific domains. For instance, joint attention can be viewed as a communication and a social skill. These team members were very interested in observing Josh's response to specific prompts that encourage early social and communication skills.

The main component of the play-based assessment was observing free play with Josh's mother. The playroom, which had a one-way mirror, was stocked with toys that were developmentally appropriate and would elicit various skills or autistic symptoms. For example, a puzzle and a shape sorter were chosen to observe visuospatial skills while blocks were used to assess construction skills in addition to fine motor skills. Cooking and serving toys were placed in the room near a doll to encourage pretend-play scripts, a telephone and a car were chosen for functional play, and a ball was used to examine possible reciprocal play skills. A couple of books, along with drawing materials, were used to assess Josh's response to visual stimuli; his attention to letters, pictures, words, and their joint attention; and his fine motor skills. A small box was placed in the room that contained assorted sensory-based items to examine Josh's affinity for or aversion to various sensory inputs. The box contained a Koosh ball, a textured hedgehog squeeze toy, a magic wand with floating stars inside of it, and a pom-pom. Also, large cushions were placed in the room to facilitate comfortable floor play. Often they are used by children and parents for hiding and tickling games or as a way to apply deep pressure to children who crawl under the cushions. Sometimes children have strong interests in items such as trains, cars, or particular characters. When this occurs, efforts are made to include these things in the assessment in order to observe the child's level of interest and flexibility around them. However, Josh's mother did not report that he had any fascinations other than letters.

Josh and his mother were asked to play together in the room with the mirror while the occupational therapist, speech-language pathologist, and psychologist observed from behind the mirror for 20 minutes. Josh's skills were assessed in a number of areas of development, including typical and atypical developmental characteristics. After the first few minutes of the observation, it was clear that Josh was overwhelmed with the number of toys in the room. He randomly ran around the room, occasionally throwing the toys. After conferring with Josh's mother, the decision was made to structure the playtime to a greater degree. His mother cleared the toys into a pile and systematically tried to engage Josh with them.

During the play-based evaluation, the clinicians observed Josh's behavior in order to assess his social, communicative, motor, cognitive, play, organizational, and sensory development. These observations were placed within a general developmental context, so that a picture of Josh's overall development could be obtained. (The reader is directed to Knox, 1997, and Linder, 1993, for descriptions of how to structure and interpret a general play-based assessment of young children.) Josh's behavior was also monitored for atypical behaviors and those that are strongly associated with autism (see Table 14.1). To a lesser extent, Josh's mother's behavior was observed to assess the general

Table 14.1.   Checklist of atypical behaviors to observe in play-based assessments for toddlers and young children with autism spectrum disorders

Dramatically reduced ability to respond to social information, such as name being called or orienting to examiner entering the room
Lack of pretend play expected for developmental age
Lack of pointing to indicate interest by 18 months of age, even when prompted
Lack of ability to follow a point by 18 months of age
Reduced eye contact
Decreased smiling, responses to smiles of others, and use of eye contact combined with smiling
Tendency to prefer solitary activities
Lack of conventional gestures
Use of others' bodies as if they are tools

Other characteristics to note:

Perseverative interests or highly repetitive activities
Intensity of focus with preferred objects
Presence of stereotypic or repetitive motor actions
Interest in visual information (e.g., letters, numbers)
Decreased ability to modulate responses to sensory input
Atypical communication patterns:
  Extended period of babbling, jargon, or unintelligible sequences that appear stereotypic
  Echoing words and phrases but not for a clear function
  Pattern of gaining and losing verbal skills

Empirically supported impairments that distinguish the social/communication skills of young children with autism, as described in Charman (2000) and Stone (1998).

quality of the mother–child relationship and the mother's ability to read Josh's cues and to provide support.

Semistructured Play Interview

After the unstructured 20-minute play observation, the speech-language pathologist and the psychologist developed a list of skills that had not been adequately observed during free play. Then attempts were made during the semistructured play interview to elicit them.

The speech-language pathologist and the psychologist worked together for 40 minutes, alternately entering the room with Josh and his mother in order to prompt for and examine specific social, communication, and play skills as well as his attention and repetitive motor behaviors. The majority of this interview involved items from the Autism Diagnostic Observation Schedule–Generic (ADOS-G; Lord, Rutter, & DiLavore, 1998). This is an empirically validated play-based diagnostic assessment of autism spectrum disorders. Ideally, a full ADOS-G would have been administered. However, due to time constraints, some portions of the ADOS-G had to be omitted. In addition to the ADOS-G elements, other prompts were introduced such as examining

Josh's response to another person's distress and the communication assessment prompts described by Wetherby and Prizant (1992, 1998).

PROCESSES AND FINDINGS OF INDIVIDUAL DISCIPLINES

After the initial play-based assessment and the semistructured interview, the psychologist and the speech-language pathologist evaluated Josh for an additional hour each. On the second day of testing, the occupational therapist and the developmental psychiatrist evaluated Josh for 2 hours each. The findings from these individual evaluations are explored next.

Psychology

The goals of the psychologist's evaluation involved assessing Josh's skills for diagnostic purposes, documenting eligibility for services, and recommending interventions. Standardized measures, both parent report and cognitive assessment, were to be used to ascertain the severity of Josh's delays compared to same-age peers and, in turn, to establish eligibility for services. The parent report of Josh's adaptive skills would give a good picture of his capabilities at home. Josh's performance on nonverbal measures would provide information on Josh's cognitive abilities when language is minimized. (A full IQ evaluation would not be performed because of time limitations, likely compliance issues, and the fact that the speech-language pathologist would perform an assessment of Josh's expressive and receptive language.) Standardized testing would also allow observation of the child's ability to comply with instruction and his flexibility, and the examiner could begin to anticipate Josh's initial response to more direct therapeutic interventions. Previously monitoring Josh in free play and semistructured play gave an opportunity for assessment of Josh's typical social, communication, and play skills as well as his use of the environment. This observation also allowed the clinician to begin to anticipate how Josh would respond to more play-based approaches and to document Josh's development for treatment planning and in measuring future progress.

Across these assessments, the clinician would develop a picture of Josh's overall cognitive abilities. Once this impression was formed, Josh's nonverbal social and communication skills could be assessed in relation to his general nonverbal cognitive level for diagnostic purposes. Thus, if Josh displayed social skills at the same level as his nonverbal skills, a diagnosis of autism would not be considered.

Assessment

The first standardized assessment tool used was the Mullen Scales of Early Learning (Mullen, 1992). It is likely that Josh would be able to demonstrate higher abilities during incidental play at home when allowed to work on tasks on his own terms. However, given that Josh was able to comply with some of the testing demands, this evaluation yielded a reasonable estimate of Josh's abilities in a standardized testing situation. Two scales of the Mullen were administered to Josh in order to assess his visuospatial and visual-motor development. On the Visual Reception Scale, Josh's accomplishments were at the 18-month-old level, which placed his skills in the average range. On the Fine Motor Scale, Josh's performance was in the average range at the 18-month-old level.

The next standardized test was the Vineland Adaptive Behavior Scales (VABS; Sparrow, Balla, & Cicchetti, 1984). Based on parent report, Josh displayed delays in communication, daily living, and social skills. In the overall Communication category, he received a standard score of 69, with receptive and expressive age equivalents being 10 and 8 months respectively. Josh received standard scores of 69 in Daily Living Skills and Socialization. The Motor Scale was not performed due to time constraints and the occupational therapist's use of parent report measures in her evaluation.

In addition to standardized assessment measures, nonstandardized techniques were used in this portion of Josh's evaluation. Play observations yielded a wealth of information. In terms of social development, Josh displayed a great deal of variation in his ability to attend and respond to his mother and the evaluator. He turned to the examiner when she entered the room but did not respond to the examiner calling his name at a later time. Josh did, however, respond to his mother the second time she said his name. In addition, before the majority of toys were removed from the room, Josh rarely attended or responded to his mother. After the toys were removed and his mother presented materials one by one, Josh took interest in his mother's actions when she was playing with toys that were enticing to him (e.g., books, puzzles). Once he obtained the appealing toy, the child tended not to look at his mother, although he did imitate her previous actions with these toys at times. As for imitation without objects, Josh clapped his hands to a game of Pat-a-cake but did not imitate any other actions, even when prompted. Josh was also able to engage in a social routine that involved tickling and swinging. He smiled and ran away when his mother introduced an "I'm gonna get you" game. After running away and hiding behind the chair, he turned and looked at her while smiling, waiting for her to catch him. Overall, however, Josh tended not to look at adults when smiling. He rarely alternated gaze between objects and adults, and this only occurred for the purpose of requesting. He did not point or show objects for the purpose of commenting, yet it appeared that Josh pointed at pictures in order to label them. When the evaluator feigned hurting her finger, Josh looked briefly at her and then returned to his activity. This suggested delays in his ability to notice and respond to emotional displays.

Josh revealed varying abilities to communicate. During free play, he did not use any intentional communication strategies. Most of the time, he ran around the room and produced repetitive vocalizations. When his mother and the evaluator presented toys in a systematic, routine, and highly structured manner, Josh was able to employ more sophisticated communication skills, especially when toys of optimal interest were used. For instance, Josh and the evaluator developed a routine in which the evaluator would hold the bubble wand up to her face and say "Ready, set . . . ," and Josh was able to state "Go" in order to request that the evaluator blow the bubbles. As the pattern became familiar, Josh sporadically combined eye contact with *go*. However, Josh was not able to engage in routines with objects if he was overly interested in them. At these times, it appeared that he had difficulty taking his eyes off or releasing possession of highly preferred objects, even when he wanted help with them. For instance, he became quickly upset when the wind-up car stopped but was unable to request help in order to get it to go again, even when given a high level of prompting and support. Josh used some repetitive vocalizations during this time as well. (See the speech-language report for a more thorough description of Josh's communication skills.)

Josh's toy play and use of the environment were also noted during the play observation. When too many objects were present in the room, Josh appeared overstimulated and his behavior became more disorganized and self-stimulatory in nature. Josh also tended to become focused on some toys to the extent that it was difficult to obtain his attention by calling his name. Nonetheless, if another highly interesting toy was presented, Josh was able to attend to this new object. In addition, when the toys were presented one at a time with no other objects available, Josh was able to play in a more organized fashion. Josh demonstrated some beginning functional play skills by rolling a car around the room and placing a telephone by his ear. Even when prompted by the examiner, Josh did not display any early pretend play, such as talking into the telephone or feeding dolls. Josh used some toys in a slightly repetitive fashion. He also tended to run around the room when activities were not structured, which his mother reported often occurred when Josh was in new environments. Overall, however, the child did not perform any clear repetitive motor actions.

Impressions and Commentary

Based on observation and testing, Josh exhibited delays or atypical development in a number of areas. For example, he presented with impairments in social development. Specifically, these included lower than average responsivity and eye contact with others, difficulty showing or pointing to objects for the purpose of sharing his interest, and trouble understanding emotional displays in others. He also evidenced delays in his ability to use gestures to communicate and a lack of pretend play. At times, Josh was highly focused in play that had a slightly repetitive quality. Nevertheless, he could be easily distracted with another preferred toy, and he often repeated actions that had a functional purpose, such as using a shape sorter a number of times.

It should be noted that Josh had a number of considerable strengths. His nonverbal abilities were near age level, and he had an early interest in numbers and letters. Josh was able to use toys functionally on his own at home, particularly puzzles and shape sorters, and this boded well for Josh's continued cognitive development. In addition, Josh was able to engage in interaction with adults when it was structured and routine. In these contexts, he demonstrated intentional and functional communication skills as well as the ability to share smiles with his mother. These qualities provided a good foundation upon which to build more complex social, cognitive, and communication skills.

Josh had a great deal of difficulty completing the cognitive assessment. He refused many items that his mother reported he could easily complete at home, and Josh displayed higher nonverbal skills during the free play when he could use toys on his own agenda. In this way, Josh's assessment may have underestimated his abilities. However, the testing was important because it established that Josh's nonverbal cognitive skills were at least near age level, ruling out a global developmental delay. In contrast, Josh demonstrated nonverbal communication and social skills that were scattered, with none higher than the 9-month-old level (e.g., use of gestures and alternating gaze for requesting, participation in ritualized games). This meant that Josh's social and nonverbal communication skills were far below what would be expected for a child at his near-age level of development. If Josh had displayed nonverbal cognitive skills below a 9-month-old level, it is unlikely that a diagnosis of an autism spectrum disorder would be considered. This diagnosis would be discussed in the team meeting after the completion of all discipline evaluations. Because a full ADOS-G could not be completed, a diagnosis based on ADOS-G algorithm could not be computed. Nonetheless, many of the tasks from the ADOS-G gave the clinician important opportunities to observe Josh's social and communicative behavior in prompted situations.

Occupational Therapy

The occupational therapy assessment was to include standardized testing, parent interview, structured play observations, and clinical observations. Standard performance scores would allow for easy identification of areas of concern. Gross and fine motor skills would be measured through standardized testing and clinical observations. Due to Josh's high need for control, it was likely that standardized test scores would not reflect abilities that Josh displayed day to day. Therefore, the goal of standardized testing was to obtain scores that could be used to establish eligibility for services, to reflect Josh's abilities relative to typically developing peers, and to provide a baseline for comparing future performance.

A structured parent interview would be used to gather information regarding self-care abilities and the functional use of fine motor skills. Interviewing could be completed while the child was playing or over the telephone if time did not permit an in-person interview. Play skills would be measured through two observation periods. First, team observations of Josh and his mother interacting with selected toys would reveal functional toy use, initiation, toy preferences, quality of movement, access to and manipulation of toys, and his mother's ability to gauge and respond to Josh's behavioral cues. Second, observation during occupational therapy assessment would include gross motor, vestibular, and sensory play experiences and focus on organizational skills, the influence of sensory experiences on organization and play, and experiences Josh sought or avoided. In addition, foundation skills such as muscle tone, movement patterns, range of motion, strength, endurance, protective responses, and soft neurological signs would be assessed through clinical observations.

Information regarding sensory processing abilities would be gathered through parent completion of a sensory history questionnaire and through structured observations. The sensory history questionnaire would be mailed to the family prior to the clinic appointment so that the therapist could review responses, identify any potential areas of difficulty or areas requiring further investigation, and develop a plan to evaluate the areas of poor processing in the clinic environment. Clinical observations would also involve watching for variations in response, indications of hyposensitivity or hypersensitivity to sensory stimuli, the impact of sensory experiences on arousal level, and Josh's ability to self-regulate his responses or the need for external support and assistance in modulation.

Assessment

Josh presented with hypotonia (low muscle tone) in his trunk and mild joint laxity in his hips and knees. He used a W-sit position for floor sitting. When placed in long sitting, his back was rounded and shoulders were slumped. Josh was fearful and clung to the therapist when placed on a therapy ball. He enjoyed slow, rhythmic bouncing but did not release his grasp of the therapist. He resisted lying on the ball. Ambulation was characterized by wide base of support and intermittent decreased dorsiflexion.

The Peabody Developmental Motor Scales (PDMS; Folio & Fewell, 1983) were utilized to assess gross and fine motor skill development. At times it was difficult to ascertain whether Josh was not capable of an activity or if he was merely resisting the requests of the therapist. Some modifications were made to standardized testing procedure in order to gain the highest level of compliance. For this reason, the scores reflected a fair estimate of Josh's abilities in a standardized testing environment but may have been different than skills he displayed at home. On the Gross Motor Scales, Josh received a total score of 157, corresponding to the 2nd percentile, 2.05 standard deviations (SDs) below the mean, and an age equivalency of 16 months. On the Fine Motor Scales, Josh received an overall score of 129, corresponding to the 9th percentile, 1.38 SD below the mean, and an age equivalency of 17–18 months.

The Self-Care Domain of the Pediatric Evaluation of Disability Inventory (PEDI; Haley, Coster, Ludlow, Haltiwanger, & Andrellos, 1992) was used to guide a structured parent interview regarding Josh's self-help abilities. Josh received a total score of 11, corresponding to a standard score of 22, a scaled score of 33, and an SD of more than 2.0, indicating delays in self-care abilities.

Josh's parents completed the Sensory Profile (Dunn & Westman, 1995), on which they rated the frequency of several sensory-based behaviors. The findings were suggested sensory sensitivity. He demonstrated mixed responses to auditory and visual input, being sensitive to intense levels of input but appearing to not notice low levels of stimulation, particularly when of a social nature (e.g., responding when his name was called). Josh turned to the sound of the overhead paging system and often covered his ears in response to loud noise. Josh also showed signs of tactile defensiveness, as his sensitivity to some textures (e.g., the feathers in a duster) caused him to avoid a variety of play and learning opportunities. Yet this sensitivity was not all-encompassing. Josh enjoyed pulling the strands of a Koosh ball and playing with a prickly squeeze toy; he responded to the sound of the squeeze toy with laughter. Josh's play skills were observed as part of team observations and in selected opportunities during occupational therapy assessment. Josh's performance was partially interpreted using the Revised Knox Preschool Play Scale (Knox, 1997). Results for the various domains are summarized next.

In terms of motor skills, the child's movements were functional but lacked fluidity, with no rotation evident. Josh was able to obtain and manipulate toys, though the quality of his movements was hindered by hypotonia. Josh enjoyed playing in the tunnel and sitting on the trampoline while his mother jumped on it. He avoided all off-ground movement, refusing the balance board and swing. When he was excited, Josh tensed his body and hands, maintaining this posture for several seconds while intensely focusing on the intriguing activity. Josh was also noted to run in circles, producing vocalizations.

Josh's attention and organization were limited. He was able to engage in play for more than 5 minutes; however, in extended play, the quality became persistent. When fixated on a toy, multiple cues and occasional physical assistance were required to help Josh shift his attention. At times, Josh allowed his mother to join him in play, and he visually attended to her toy use when she utilized his preferred toys.

Josh's limited gross motor skills did not significantly affect his use of space in the assessment room. He stood without support, walked with a wide stance, and threw a ball. His space management skills were similar to those demonstrated by children 12–18 months of age. Material management skills were also similar to those of children 12–18 months old. Josh threw, inserted, carried, opened, and shut toys. He did not string beads, separate pop beads, or use tools.

Josh's toy play showed a preference for dump and fill activities, and he often repeated this sequence. He poked his fingers into the holes of a pegboard but required assistance to place pegs in the board. Josh stacked blocks vertically, pushed the buttons of a toy telephone, and completed a shape sorter. He did not use markers.

Impressions and Commentary
Josh demonstrated some hypotonia, and gravitational insecurity was also evident. His hypotonicity and weak abdominal musculature contributed to delays in gross motor skills and the use of compensatory movement patterns. Fine

motor skills were well within typical limits. Self-care skills were delayed and influenced by sensory defensiveness.

Josh demonstrated fluctuating responses to auditory and visual input, suggesting difficulty integrating information through these sensory systems. His hypersensitive responses to movement and vestibular stimuli were consistent with gravitational insecurity, causing him to avoid many activities involving movement. Josh's negative reactions to unexpected touch and avoidance of a variety of textures were indicative of tactile defensiveness.

Play skills were fair, as Josh demonstrated a predominance of skills typical of children 6 months younger than his chronological age. Hypotonia and gravitational insecurity impeded engagement in functional motor play. Material management was a relative strength because Josh demonstrated functional skills for manipulation of objects; however, he had a tendency toward persistent use of objects. Inconsistency in imitation, interaction, and symbolic use of toys affected Josh's ability to engage in functional play.

Minor procedural modifications were required for Josh to tolerate standardized testing. It appeared that his resistance to some items reflected his difficulty in tolerating imposed structure and transitions. Utilizing small toys and increasing the use of routine were helpful in increasing his cooperation, and these modifications to testing procedure were documented in the testing report. The play observations provided a snapshot of Josh's abilities to gain access to play materials and apparatus and to manipulate tools and toys; ideation and flexibility in use of toys; participation in collaborative play; and skills in imaginative play, sensory exploration, and gross and fine motor activities.

Josh's case depicts the importance of assessing sensory processing and the impact of poor sensory processing on arousal level. Completion and return of the sensory history questionnaire prior to the clinic appointment allowed the therapist to identify potential areas of lower processing. The therapist was then able to create opportunities during the testing situation to elicit some of the reported behaviors by including relevant toys and setting up the testing environment to contain significant sensory experiences. Thus, the quality and intensity of responses, as well as effective and ineffective methods of recovery, could be compared.

These play situations were important for observing the effect of sensory stimulation on Josh's arousal level. The physiological state of Josh's nervous system influenced how organized he could be in his interactions with the environment and the people and objects in it, as changes in sensory stimulation can cause fluctuations in arousal level. Therefore, it was crucial to assess each sensory system and determine which types of sensory stimuli caused such extreme fluctuations that he was unable to modulate his responses to the stimuli, resulting in behavior that was inappropriate for the situation. It was evident that Josh was easily overstimulated by the visual input of the toys scattered throughout the room. When the toys were gathered into one location, he was able to calm himself, leading to increased organization and the ability to engage in purposeful toy play.

On a similar note, it was necessary to assess the parent's ability to interpret her child's state of arousal and her effectiveness in helping him to modulate his responses to sensory stimuli. Most of the time, Josh's mother was able to modify her style of interaction according to her son's level of arousal. She decreased the level of auditory input by using short sentences, incorporated familiar games when Josh did not initiate functional play, and attempted to redirect his attention when he demonstrated signs of overexcitement.

Speech-Language Pathology

The aims of the speech-language assessment were to assist in determining a diagnosis, to document a need for services, and to develop appropriate recommendations for intervention to foster social-communication skills. Parent report would be important for determining a diagnosis and skills and behaviors seen at home. Although Josh was very young, report of his development to this point (and any changes in development) would be needed for diagnosis. A description of current skills in a more familiar environment would be compared to skills and behaviors observed during testing in a less familiar environment. Standardized testing of language comprehension and expressive language skills would offer a standardized score or age equivalency and an opportunity to observe Josh's interaction with materials and tasks that could not be modified. Semistructured tasks and observation of play with his mother would be used to assess and observe auditory attention and comprehension of language with varying levels of contextual, gestural, and visual supports. These settings would also be employed to ascertain expressive communication across the continuum from physical behaviors and vocalizations to gestures and words. Communicative intent would be evaluated along with other nonverbal social skills. Speech development, generally assessed through nonstandardized approaches at this age, could be observed in spontaneous as well as imitative interactions.

Assessment

Although many of Josh's social and communication skills were exhibited during the observed sessions, additional information was needed to complete the assessment of communication skills. A standardized test of language skills, the Preschool Language Scale–3 (PLS-3; Zimmerman, Steiner, & Pond, 1992), was attempted but could not be completed due to noncompliance.

The play assessment yielded greater results. Based on earlier observations, toys and materials were brought into the room in closed, opaque containers and presented one at a time in small sets. Josh's mother remained in the room and was asked to participate in some of the activities. A semistructured play-based assessment of language comprehension, expressive language, nonverbal social-communication, and speech-phonology skills was completed. Sensorimotor toys, thematically related toys, and toys that could be used to support social interactions were presented to elicit behaviors. The observations and behaviors obtained during the play-based assessments formed the basis for evaluations in the domains described next.

Language Comprehension

Josh exhibited decreased attention to auditory and verbal information. His focus increased when toys were presented individually into his visual field and when he was strongly motivated by the toy or activity. It was difficult to get his attention by calling his name when he was involved in a preferred activity. Josh showed no response to a loud sound outside in the hallway, and he generally required physical prompting to follow a direction. He also used context and routine to support comprehension of directions, sometimes making it unclear whether he understood key words in the verbal prompt or was using a strategy based on familiar routine. (For example, at home, he showed a consistent response to the words "bottle" and "up.") Josh paused when the evaluator warned him, with a loud "no," to stay away from an electrical outlet but continued to touch it.

Expressive Language

Josh appeared to be presymbolic, though he had been using some protowords (e.g., "da," "ba") and one-word approximations, such as "baba," for *bottle*. Josh primarily vocalized a series of consonants and vowels that appeared to be self-stimulatory in nature. He produced one true word, "go," in a verbal routine associated with a motor-based activity (e.g., "ready, set, go") during the session. His mother reported he used this word consistently at home, and "uh-oh" was heard sporadically at home. In addition, Josh's mother stated that he would use a word a few times and then never use it again.

Social-Communication

Josh primarily demonstrated preintentional communication. He vocalized, fussed, or screamed to protest when toys were put away or when limits were set. He pointed proximally to pictures in books and to some objects but did not call the adult's attention to the item in any way. These behaviors suggested that Josh may have been beginning to use a point to label. During the sessions, Josh was prompted to give the bubble wand to the evaluator to request more bubbles, but he resisted giving other objects when prompted. He seemed to lack the understanding that the object would be returned. Josh displayed reduced eye contact except when a motivating toy was held close to the evaluator's eyes, and he glanced at her eyes when an action was delayed. He also rarely appeared to look at adults as he played with other toys. Josh protested and showed very early requests for the continuation of an appealing activity with significant structuring of the activity. He also used proximity to an object or container to signal interest in something. He attempted to get most things himself at home and was just beginning to take an adult's hand and pull the adult toward a desired object.

Speech Phonology

Josh produced strings of consonants and vowels in a babbling-like sequence that appeared to be self-stimulatory. Consonants included *b*, *d*, and *g*. He showed some evidence of syllable formation in his protowords ("ba," "da," and sometimes "baba") and one true word ("go").

Impressions and Commentary

At age 20 months, Josh presented with significant delays in the development of language comprehension, expressive language, nonverbal social-communication, speech phonology, and play skills. He also exhibited atypical development in regard to his 1) decreased attention to auditory and verbal information, 2) difficulty shifting attention from a preferred activity to the source of a voice, 3) reduced eye contact and number of social-communicative interactions, 4) very limited use of conventional gestures to communicate intent, and 5) extended period of babbling with the production of self-stimulatory sound sequences.

Standardized assessment procedures could not be used to assess Josh's skills for various reasons. First, testing was limited by materials that did not motivate Josh or hold his attention. Second, most receptive language items rely on the child's motivation to follow directions. Given Josh's high need for control, he found this test very frustrating. In addition, no modifications to the testing would engage Josh. The observations of play with his mother, along with the semistructured play-based assessment, offered the opportunity to use motivating toys and activities. It also allowed the examiner to observe Josh's response to varying levels of support and prompting. The use of these approaches resulted in information that could be used to consider a diagnosis of an autism spectrum disorder. As this diagnosis was being considered, it was important to look at Josh's atypical development as well as his delays.

Psychiatry

Much of the psychiatrist's assessment was based on Josh's past. The next section examines in detail information from different categories in the child's history.

Developmental History

Josh was an "easy" baby who fell into a routine of eating and sleeping by his second month. Although Josh grew typically throughout his early life, since 15 months of age he had refused to eat meat. His mother had supplemented the child's diet with multivitamins but Josh inconsistently took these as well. The parents noted some tactile and auditory sensitivities early on. Josh's early motor development was slightly delayed but within typical limits. During infancy, Josh responded to face-to-face interaction at times, such as smiling when his parents spoke to him, and he engaged in physical baby games (especially if tickling was involved) by 10 months of age. However, it was more difficult to get Josh involved in nonphysical games such as Peekaboo.

Josh began using simple instrumental gestures, such as reaching his hands up to get out of his crib, by 12 months of age. At approximately 15 months of age, Josh began pointing to request foods that he wanted, and he started using a word to request actions. By approximately 18 months of age, Josh began pointing at objects that he obviously was not requesting, such as items in books. Yet he did not reference his parents when pointing; instead, his parents reported that this pointing appeared to have a more routinized quality. Josh would engage in rough-and-tumble play with his siblings, such as tickle games and chasing games. He did not display interest in peers, although he would engage in parallel play with a group of peers if the activity was motivating to him.

During periods of Josh's intense interest, his mother noticed that he seemed even less responsive to his name. Although no one in the family ever observed any behavior that could clearly be called a seizure, these episodes of unresponsiveness, lasting 20–30 seconds, were a source of worry. There had been no loss of skills, vomiting, birthmarks, loss of vision, or visual impairment. Josh's parents also reported their son's sleep had been increasingly discontinuous at night. On some nights he slept no more than 5–6 hours, even though, with naps, he slept about 8–10 hours per 24-hour period.

Medical History

Josh was born as the fourth child to a 36-year-old, healthy female after a 44-week pregnancy, which ended in a vertex vaginal delivery after an 18-hour uncomplicated labor. His birth weight was 7 pounds 11 ounces, and he was $20^{1}/_{2}$ inches in length. His Apgar scores were approximately 8 or 9. Josh went home and was believed to be well at 2 days of age.

Growth and developmental milestones were smiling at 1 month of age, rolling at $4^{1}/_{2}$ months old, sitting at $6^{1}/_{2}$ months of age, crawling at 8 months old, and walking at 14 months of age. Josh produced a few words, which he used sporadically, by the time he was 15 months old. Toilet training had not occurred at the time of this assessment. Tantrums were present.

There were no indications of heart disease, hypertension, diabetes, convulsions, strokes, meningitis, encephalitis, brain injuries, or abuse. Two bouts of otitis media resolved easily with antibiotics. No past surgeries, hospitalizations, allergies, or current medications were noted, and immunizations were up to date.

Social History

Josh lived with his parents and three siblings. His 12-year-old brother had autism and Josh's two sisters had average or above-average intellectual abilities, although one had a mild learning disability. Josh's family had private insurance, and their eldest son received Division of Developmental Disabilities (DDD) respite services. The mother was trying to obtain Supplemental Security Insurance for her older son. The parents described their relationship with each other as good, but it was strained at times by stresses involving their eldest son's problems. Consequently, Josh's parents had sought counseling once in the past and found it very helpful. They stated that they moved to the area 4 years ago and that they had good social supports through their church. Nevertheless, Josh's parents reported being very concerned about his development.

The mother, who was not employed outside of the home, was experiencing a high level of stress; the father, although concerned, seemed less stressed.

Besides an exploration of Josh's history, certain on-site evaluations provided pertinent information. One of these was a mental status examination. Josh presented as a healthy child with no obvious dysmorphic features. He made repetitive utterances but used no discernible words. During the interview with his parents, he occasionally looked up but showed no distress when his parents left him alone with the interviewer. Instead, he played intensely with a brightly colored toy he brought from home. In fact, the child also was extremely difficult to engage and would not accept other toys offered him during the evaluation. At the end of the interview, when his plastic toy was put aside, he cried inconsolably. Aside from that episode, which was quickly resolved when the toy was given back, Josh appeared generally cheerful. There seemed to be no evidence of hallucinatory experience or staring spells, but he did exhibit other autistic-like characteristics. For instance, he withdrew from touches on the arm to get his attention. Furthermore, at one point in the interview, he climbed a chair to a paper towel dispenser in the exam room and repeatedly pulled out paper towels. When redirected, he ran around the room looking for his plastic toy.

A physical examination showed that Josh was at the 25th percentile for height and weight but at the 95th percentile for head circumference; these measurements were consistent with previous measures obtained by his family physician. His vital signs were normal. There were no birthmarks on his skin. Some of his physical features were marginally atypical (e.g., clinodactyly; small, slightly rotated ears; a high-arched palate). There were no cardiac murmurs or other physical findings. Josh's neurological examination revealed no focal difficulties, but he had trouble running and jumping and tended to fall, although to no consistent side.

Impressions and Commentary

This 20-month-old boy presented with delays in language acquisition, gross motor development, and social behaviors. In addition, he demonstrated some atypical behaviors, including self-directed behaviors, developmentally inappropriate activity, and the inability to regulate attention. His mental status examination corroborated these historical findings as well as the fact that his play was nonsymbolic and would be repetitive at times. His sensorium was clear, and he did not evidence a psychotic process. Although he did not appear to have staring spells, this feature as the result of seizures had to be ruled out. At this time, the DSM-IV Axis 3 had to be tested to eliminate a diagnosis of fragile X syndrome, some other karyotypic irregularity, epilepsy, or an inborn error of metabolism. Also, a secondary nutritional deficiency from his restricted diet needed to be considered. On Axis 4, he probably was experiencing mild stress from his parents' hypervigilance and marital difficulties. On Axis 5, he was globally functioning with mild to moderate impairments. This level of functioning was consistent over the previous year. Axis 1 and 2 DSM-IV diagnoses would be postponed until the multidisciplinary team meeting, once all the discipline evaluations had been completed.

Research shows a strong genetic component in autism is indicated by an increased concordance rate in monozygotic versus dizygotic twins (Bailey et al., 1995), and the risk to siblings of idiopathic cases is 75 times greater than that of the general population (Bolton et al., 1994). According to Folstein and Rutter (1977), about 2% of siblings are affected, and speech-language delay is common among siblings of children with autism. A later review by Smalley (1997) found that the sibling recurrence risk is 3%–5%. The implications of these statistics would be discussed with Josh's parents, as it was likely that a strong genetic component for autism existed in this family. This point was upheld by the fact that Josh appeared to have and his brother did have an autism spectrum disorder; also, one sister had a learning disability.

Diagnostic tests were ordered to test for conditions based on symptom presentation and those known to co-occur with autism. A complete blood count (CBC)/differential test was ordered because of Josh's restricted intake of meat proteins. If this lab test indicated iron deficiency anemia, Josh would be prescribed iron supplements in addition to a multivitamin. Karyotype was ordered to screen for any obvious chromosomal abnormalities, while DNA was examined for X-linked mental retardation syndromes such as fragile X. This test was necessary because the signs of fragile X syndrome in early childhood are nonspecific; developmental delay is an almost universal manifestation. Thus, any child (male or female) with a speech-language or motor delay of unknown etiology should be evaluated for fragile X syndrome, particularly in the presence of a positive family history and a consistent physical and behavioral phenotype and the absence of especially atypical structural features (Curry, Stevenson, & Aughton, 1997). When fragile X DNA-based testing is used regularly in this large and loosely defined group of children, the yield of positive test results is relatively low; approximately 3%–6% of unselected males have mental retardation (Curry et al., 1997). Urinalysis and an inborn errors of metabolism (IEM) screen were ordered to rule out phenylketonuria (PKU) and other metabolic disorders. The risk of these disorders is less than 1%; however, if present, they can significantly affect a child's presentation.

INTEGRATION OF DISCIPLINARY INFORMATION AND RECOMMENDATIONS

The team met to discuss each member's findings and to draw conclusions regarding diagnostic impressions and recommendations. Based on these evaluations, the following information was obtained in each of the areas:

1. A physical exam revealed no significant findings. Nonetheless, tests were ordered to rule out the possibility of any other medical conditions that could contribute to Josh's overall delayed and atypical development. These results would be discussed with Josh's parents when tests were completed.

2. Josh showed atypical development in the use of nonverbal social behaviors such as making eye contact, orienting and attending to social information, producing reciprocal interaction with adults, using joint attention techniques (e.g., pointing, showing) to share information, and understanding emotional displays.

3. In terms of communication, the child's development was atypical regarding utilizing gestures, employing expressive and receptive language, engaging in pretend play skills, and vocalizing.

4. Delays in gross motor development and the ability to regulate sensory input in a number of domains impaired Josh's capacity for organization and focusing attention.

5. The child's attention span was limited; in fact, he possessed higher than average levels of distractibility and inability to focus when presented with competing stimuli. Josh also had the tendency to overfocus on some tasks.

Diagnostic Process

Given the preceding characteristics, a diagnosis of an autism spectrum disorder was likely indicated. Yet before confirming this diagnosis, the team discussed possible differential diagnoses. The psychologist's testing showed that Josh's nonverbal skills were within the average range. Ruling out a global developmental delay, the question arose whether Josh had an isolated language impairment. The assessment information, however, did not suggest this to be true. Josh displayed an inconsistent response to auditory and verbal information; he also had an extended period of babbling, and this babbling appeared to be self-stimulatory in nature. In addition, the child's development of communicative gestures was delayed, and the communicative intentions expected by 20 months of age (especially "give to request" and pointing or showing to comment) were absent. The absence of complex and sequenced gestures implied that this was not a speech disorder, as most children with average nonverbal abilities and an absence of oral communication generally find a way to communicate nonverbally.

If Josh's development remained consistent, his current profile suggested a diagnosis of a high-functioning autism spectrum disorder. Over time, a clearer picture would emerge regarding his specific diagnostic status. Because of his delays in language at the time of assessment, a late diagnosis of Asperger syndrome would be unlikely. However, at this point it was difficult to diagnose PDD not otherwise specified (NOS) versus autism due to issues of diagnostic instability at Josh's young age. A future differential diagnosis would need to pay particular attention to the third category of behaviors that included Josh's development of repetitive behaviors and restricted interests.

Recommendations

After the team deliberated on their individual findings, they jointly designed a set of intervention recommendations. These items are described in the following section.

Educational Programming

Research suggests that early intervention can be highly effective for young children with autism when it is systematic and intense. The team strongly recommended that Josh receive early intervention services, with the majority of these services delivered in a one-to-one, structured, therapeutic context for the next year. His intervention program might also incorporate a few different approaches, including classroom time, speech-language therapy, occupational therapy, and individual therapy in a structured or play setting. Specific recommendations in each of these areas are listed next.

One-to-One Intervention

Josh would likely benefit from working with a therapist in a personalized home-based or school setting. Typically, home programs can incorporate strategies from discrete trial behavioral interventions, structured teaching approaches such as TEACCH (Treatment and Education of Autistic and related Communications Handicapped Children; Cox & Schopler, 1993), natural language therapy methods, or highly systematic developmental play therapy. It is important that the intervention consists of structured and consistent teaching and involves specific strategies for generalizing the skills learned in this environment. Also, it is imperative that this program is supervised by an expert in the field of early treatment for children with autism. Given Josh's tendency to be easily overstimulated with too many items, he would likely respond well to a program with a discrete trial component. In order to optimize Josh's engagement and motivation, it would be best if this program first incorporated highly motivating objects with a great level of reinforcement for the completion of tasks. Then, gradually, his programs could include activities requiring more compliance and attention. Josh also responded well to ritualized social interaction, so a Natural Language approach might help the development of early social and communication skills. These approaches were described and discussed with Josh's parents, and community referrals were made.

Birth-to-3 Program

Josh would benefit from receiving services from a birth-to-3 program. It was suggested that Josh's mother connect with a family resource coordinator at the birth-to-3 center in her area to enroll Josh for DDD services.

Speech-Language Pathology and Occupational Therapy Consultation

If Josh's parents decided to implement a home program for Josh, it was recommended that they receive periodic consultation from a speech-language pathologist and an occupational therapist to incorporate activities that promote development in these areas.

Speech-Language Pathology

The team recommended that Josh receive speech-language pathology services, in a clinical or birth-to-3 center, with emphasis on the following areas:

Language Comprehension

Increasing Josh's ability to attend to auditory information was necessary. He also required assistance in utilizing visual cuing for comprehension and focusing attention. His increasing use of key words and phrases in context needed to be continued, and a receptive vocabulary with functional words related to daily activities and interests had to be fostered.

Expressive Language

The initial focus in this domain was on the development of nonverbal communication skills. As Josh's comprehension improved, the use of visual communication systems such as the Picture Exchange Communication System (PECS; Frost & Bondy, 1994) should be considered. Another means of helping the child was to utilize verbal routines with rhythm and predictability.

Social-Communication

Expanding Josh's utilization of proximal and distal pointing to request was a primary goal. In addition, the following needs were identified: developing his use of the "give for help" gesture, increasing his employment of eye contact in coordination with gestures, and augmenting his commenting behavior through point-and-show gestures.

Speech Phonology

Josh's attention to sounds and voices, as well as the frequency of his vocalizations, needed to be augmented. In addition, attempts to increase vocal play, turn-taking, and imitating sounds and words should be made. Furthermore, a focus on words beginning with the letters m, b, p, t, d, n, and w was recommended.

Play

Josh's caregivers needed to nurture functional pretend play and relational play, with the goal of using play to support language comprehension and expression (e.g., two-word combinations—"push car," "wash face").

Occupational Therapy

Josh would benefit from clinical occupational therapy services to focus on gravitational insecurity, immature movement patterns, and self-care impairments. In addition, specific foci would strengthen this occupational therapy treatment.

Sensory Processing

Josh's mother would greatly benefit from education and training regarding sensory processing issues. A sensory diet, including deep tactile pressure and an emphasis on decreasing tactile defensiveness, should be established for Josh. His mother could begin to address these needs by using deep pressure touch (e.g., tight bear hugs, firm back rubs) when interacting with her son. Tickling, as long as it was tolerated, could occur in conjunction with rough play or other games familiar to Josh.

Physical Therapy Consultation

Josh might benefit from a physical therapy consultation to address decreased dorsiflexion.

Birth-to-3 Program

Josh would benefit from occupational therapy services provided though the birth-to-3 program to ensure optimal outcomes from the educational opportunities available to him in that environment.

Medical

Josh needed to be tested with a CBC, a karyotype and a DNA test for fragile X syndrome, general urinalysis, and urinalysis for inborn errors of metabolism. A baseline of staring spells also needed to begin, and a consultation from a pediatric neurologist to rule out seizures was ordered. An electroencephalogram (EEG) and advanced brain imaging studies would be reconsidered after this consultation. The team would request follow-up appointments with Josh's parents once the tests were completed to discuss the results and any further treatment.

Community Resources

Josh's parents were already aware of the Autism Society, and it was likely that his mother would continue to find that group a helpful resource. In addition, Josh's parents could also contact the local Families for Early Autism Treatment (FEAT) group to obtain support in assembling and maintaining Josh's home program. The clinic provided Josh's parents with brochures from both organizations.

Problem Behaviors

It was likely that a number of Josh's tantrums stemmed from either his frustration in not being able to communicate his needs or from his need for more structure. As Josh's communication program became more systematized and incorporated into everyday situations, his tantrums would probably decrease. Furthermore, Josh appeared to become easily overstimulated by his environment, but he responded well and quickly to increased structure. The team members shared specific strategies with Josh's parents for augmenting structure, and they included a handout on how to use visual supports (e.g., picture schedules, picture cue cards).

Reevaluation

The interdisciplinary team wanted to reassess Josh in approximately $1^1/_2$ years to ascertain his levels of development and progress. In addition, his response to intervention would be assessed and subsequent treatment recommendations would be offered. A more specific diagnosis would probably be made at that time.

Discussion with Parents

A specific diagnosis (autism versus PDD or Asperger syndrome) at 20 months could not be established. Nevertheless, although a definite diagnosis was not provided for the parents, they were told that Josh clearly evidenced autistic characteristics. These features were described to the parents, including specific information regarding the severity of their son's impairments. The parents were informed that although these characteristics would likely remain with Josh throughout his life, the team expected him to respond well to intervention. The clinicians also outlined Josh's strengths, such as his ability and interest in interacting with others in structured predictable environments, his relatively strong nonverbal cognitive skills, his ability to engage in functional activities without parental support at home, and his emerging use of communication through words and gestures. In addition, the family's strengths were noted: Josh's parents were quite knowledgeable regarding autism spectrum disorders, and they were sensitive to Josh's need for structure and predictability and his tendency for sensory overstimulation. All of these factors boded well for his future.

In the feedback session, the recommendations, as well as various intervention approaches, were discussed with Josh's parents. Because his parents were already familiar with some interventions for children with autism, they were able to discuss the various approaches and the types of empirical and clinical support associated with each method. However, for many families that are first receiving a diagnosis of an autism spectrum disorder, specific information regarding intervention is often too overwhelming. In such cases, families need to be prepared for the wide array of interventions that are available for children with autism and the strong and often contradictory opinions regarding which types of interventions are most appropriate. One way to assist parents is to give them an overview of the major types of interventions that are available. Breaking them down into categories of those that have empirical support and those that do not can often be useful. (Freeman, 1997, provided guidelines for families that are evaluating intervention programs for children with autism.) Furthermore, a discussion of the general principles that constitute effective intervention is helpful. Dawson and Osterling (1997) furnished a review of the important elements in a child's early intervention programming, and Rogers (1998) surveyed the literature on empirically supported interventions for young children with autism.

Finally, although Josh's parents did not plan to have more children, their genetic risks were discussed. The team also presented the potential genetic risks of Josh's typically developing siblings having a child with an autism spectrum disorder.

CONCLUSION

Through this interdisciplinary evaluation, the team was able to offer Josh's parents a comprehensive and integrated picture of their son's current development and characteristics. By combining results across disciplines, his skills could be understood within the context of his overall development. For instance, his social, cognitive, and communication abilities were greatly influenced by his difficulty in sensory processing. This information would likely be useful to those working with Josh in the future. This case study provides the reader with information regarding assessment and diagnostic formulation of autism spectrum disorders in very young children as well. In addition, it illustrates one way of providing families with information that is coherent and useful while acknowledging what is not known in the field of early identification of and treatment for this disorder.

Given the importance and efficacy of early intervention for children with autism, an interdisciplinary team renders a crucial service. By providing families with information regarding the components of effective early intervention programs and by connecting families to appropriate services, the interdisciplinary team has an important role in changing the course of a child's development for the better.

REFERENCES

American Psychiatric Association. (1994). *Diagnostic and statistical manual of mental disorders* (4th ed.). Washington, DC: Author.

Bailey, A., Le Couteur, A., Gottesman, I., Bolton, P., Simonoff, E., Yuzda, E., & Rutter, M. (1995). Autism as a strongly genetic disorder: Evidence from a British twin study. *Psychiatric Medicine, 25,* 63–77.

Baranek, G.T. (in press). Autism during infancy: A retrospective video analysis of sensory-motor and social behaviors at 9–12 months of age. *Journal of Autism and Developmental Disorders.*

Baron-Cohen, S., Allen, J., & Gillberg, C. (1992). Can autism be detected at 18 months? The needle, the haystack, and the CHAT. *British Journal of Psychiatry, 161,* 839–843.

Baron-Cohen, S., Cox, A., Baird, G., Swettenham, J., Nightingale, N., Morgan, K., Drew, A., & Charman, T. (1996). Psychological markers in the detection of autism in infancy in a large population. *British Journal of Psychiatry, 168,* 1–6.

Bolton, P., MacDonald, H., Pickles, A., Rios, P., Goode, S., Crowson, M., Bailey, A., & Rutter, M. (1994). A case-control family history study of autism. *Journal of Child Psychology and Psychiatry, 35,* 877–900.

Charman, T. (2000). Theory of mind and the early diagnosis of autism. In S. Baron-Cohen, H. Tager-Flusberg, & D. Cohen (Eds.), *Understanding other minds: Perspectives from developmental cognitive neuroscience.* (2nd ed.). London: Oxford University Press.

Cox, R.D., & Schopler, E. (1993). Aggression and self-injurious behaviors in persons with autism: The TEACCH (Treatment and Education of Autistic and related Communications Handicapped Children) approach. *Acta Paedopsychiatrica, 56,* 85–90.

Curry, C.J., Stevenson, R.E., & Aughton, D. (1997). Evaluation of mental retardation: Recommendations of a consensus conference: American College of Medical Genetics. *American Journal of Medical Genetics, 72,* 468–477.

Dawson, G., & Osterling, J. (1997). Early intervention in autism. In M.J. Guralnick (Ed.), *The effectiveness of early intervention* (pp. 307–326). Baltimore: Paul H. Brookes Publishing Co.

Dunn, W., & Westman, K. (1995). *Sensory Profile.* Kansas City: University of Kansas Medical Center.

Fenske, E.C., Zalenski, S., Krantz, P.J., & McClannahan, L.E. (1985). Age at intervention and treatment outcome for autistic children in a comprehensive intervention program [Special issue: Early intervention]. *Analysis and Intervention in Developmental Disabilities, 5,* 49–58.

Folio, M.R., & Fewell, R. (1983). *Peabody Developmental Motor Scales and Activity Cards (PDMS).* Itasca, IL: The Riverside Publishing Co.

Folstein, S., & Rutter, M. (1977). Infantile autism: A genetic study of 21 twin pairs. *Journal of Child Psychology and Psychiatry, 18,* 297–321.

Freeman, B.J. (1997). Guidelines for evaluating intervention programs for children with autism. *Journal of Autism and Developmental Disorders, 27,* 641–651.

Frost, L., & Bondy, A. (1994). *The Picture Exchange Communication System (PECS) Training Manual.* Cherry, NJ: PECS.

Haley, S.M., Coster, W.J., Ludlow, L.H., Haltiwanger, J.T., & Andrellos, P.J. (1992). *Pediatric Evaluation of Disability Inventory (PEDI).* San Antonio, TX: Therapy Skill Builders.

Knox, S. (1997). Revised Knox Preschool Play Scale. In L.D. Parham & L.S. Fazio (Eds.), *Play in occupational therapy for children* (pp. 47–51). St. Louis, MO: Mosby.

Linder, T.W. (1993). *Transdisciplinary play-based assessment: A functional approach to working with young children* (Rev. ed.). Baltimore: Paul H. Brookes Publishing Co.

Lord, C. (1995). Follow-up of two-year-olds referred for possible autism. *Journal of Child Psychology and Psychiatry, 36,* 1365–1382.

Lord, C., Rutter, M., & DiLavore, P. (1998). *The Autism Diagnostic Observation Schedule–Generic (ADOS-G).* Chicago: University of Chicago Press.

Mars, A.E., Mauk, J.E., & Dowrick, P.W. (1998). Symptoms of pervasive developmental disorders as observed in prediagnostic home videos of infants and toddlers. *Journal of Pediatrics, 132,* 1–5.

Mullen, E.M. (1992). *Mullen Scales of Early Learning.* Cranston, RI: T.O.T.A.L. Child.

Osterling, J., & Dawson, G. (1994). Early recognition of children with autism: A study of first birthday home videotapes. *Journal of Autism and Developmental Disorders, 24,* 247–257.

Rogers, S. (1998). Empirically supported comprehensive treatments for young children with autism. *Journal of Clinical Child Psychology, 27,* 168–179.

Simeonsson, R.J., Olley, J.G., & Rosenthal, S.L. (1987). Early intervention for children with autism. In M. Guralnick & F. Bennett (Eds.), *The effectiveness of early intervention for at-risk and handicapped children* (pp. 275–296). San Diego, CA: Academic Press.

Smalley, S.L. (1997). Genetic influences in childhood-onset psychiatric disorders: Autism and attention-deficit/hyperactivity disorder. *American Journal of Human Genetics, 60,* 1276–1282.

Sparrow, S.S., Balla, D.A., & Cicchetti, D.V. (1984). *Vineland Adaptive Behavior Scales (VABS).* Circle Pines, MN: American Guidance Service.

Stone, W. (1998). *Early behavioral indicators of autism.* Paper presented at the NIH Meeting on the State of the Science in Autism: Screening and Diagnosis, Washington, DC.

Stone, W.L., Lee, E.B., Ashford, L., Brissie, J., Hepburn, S.L., Coonrod, E.E., & Weiss, B.H. (1999). Can autism be diagnosed accurately in children under three years? *Journal of Child Psychology and Psychiatry, 40,* 219–226.

Wetherby, A.M., & Prizant, B. (1992). Facilitating language and communication development in autism: Assessment and intervention guidelines. In D. Berkell (Ed.), *Autism: Identification, education, and treatment* (pp. 107–134). Mahwah, NJ: Lawrence Erlbaum Associates.

Wetherby, A.M., & Prizant, B. (1998). *Communication and Symbolic Behavior Scales* (Developmental profile–research ed.). Chicago: Applied Symbolix.

Zimmerman, I., Steiner, V., & Pond, R. (1992). *Preschool Language Scale-3 (PLS-3).* San Antonio, TX: The Psychological Corp.

Chapter 15

A Child with
Fetal Alcohol Syndrome

*Sterling K. Clarren, Heather Carmichael Olson,
Sandra G.B. Clarren, and Susan J. Astley*

Alcohol is a common human teratogen that, when ingested by a pregnant woman, can produce a wide array of fetal complications. The fetus's developing brain seems most sensitive to prenatal alcohol exposure: Alcohol-related brain damage can be quite diffuse, ranging from microcellular, neurochemical aberrations to macroscopic malformations (Stratton, Howe, & Battaglia, 1996). The neurological, cognitive, and behavior problems that arise from prenatal alcohol exposure are protean in their severity and diversity. Other prenatal determinants—for example, genetic factors or teratogenic exposures that lead to specific conditions, such as attention-deficit/hyperactivity disorder (ADHD) or

The authors wish to thank our colleagues who have helped us develop and use the model described in this chapter: Sharon Beck, M.Ed., Educational Counselor; Tracy Jirokowic, M.S., OTR/L, Occupational Therapist; Truman Coggins, Ph.D., Speech-Language Pathologist; Robin LaDue, Ph.D., Clinical Psychologist; and Julie Gelo, Family Advocate.

307

learning disabilities—can further affect the developmental outcome of a child prenatally exposed to alcohol. Aversive experiences after birth and throughout life also can have a profound influence on an individual's performance in these domains. Complexity in etiology and outcome is the rule, not the exception, in working with children who have been exposed to alcohol.

Fetal alcohol syndrome (FAS) does not represent the totality of individuals exposed to alcohol in gestation or the entire group of people with impairments related to prenatal alcohol exposure. Rather, FAS is defined by specific aberrations in growth, facial form, and central nervous system (CNS) functioning (Stratton et al., 1996). FAS is noteworthy because it can be specifically identified as a condition due to gestational alcohol abuse. Thus, it is an important starting point for outreach to women who are at high risk of having other children with disabilities. In addition, this designation assists government systems related to education, social service, and criminal justice in planning for service needs.

The label *FAS* is actually less helpful for individuals who have the disorder themselves as it does not, in and of itself, guide parents or professionals in proceeding with interventions specific to the child. Moreover, the term excludes many individuals with the same degree of developmental delays related to alcohol exposure who do not have the diagnostic markers of FAS.

Nevertheless, there are two important reasons to examine whether a child's impairments are related to alcohol teratogenesis, especially to FAS. First, knowing that alcohol exposure occurred during pregnancy helps a clinician understand that if the child has a complex profile of cognitive or behavior difficulties, then alcohol-related damage may be one antecedent in a larger set of etiological factors. Children with FAS or related conditions may generally have some combination of ADHD, learning delays, language processing and usage difficulties, problems in planning and judgment, or increased soft neurological signs. In addition, if the child is school-age or older, "secondary disabilities" may have emerged from experiences of frustration, failures, and lack of acceptance by peers and adults, particularly if the full extent of the child's disability has not been recognized.

Clearly, a team approach to assessment and intervention is necessary for understanding such complex problems. A diagnosis often initiates an important spontaneous intervention by changing the attitude of family members and teachers working with the child, so they can see that the child "can't" rather than "won't" behave in an acceptable manner. Members of the child's community can then understand that the child is disabled and not simply disobedient (Streissguth, Barr, Kogan, & Bookstein, 1996).

Second, recognizing that a child has FAS may help prevent prenatal alcohol exposure in the biological mother's future pregnancies. In an assessment of FAS, both the biological mother and her child are the focus of the team's efforts. Women who have children with FAS usually drink regularly and in high volume during pregnancy. Although it is true that women who consume alcohol in the gestation period may be committing "fetal abuse," the case of a woman drinking purposefully during pregnancy to harm her child is rare. It is therapeutic to inform biological mothers of this problem so that they know that the child is receiving appropriate supports and everyone can proceed in a positive manner. Although the process of working with the biological mother can be complex and involves a different group of professionals than those needed to assess the child, it is critical and ethically necessary that these diagnostic and intervention efforts be linked (Astley, Bailey, Talbot, & Clarren, 1998).

ASSESSMENT FOR DIAGNOSIS OF FETAL ALCOHOL SYNDROME

The features of FAS are not dichotomous (present or absent) but, rather, each feature is on a continuum from clearly within the normal range to clearly the feature of FAS. Without suitable guides and standards, this leads clinicians to variable judgment in final diagnosis. To minimize clinical variability, the diagnosis of FAS or related conditions is made using a sequence of four 4-digit Likert scales (Astley & Clarren, 1997) in the clinics of the Washington State FAS Diagnostic and Prevention Network. Delays in growth, facial morphology, organic brain damage, and teratogenic exposure to alcohol are each evaluated separately. A "1" on any scale means a finding within the normal range. A "4" on any scale represents a finding that corresponds with accepted cases of FAS. A score of "2" or "3" specifically defines intermediate steps between clearly typical and atypical. It is important to note that these scales do not necessarily measure increasing severity; rather, they are scales of greater clinical confidence that the sought FAS characteristic is present. A child with a "4" for brain damage, for example, meets the medical criteria for a structurally altered brain but may be more cognitively or behaviorally within the normal range than a child with a score of "2" in whom the etiological relationship between brain structure and brain function is diagnostically indeterminate. Similarly, a child with a "4" for facial morphology has all of the facial diagnostic features of FAS yet may be somewhat more attractive than a child with a score of "2"—who has an unusual face, but not the facial features common to FAS. The final category based on examination of the child is whether he or she has delayed growth. Establishing if a person's height or weight is "blunted," due to prenatal reasons, from its genetic potential is actually the most difficult part of diagnosis. Growth retardation is defined as a "4" when a child's measurements are less than 2 standard deviations (SD) from the mean after height (adjustment for mean parent height) and for weight.

The alcohol exposure scale is judged by whether the dose exposure pattern approaches one that causes fetal damage in animal models and whether the information is documented or speculative. Dose response relationships between maternal alcohol intake and fetal outcomes remain complex and somewhat vague for various reasons. Obtaining accurate information on alcohol intake during pregnancy is difficult because it is almost always recorded in retrospect, with the potential problems of the mother's poor memory or denial. Many maternal and fetal factors also play key roles in determining if any specific dosing pattern is damaging to that individual. In the majority of animal studies in multiple species, it has been necessary to give high dosage exposures, with peak blood alcohol concentrations (BAC) in the 100–200 milligrams per kilogram (mg/kg) range, and to deliver them at least weekly for the first several weeks of pregnancy. Even these high doses are not uniformly teratogenic; they are "high risk." When women report consumption likely to cause drunkenness (an approximate BAC = 100 mg/kg or higher) on a weekly basis, this is considered a "4." Any other pattern of definite exposure is judged a "3" because no dose is guaranteed to be absolutely safe.

The term FAS applies to children who have all "4"s or combinations of at least two "4"s and no more than two "3"s on the four scales. Other scores are converted to words in combinations of the descriptive terms: sentinel physical findings; static encephalopathy or neurobehavior disorder; and alcohol exposed, alcohol unexposed, and alcohol exposure unknown. A full explanation of this approach and its diagnostic terms and definitions, as well as a method for judging the importance of these comorbidities, are available in the *Diagnostic Guide for Fetal Alcohol Syndrome and Related Conditions* (Astley & Clarren, 1997). The fetal alcohol diagnosis must be considered in the context of other prenatal and postnatal factors that contribute to the unique findings for each individual.

CASE STUDY INVOLVING AN INTERDISCIPLINARY TEAM ASSESSMENT

The FAS clinic team is comprised of individuals who help collect and interpret the data needed for diagnosis, assist in developing a comprehensive intervention plan, or both. Professionals are needed from the disciplines of medicine, psychology, speech-language pathology, occupational therapy, social work, public health nursing, and family advocacy. It is also helpful to have a staff epidemiologist who can create data forms and databases and direct clinical research efforts based on these data.

The remainder of this chapter presents the composite case of Anna, a child with FAS. This case illustrates the following steps in the diagnostic interdisciplinary team process: 1) preliminary team conference; 2) team assessment, including caregiver interview, physical examination of the child, and assessments of the child by occupational therapy, speech-language pathology, and psychology team members; 3) team deliberation; 4) case discussion and feedback to the parents; 5) additional case discussion and a therapeutic debriefing with the parents; 6) further case discussion and a therapeutic debriefing with the child (when appropriate); and 7) staff debriefing. Beside preserving patient confidentially, employing a composite case permits discussion of a combination of FAS characteristics that would not necessarily be found in any one case. Exploring the case of a primary school-age child allows a more extended developmental perspective. It also sensitizes the reader to the full scope of difficulties that children with FAS have by the time they reach elementary school, which generally are not clear in preschool. Overall, although Anna is fictitious, she presents the typical challenges in FAS diagnosis, treatment, and family support.

Record Review and Preliminary Team Conference

Anna's adoptive parents initially called the FAS clinic for an appointment. The family had been referred to the clinic by Anna's teacher, who had taken a workshop on FAS, and by her physician. As is frequently the case, Anna's doctor had not previously considered an alcohol-related diagnosis but agreed to the assessment when Anna's parents sought his advice (Clarren & Astley, 1998). The family had been sent an extensive intake form. This form was specifically designed to obtain historical data from the family that would help the clinic team reach a fair and complete conclusion. These data included 1) growth records; 2) childhood photos; 3) medical records of congenital abnormalities; 4) neurological problems and ongoing health issues; 5) previous evaluations of cognition and behavior; 6) reports of response to psychotropic medication; 7) specific documentation of alcohol exposure in pregnancy; 8) exposure to other drugs or additional complications during pregnancy; 9) academic problems or cognitive delays of the biological parents or their families; 10) a general overview of the family's genetic background; 11) reports of multiple placements and issues of caregiver attachment; 12) abuse or neglect; and 13) a general record of problems or difficulties with family, peers, and school. This intake form is available in the *Diagnostic Guide for Fetal Alcohol Syndrome and Related Conditions* (Astley & Clarren, 1997).

At the preliminary team conference, these extensive past records were reviewed, and the following summary was presented to the clinic staff by the physician and the psychologist. Anna was 8 years and 1 month old. She was born to married, Caucasian parents when her mother was 28 years of age and her birth father was 35 years old. This was the third live born infant for Anna's birth mother. Her pregnancy was complicated by extensive alcohol use. The birth father reported that he would generally buy one case of beer daily and that when it was available he and his wife would each drink about half of this amount in the evening. This level of drinking persisted through the first half of the pregnancy. During the second half of Anna's gestation, Anna's birth father drank more while her mother drank less, although she still probably ingested about a six-pack daily until delivery. Anna's mother also used marijuana about once a month and smoked half a pack of cigarettes each day. The pregnancy was further complicated by physical abuse of the mother by her husband, although this abuse never led to a medical assessment during the pregnancy. Both biological parents reported that their own fathers, but not their mothers, had been heavy drinkers. Neither biological parent reported significant academic problems, and both had finished high school.

Anna was born at term, and her delivery was described as typical. At birth, she weighed 2.2 kilograms (kg) and her length was 4.4 centimeters (cm). Anna was always described as small. While in foster care, Anna received a nutritional evaluation and a thyroid screen. Anna grew steadily but more slowly than typically developing children. One previous foster parent repeatedly asked her physician to hospitalize the infant because she ardently believed that her inability to "fatten the baby up" meant that the baby was ill. Anna had an inguinal hernia that was repaired when she was 9 months old. She had chronic problems with otitis media until she reached age 3, though she never had a documented hearing loss. Despite these problems, she had been in good health overall.

After Anna was born, she lived with her parents for about 6 months, then she was removed from parental custody after the biological mother was severely beaten by her husband. In addition, investigators found that the child was living in an unclean apartment without food or appropriate clothing. Six-month-old Anna was placed in foster care and moved periodically over the next $2^{1}/_{2}$ years while social service agencies determined that neither parent could control their drinking and regain custody. Anna was then made available for adoption and was retained by her last foster family (mother, father, and a brother 3 years older than Anna) when she was about 3 years of age. The adoption was legalized when Anna was almost 5 years old.

At the time of the clinic visit, Anna's adoptive parents reported that she had shown behavior problems since 30 months of age. Sometimes Anna was very negative and aggressive, especially with family members, while at other times she was cooperative and pleasant. Upon entering preschool, she was reported to be quiet but soon showed qualities similar to those observed at home. In fact, she was so aggressive with her peers that she was unsuccessful in two preschool programs. Her parents said that these behavior problems continued but had grown less frequent and violent since Anna started kindergarten.

Anna was evaluated by a developmental pediatrician at 6 years and 11 months of age, and she was diagnosed with severe ADHD. Anna was placed on methylphenidate but had an unanticipated response with a dramatic increase in irritability. Her parents stopped giving her the medication. Anna's reaction distressed her whole family, and her parents declined to try other medications, but they did attempt to reduce the amount of sugar in her diet with no apparent positive effect. A psychiatric evaluation produced a further diagnosis of oppositional defiant disorder, and Anna was described as "anxious."

At age 7 and midway through first grade, Anna was made a "focus of concern" by her school district because of poor academic progress and increasingly problematic behavior. As part of her school assessment she was evaluated using a standardized test of intelligence, the Wechsler Intelligence Scale for Children–Third Edition (WISC-III; Weschsler, 1991). On that test, her verbal

IQ score was a standard 68 (below expectations), and her performance IQ score was a standard 90 (within normal limits). A full-scale IQ score was not calculated because of the discrepancy between Anna's verbal and performance scores. Factor scores in the areas of verbal comprehension and freedom from distractibility revealed significant difficulties while Anna's factor score in the area of perceptual organization was in the low-average range. On an individually administered academic skills measure, the Woodcock-Johnson Test of Achievement–Revised (Woodcock & Johnson, 1989), Anna received the following scaled scores: Broad Reading (75), Broad Mathematics (71), Broad Written Language (80), and Broad Knowledge (86). Her standard score on the Vineland Adaptive Behavior Scales' (VABS; Sparrow, Balla, & Cicchetti, 1984) Adaptive Behavior Composite was 52, and the subdomain scores were Communication (50), Daily Living Skills (45), and Socialization (64). School district recommendations were to provide resource room assistance given her ADHD diagnosis, but no specific educational plan was developed to address her cognitive and academic difficulties.

At the time of the FAS assessment, Anna's adoptive parents were confused and exhausted. They wished to understand how Anna's multiple diagnoses related to each other and how to maximize the effectiveness of her academic and mental health interventions.

Team Assessment

The FAS clinic evaluation included an hour-long interview of Anna's adoptive parents and several assessments of the child (whose chronological age was 8 years and 1 month), which included a physical examination, an occupational/ physical therapy assessment for soft neurological signs and fine motor problems, a specialized speech-language evaluation, and a limited amount of additional psychological testing. The goal of conducting these assessments was not necessarily to evaluate the full extent of Anna's development. Rather, it was to gather sufficient information to reach a diagnostic conclusion regarding the diversity and nature of her developmental functioning.

Caregiver Interview

A team physician and psychologist conducted an interview with Anna's adoptive parents. The interviewers guided the session to determine if Anna had the related conditions and functional impairments common in cases of FAS. These questions probed the arenas of planning, behavior regulation, abstract thinking and judgment, information processing and verbal memory, spatial skills and memory, social skills and adaptive behavior, sensorimotor integration, and both oral-motor and motor control skills.

Anna's parents seemed appropriately concerned but confused about the many previous assessments of their daughter that had apparent nonoverlapping diagnoses. They commented that they sometimes understood the antecedents of her angry outbursts (but often did not) and that Anna was basically loving and caring. Nevertheless, Anna had never enjoyed being held or hugged for more than a brief period of time. Furthermore, her parents said that she had always been very sensitive to loud noise and to rough or scratchy clothing.

Anna's parents noted that their daughter had difficulty organizing spaces; for example, she tended to crowd the letters of her name into one corner of a page and she could not put her toys away in their proper places. Her parents also agreed that their daughter had tremendous difficulty following directions. They reported that she generally failed to remember an instruction if more than a few minutes elapsed between the time the instruction was given and when she was expected to carry it out. Anna also could not successfully follow more than a one-step instruction. She could repeat instructions if she practiced saying them many times (e.g., Question: "Anna, what do we do before we eat?"; Answer: "We wash our hands"). Yet Anna usually forgot the rule without a direct reminder at the time the instruction was to be implemented. In fact, she did not understand lengths of time (e.g., the difference between an event taking place in a few minutes or one that was a few days away).

In the domain of social skills, Anna's parents described her as isolated with no friends. She seemed to enjoy the company of other children but often tried to direct all activities. This behavior usually led to marginalization by her peer group. When rejected, Anna sometimes played alone, but she usually responded to peer rejection or noncompliance with anger or physical aggression. Anna played well with younger children (ages 3 or 4 years) and was kind to animals.

In physical terms, Anna had trouble going to bed and often awoke in the night, but then she generally tired during the later part of the day. Her mother commented ruefully that Anna could climb, in-line skate, and do other age-appropriate outdoor activities but did them in a frighteningly reckless and somewhat clumsy way. In general, Anna was described as having problems with self-regulation. Her parents had learned to send their daughter to her room when she was out of control. In time out, Anna quickly calmed down and seemingly forgot the entire event within minutes. Such outbursts could occur daily or even several times per day.

During the interview, Anna's parents confirmed the history of alcohol exposure that had been reported to them by the biological father. Apparently, Anna's biological mother had been in recovery at the time of the adoption and had given the adoptive parents the same facts. Anna's adoptive parents thought her biological mother was still living in the area and was once again drinking. They had not been in contact with her for several years.

Pediatrics

The results of the physical examination conducted by the team physician revealed that Anna's height was 115 cms, her weight was 18 kgs, and her head circumference was 48.5 cms. The three facial features that define the dysmorphic face of FAS were each carefully assessed. Her palpebral fissures (the horizontal length of the eyelid slit opening) measured 2.3 cms. Her philtrum (the vertical furrows between the nose and border of the red portion or vermilion border of the upper lip) was judged to be "flat" when compared to standard photos of philtrums of variable fullness. Similarly, the vermilion border was judged to be "very thin" using the photographic guide (available in the *Diagnostic Guide for Fetal Alcohol Syndrome and Related Conditions* [Astley & Clarren, 1997]). In addition, Anna had a small jaw and a mild overbite of her new secondary upper incisors. The rest of Anna's physical examination was unremarkable.

Occupational Therapy

Fine and gross motor skills were within normal limits using the Bruininks-Oseretsky Test of Motor Proficiency (Bruininks, 1978). Although Anna's parents had concerns about "clumsiness," that problem was not identified with this tool. The Quick Neurological Screening Test–Revised (QNST-R; Mutti, Sterling, & Spalding, 1978) was also administered. This tool is generally more useful to screen multiple areas of neuromotor integration and soft neurological signs. A normal score is less than 20; an abnormal score is more than 50. Anna's score was 45, in the "suspicious" range. Particularly difficult for Anna were coordinating rapid controlled movements, balance, and tasks involving spatial awareness of her body. These results fit with findings on the Beery-Buktencia Developmental Test of Visual-Motor Integration (VMI; Beery, 1997), signifying that Anna had below-average abilities in figure copying and a very disorganized approach to more complex visual information. A short sensorimotor history questionnaire completed by Anna's adoptive parents revealed sensitivities to tactile and auditory information, echoing descriptions from the caregiver interview. This sort of nonstandardized checklist is used in FAS clinics when there are concerns about sensory processing.

Speech-Language Pathology

Impairments with language, cognition, and social behavior are not unusual for children with FAS and related conditions, and they underlie difficulties in social competence and some aspects of academic performance. Research measures of social communication and social reasoning are used in FAS clinics to tap this common area of concern, and the results these measures produce capture something of the day-to-day problems that parents of children affected by alcohol describe. In addition, age- and developmentally appropriate standardized measures of receptive and expressive language are also employed in clinics to conduct a brief assessment of language development.

Anna's receptive and expressive language skills were broadly within the typical range; she nonetheless showed notable delays in storytelling and mental-state reasoning, two aspects of social communication and social reasoning. Anna was asked to retell a story she had just heard, using a picture book without words as a cue. Anna's narrative was vague and poorly connected; in effect, she described elements in each picture without linking them into a story line. She could not take her listener's perspective into account in communicating the story. Anna understood the facts of the story but could not mentally "step into another person's shoes" when asked questions that required understanding another person's perspective. In these tasks, Anna did not give clear evidence that she understood what other people were thinking. These observations were congruent with reported information from the caregiver interview.

Psychology

As is often the case, the clinic was provided with valid and relatively recent testing by school and community professionals. To supplement these data, Anna was given the core assessment from the NEPSY, a Developmental Neuropsychological Assessment (Korkman, Kirk, & Kemp, 1998), a standardized battery of tasks that provides a developmental neuropsychological assessment for children ages 3–12 years. Anna's scores on the test's Core Domains of Language and Sensorimotor Function were low-average while visuospatial processing was in the borderline range. She scored well below average on Attention/Executive Function and Memory and Learning. Her scores on individual subtests were uneven and provided considerable insight regarding her problem-solving and learning styles. Of particular interest was Anna's very poor performance on a narrative memory task similar to one given in the speech-language assessment. In this task, which resembles school activities, the child listened to a story read aloud, attempted to tell it on her own, and then answered comprehension questions. Again, Anna's version of the story was vague and sparsely detailed. Even when cued, Anna often could not always remember the information offered in the story. When asked a question she often started to give an answer, then seemed to lose the aim of the task, and finally made unrelated responses that suggested she was guessing just to give an answer. She appeared very anxious during this task, shifting around in her chair, commenting on noises outside the room, and asking whether the testing was almost done.

To provide an estimate of behavioral function, Anna's adoptive mother completed the Child Behavior Checklist for 4- to 18-year-olds (CBCL; Achenbach, 1991). Her second grade teacher completed the Teacher's Report Form (TRF; Achenbach, 1991). Parent report on the CBCL revealed overall behavior difficulties, with a Total Behavior Problems T score of 79, which is within the clinically significant range. The realm of internalizing problems was also clinically significant due to an elevated score suggesting anxiety. Externalizing behavior problems were also rated in the significant range, with elevated scores on scales of aggressive and "delinquent" behavior as well as difficulties with thinking, social skills, and attention span. Anna's Total Competence T score was 32, falling below the clinical cutoff, with poor scores on scales of social and school competence. This resonated with the mother's concerns about her daughter's inability to learn right from wrong: Anna sometimes attempted to hurt family members, yet she had a sense of humor and the ability to be loving and caring.

On the TRF, Anna's teacher expressed concern about behaviors in both Internalizing and Externalizing scales. Again, Anna's overall Internalizing problem score was elevated primarily because of her anxious behavior. Her Externalizing behavior problem score was elevated mostly due to her overactive and aggressive behavior. Anna's teacher reported that the child would destroy her own and others' possessions when angered. However, her ratings showed that she could occasionally work hard and seem happy. Overall, Anna's teacher's ratings also indicated that her student was having some difficulty behaving appropriately and learning. She noted that Anna did better in small, highly structured environments than in the larger classroom setting. The teacher thought that Anna was very hard on herself, with very high expectations and a tendency to become very upset (even self-abusive) if she did not meet her own expectations.

For many children in the FAS clinic, only brief screening is carried out by the psychologist to supplement available test results from community professionals. For children who are old enough and have sufficient intellectual capability, the child and adult versions of the California Verbal Learning Test (CVLT; Delis, Kramer, Kaplan, & Ober, 1994) and the Rey Complex Figure Test (RCFT; Meyers, Meyers, & Kelly, 1995) are highly informative. Used together, these tools assess verbal learning and memory, nonverbal memory and visuospatial skills, the child's ability to organize his or her behavior toward a complex end, and his or her behavior when carrying out demanding tasks. Literature on fetal alcohol effects suggests these might be areas of concern for individuals affected by prenatal alcohol ingestion. Findings from the CVLT and RCFT are often supplemented by several informal drawing tasks and a short interview. For children from preschool to late elementary school age, behavior observations are often carried out while the child is receiving the physical examination or other on-site testing and when the child is in an unstructured, highly stimulating environment (e.g., in the waiting room, on an elevator ride, during a walk through the building). Because a formal adaptive behavior assessment is often not part of a child's file, the psychologist will sometimes give the Summary Version of the VABS (Sparrow et al., 1984) prior to the caregiver interview.

Team Deliberation

Anna met the criteria for FAS in that she had been exposed to alcohol and had confirmed growth delays, specific atypical facial features, and evidence of CNS dysfunction. Details for these and other factors are provided as follows:

Growth

Anna's growth was considered definitely atypical, as her height and weight were both below the 3rd percentile after a height adjustment for mean parental height. Anna's height of 115 cms was at the 2nd percentile. The height of her biological parents averaged 174 cms. Adjusting for mid-parental stature determined that Anna was actually 3 cms smaller than would be predicted from her genetic background. Therefore, her atypical growth pattern was independent of her genetic background.

Dysmorphology

Those with FAS have short palpebral fissures ("short" when more than 2 SD below the mean) and a flat philtrum and thinned vermilion border. The philtrum and lip must each be judged a "4" or "5" on a 5-point rating scale in comparison to a standard set of five photos. Anna's palpebral fissures were measured at 3.5 SD below the mean. Her lip was judged a "5" while her philtrum was given a rating of "4." Her dental malocclusion, although not of relevance to the FAS diagnosis, was a common associated finding. Overall, she had the distinctive facial features that characterize FAS.

Central Nervous System Dysfunction

Evidence for CNS dysfunction can be defined structurally, neurologically, or by examining psychometric evidence. Anna had positive findings in all of these areas. Her head circumference was below the 2nd percentile. By itself, microcephaly is a sufficient finding for FAS diagnostic purposes, but Anna also had an atypical neurological exam, with a QNST score above the usual cutoff and evidence of visual-motor difficulties on the Developmental Test of Visual-Motor Integration. Anna's behavior was characterized by severe ADHD, adaptive behavior problems, clear social-communication impairments, a learning disorder, a significant verbal-performance discrepancy shown in IQ testing, and evidence of memory and attention/executive function problems in neuropsychological assessment. The descriptive diagnostic term *static encephalopathy*, with evidence of diffuse CNS dysfunction, applied to Anna.

Alcohol Exposure History

The history of alcohol exposure in utero was judged to be definite, as it was independently confirmed by both birth parents. Consumption of 6–12 beers or more, on a daily or nearly daily basis, would place a fetus at definite risk for damage due to alcohol exposure.

Comorbidities

There were no additional physical findings, problems in the genetic background, or other teratogenic exposures that suggested an alternate or additional prenatal etiological diagnosis. Based on record review, interview, and behavioral observations, the team was in agreement with the psychiatric diagnoses of oppositional defiant disorder and moderate anxiety. In part, these conditions were hypothesized by the team to be situational, arising from Anna's prolonged frustration from criticism by others as well as herself regarding her poor performance. In other words, these would be secondary disabilities.

Recommendations

After discussion to establish the diagnosis, the team began to develop a tentative list of recommendations to be shared with the family during the case conference. It is useful to divide suggestions into at least four categories: medical, mental health, formal/informal education, and social services. In certain cases, additional categories (e.g., legal, correctional) are needed.

Medical

Anna had a classic presentation of FAS. No further specific medical diagnostic evaluations were necessary in this case. However, this is not always the case. Individuals with prenatal alcohol exposure can have alcohol-related and other conditions or simply alternate conditions. Differential diagnosis often needs to consider relatively common genetic conditions like fragile X syndrome or Turner syndrome as well as obscure dysmorphic syndromes of genetic or alternate teratogenic cause. Any FAS program must always be alert to the possibility of alternate diagnoses involving other syndromes.

Another noteworthy medical issue was that there was a strong history of familial alcoholism. Both of Anna's parents and her grandfathers were alcoholics. Thus, there was a chance that Anna carried a genetic propensity for alcoholism independent of her condition of FAS. The team felt that Anna would need clear and regular warnings throughout childhood and adolescence that drinking could cause her to become an alcoholic. Such direct messages help some children withstand peer pressure to begin alcohol use in adolescence.

In addition, Anna was small but had consistently grown parallel to typical parameters. This fact, along with her generally unremarkable physical examination, meant that there was no reason to recommend further medical evaluation of her growth. (Intriguingly, many children with FAS have a robust growth spurt at the time of puberty, moving into the typical range for height at that time.) On this note, it is not surprising that Anna's physician had not considered an FAS diagnosis or referral, because Anna's physical health was good and her problems were in areas not usually considered as health care problems.

Mental Health

Anna had clinical evidence of distractibility and inattention and had had an unexpectedly adverse reaction to methylphenidate. At the time of the clinic visit, it remained possible that Anna fit the diagnostic criteria for ADHD within the broader diagnosis of FAS. Thus, Anna might still respond to methylphenidate prescribed at a lower dose or to an alternate stimulant medication. It was also possible that her inattention and distractibility were due to anxiety and could be resolved if her anxiety and other problems were addressed, perhaps with an alternative, nonstimulant pharmacological approach as well as situational remediation.

Some families are concerned by the use of medications with children already affected by prenatal alcohol exposure. It was important that Anna's family be reassured of the general safety and potential benefits of medications. Nevertheless, the team felt it better for Anna's overall emotional state to be judged and the adjustments in her educational program and family expectations to be evaluated before further drug trials. Based on the outcome of such monitoring, a psychiatrist might then be better able to prescribe psychotropic medications.

Making those additional changes would be difficult. Anna's parents were already frustrated and fatigued by caring for a child whose behavior problems had escalated while her adaptive function had declined. Anna demonstrated complex cognitive and behavior impairments. Managing the child's behavior and helping her to learn would require expert assistance. The team decided to encourage Anna's parents to work with a counselor in developing appropriate parenting strategies and addressing the stresses inherent in raising a child with FAS. However, it is difficult to find such counselors and to fund this type of on-going counseling assistance. If the parents did find a counselor, the team felt it would be ideal if that person or Anna's psychiatrist functioned as a service co-ordinator. The case management goal would be to align home and school be-havior programs, with dual foci on eliminating aggressive behaviors and build-ing anger management and socialization skills.

Another possible source of assistance was parent networks. Such support groups are remarkably useful resources for families raising children with FAS. In the 1990s, parents increasingly began joining together to support and edu-cate one another, to advocate for funding and missing services, and to promote societal recognition of and research on FAS and related conditions. The team planned to augment the parents' access to information and self-help advice by providing them with a telephone hotline number for FAS and copies of recent issues of FAS community education newsletters.

Formal/Informal Education

In some states, Anna would qualify for special education under the category of "health impaired" given either her diagnosis of FAS or of ADHD. She might also qualify as "neurologically impaired" based on microcephaly coupled with atypical neurological findings of fine motor delays and a significant number of soft neurological signs. In addition, Anna could qualify as "learning disabled" because of her psychological evaluation. Anna clearly met the criteria for, and needed, an individualized education program (IEP).

Most school districts have an approach to children with complex needs, such as Anna, that involves special education classes or resource room help for academic work; supplemental speech-language, occupational, and physical therapy services; and inclusion with typically developing peers during certain activities (e.g., recess, lunch, library time). These qualifying children may also be accompanied by a paraeducator for a portion of or the entire school day. This general plan seemed reasonable for Anna, although her pattern of special needs did not completely fit interventions such as those designed for children with mental retardation, learning disabilities, or severe behavior disorders. Therefore, individualized and flexible intervention planning at school was needed. Based on Anna's profile of test results, specific classroom techniques included 1) repeating practice of learning materials; 2) using less abstract materials; 3) limiting the need for Anna to remember spatial information; 4) breaking long instructions, stories, or lessons into smaller parts; 5) encouraging Anna to work slowly and carefully; 6) allowing time during transitions for Anna to become self-motivated and interested in the next activity; 7) analyzing strategies Anna used on her own during learning activities and offering more effective strategies as appropriate; and 8) informing Anna when she was doing well by rewarding effort and not achievement.

The team felt that Anna would benefit from occupational therapy services designed to assist her in better modulating incoming stimuli and to decrease performance anxiety by altering her classroom environment. If occupational therapy services could be provided at school, a private occupational therapist might be a useful addition to Anna's service team. Finally, speech-language consultation was recommended to enhance Anna's social-communication skills.

Furthermore, Anna would benefit from participation in extracurricular activities that she enjoyed and did well. Such activities could help raise her self-esteem and would be less likely to promote performance anxiety. Nevertheless, it was important to emphasize that Anna should only be enrolled in activities supervised by adults accustomed to working with children with special needs.

Social Services

At the time of Anna's adoption, fetal alcohol effects and the possibility of a lifelong disability were not raised with the family. Given the documented history of voluminous alcohol exposure during gestation and the history of growth problems from birth, the team believed that the issue of FAS should have been evaluated at the time of adoption. It would have been reasonable then to offer a subsidized adoption to offset added educational and mental health services that Anna would probably need. The team recommended that this issue be revisited with the appropriate social service agency. Subsidized adoption should include medical coverage, psychiatric benefits for the future if preapproved, and a monthly cost supplement. In addition, because Anna had permanent disabilities, she should qualify for Supplemental Security Income (SSI) coverage. As a child, eligibility is based primarily on functional ability, and the receipt of benefits is dependent on parental income. The issue of SSI funding could be reexamined later when Anna neared adulthood. The Division of Developmental Disabilities was another agency to contact for possible resources or benefits. The agency has strict qualifying criteria, but this option was worth pursuing.

Case Discussion: Feedback to Parents

The case discussion actually occurred in two phases. The first part consisted of elements typically discussed with parents during an assessment feedback session. The second phase, however, was a unique feature of the particular clinic that evaluated Anna.

Part I

Diagnosis and treatment recommendations were shared with Anna's parents in a roundtable forum. Each team member who had tested Anna briefly stated his or her specific findings, gearing discussion of test results to support the recommendations that would be mentioned later. For example, the physician articulated the medical diagnosis of FAS, and then the occupational therapist, the speech-language pathologist, and the psychologist who had tested Anna all stated their findings. The psychologist who interviewed the family then gave the team's recommendations in broad outline. All feedback was provided with careful sensitivity to the parents' emotional state and apparent level of comprehension.

In this large group setting, with all team members and some observers, the parents appeared fairly composed and quietly accepting of the diagnosis and intervention ideas. Nonetheless, their emotional responses were complex. On one hand, Anna's parents seemed pleased and relieved to receive an overall explanation for Anna's primary problems. On the other hand, they were troubled that Anna's complex neurological problems and her reactions to the accompanying difficulties had not previously been made clear. They also felt despair because they believed they had floundered for so long in caring for their daughter. Finally, they mentioned some fleeting anger at Anna's biological mother for causing these problems.

Part II

At this particular clinic, after clients have discussed the situation with the whole team, they have a quiet time when they can talk privately with one person on the team, usually the psychologist involved in the initial interview. This final phase with the caregivers provides a time for parents to catch their breath, express their feelings about the events of the day, and share their reaction to the diagnosis. Thereafter, they can hear and discuss the diagnosis and recommendations again to clarify their understanding and to begin initial planning for interventions based on clinic referrals. This final period honors the caregivers' and child's needs for a limited emotional closure to a stressful experience and for a way to review the many concepts and ideas they have just heard. Families often report how important this final time of consolidation is for them.

Anna's parents had endured an emotionally intense morning. At this second phase of the discussion process, the psychologist asked, "How are you doing? Does Anna's diagnosis make sense to you?" Then she waited and listened. Tears welled up in Anna's mother's eyes; her father let out a deep sigh. Finally, the father said how hard it was to hear that Anna did have FAS. The mother said she thought all along that Anna had FAS; Anna was so like the descriptions she had read. However, she kept wishing she would wake up and Anna would be just like her cousins and the kids next door. But now the mother knew Anna would never be an ordinary little girl, teenager, or adult.

For several minutes the parents quietly cried, but they eventually regained their composure. The psychologist expressed her support. Then, Anna's mother asked what the family's next step should be.

The psychologist began to help the parents make sense of the diagnosis and recommendations. The psychologist read the diagnostic information and suggestions aloud to the parents to make sure the wording was clear and sufficiently informative. She clarified the meaning of a diagnosis of FAS. Using schematic drawings and straightforward descriptions the psychologist reviewed the word *syndrome* and each of the three basic aspects of the fetal alcohol syndrome: growth, facial features, and organic brain damage. She discussed how Anna met the growth criteria, as she had always been small, and her height and weight measurements during the assessment were below the 5th percentile compared to those of her peers. The psychologist explained the importance of small eyes and a thin upper lip and philtrum as physical markers for FAS and briefly described the embryology of these features. She also pointed out that Anna was a very pretty child and these facial characteristics did not stand out or negatively affect her looks. Then the psychologist explained the organic brain damage portion of the syndrome and how Anna demonstrated this characteristic. This was the time when the old and the new test data were analyzed. The parents asked many questions, and time was given to explain to them how Anna's profile of test results related to her learning and behavior problems. In particular, the results of the QNST, which had indicated an atypical pattern of neurological soft signs and motor weaknesses, and her low scores on adaptive problem solving on the VABS were reviewed because both lent support to the finding that Anna was functioning at the level of a child half her chronological age. Also, her limited linguistic understanding of another's point of view and the discrepancy between her verbal and average nonverbal reasoning were discussed to help the parents understand why Anna seemed well adjusted at one moment and then had such great difficulties and frustrations the next.

Specific telephone numbers were provided, and referrals to three possible counselors/behavioral consultants were made. The parents also signed a mutual exchange of information form so the psychologist could talk to Anna's teacher and school counselor at a future date. In addition, the psychologist provided handouts from the resource box of articles on FAS, copies of the most recent newsletters, and ordering information for books that might be of value to Anna's teachers.

The psychologist next asked if the parents thought Anna needed to talk about the diagnosis, and the parents said they did not think she would understand. To Anna, this day of testing was similar to her assessment process at school. In the future, they thought they could explain her diagnosis or they would contact the clinic for assistance. As a rule, feedback is given to an older child, a teenager, or an adult. If the child is briefed, there are several topics that generally should be considered for discussion with the child and the caregivers together. The feelings the child or caregivers may have about the biological mother's role and the frustration of ongoing problems in learning, behavior, and growth need to be recognized. The team should emphasize that they know the child works hard but has difficulties and may have been misunderstood over the years. In addition, the professionals need to clarify that the diagnosis explains why learning and being calm have been hard. Also, the child must be encouraged that he or she can learn and work but may need extra time and assistance. Again, the child also needs to be informed of his or her risk of becoming alcoholic. Finally, definite closure of the team assessment has to be made. This is the time to determine if the child requires follow-up with the clinic. In Anna's case, the psychologist closed the session by expressing her appreciation to the caregivers for their courage, good parenting, and cooperation as well as acknowledging how difficult the process had been. She stated she would be available to telephone Anna's teacher if necessary. Then the psychologist walked to the area where Anna was playing and shook the child's hand, told her what a good job she had done, and thanked her for coming to the clinic.

CONCLUSION

The reader may wonder why a school-age child was used as a case example when the primary focus of this book is assessment in the early childhood years. Although younger children are assessed for FAS and related conditions, an older child's case demonstrates the richness and complexity of the accompanying performance problems that are not well described or measured until elementary school. Yet early diagnosis is important. It is likely that proper planning will reduce secondary disabilities and perhaps even improve cognitive performance when a diagnosis is made at the earliest possible time. Furthermore, the younger the child at the time of diagnosis, the more probable it is that the biological mother is still of childbearing age and would ingest alcohol during future pregnancies.

Unfortunately, the diagnosis of FAS cannot always be established conclusively in young children; even if the diagnosis is established in the preschool years, it is rarely clear what specific cognitive and behavior problems will follow. After all, the diagnosis of FAS relies on independent evidence of growth delays, a cluster of specific atypical facial features, organic brain damage, and a history of prenatal exposure to alcohol. The physical findings of poor growth and facial alteration and the history of alcohol exposure can all be fairly assessed in preschoolers, but detecting subtle levels of brain damage is much more problematic. If the child has microcephaly, hard neurological signs, or has had a brain image that discloses structural aberrations, this component of the diagnosis can be confirmed. If these observations are typical, alcohol-related brain damage could still be present at a microscopic level that can only be detected with late 20th century clinical techniques through a battery of psy-chometric testing. Reliable and valid testing of this type is not available for very young children. Furthermore, even if the diagnosis can be established through physical observations, the child's functional problems could be wide ranging and only well understood through formal assessments done over sev-eral subsequent years. As of 2000, there is no solid evidence that the facial characteristics and growth delays in children with FAS predict that there will be definite brain impairments or any specific level of delay. These findings cannot be used as proxy measures for brain performance itself. For infants, toddlers, and preschoolers, a sensorimotor history questionnaire, developmen-tal screening (e.g., the Bayley Infant Neurodevelopmental Screener [Aylward, 1995] or the Miller Assessment for Preschoolers [MAP; Miller, 1988]), and ob-servation of parent–child interactions are often carried out by the FAS clinic occupational therapist and psychologist working together. Although these as-sessments are useful, they can rarely predict the types of processing difficulties that are at the heart of the ongoing FAS disability. Anna was noted to have had problems with anger and socialization in preschool although the cause was not understood at that time. Actually, many children who are later found to have significant cognitive and behavior problems seemed, to both their parents and teachers, to be developing typically before the age of 4 or 5 years.

As of 2000, the approach to the problem of FAS diagnosis in young chil-dren is twofold. First, the most complete assessment possible is conducted along the lines discussed in this chapter. Then the interdisciplinary team as-sesses the risk factors of each client (i.e., the biological mother and the child). If the mother drank substantially during this child's gestation and is still drink-ing and of childbearing age, she needs direction toward appropriate interven-tions to prevent subsequent adverse birth outcomes. She also needs support in rearing her child if she has custody. The child is considered at risk as well, based on the exposure history itself. Whether the child meets criteria for FAS, a related condition, or is found to be typically developing at the time of as-sessment, he or she needs appropriately stimulating home and preschool ex-periences and reassessments in the age period from kindergarten to second grade. As of 2000, few specific preschool programs have been specifically de-veloped for children with FAS and related conditions (see Olson & Burgess, 1997). The need for more such programs is imperative for improving the qual-ity of these children's lives.

REFERENCES

Achenbach, T.M. (1991). *Manual for the Child Behavior Checklist/4–18 and 1991 Profile.* Burlington: University of Vermont Department of Psychiatry.
Astley, S.J., Bailey, D., Talbot, T., & Clarren, S.K. (1998). Primary prevention of FAS: Targeting women at high risk through the FAS Diagnostic and Prevention Network. *Alcoholism: Clinical and Experimental Research, 22,* 104A.

Astley, S.J., & Clarren, S.K. (1997). *Diagnostic guide for fetal alcohol syndrome and related conditions.* Seattle: University of Washington Press.

Aylward, G.P. (1995). *Bayley Infant Neurodevelopmental Screener.* San Antonio, TX: The Psychological Corp.

Beery, K. (1997). *The Beery-Buktencia Developmental Test of Visual-Motor Integration (VMI) with Supplemental Developmental Tests of Visual Perception and Motor Coordination.* Parsippany, NJ: Modern Curriculum Press.

Bruininks, R.H., (1978). *Bruininks-Oseretsky Test of Motor Proficiency.* Circle Pines, MN: American Guidance Service.

Clarren, S. K., & Astley, S.J. (1998). Identification of children with fetal alcohol syndrome and opportunity for referral of their mothers for primary prevention. *Morbidity Mortality Weekly Report, 47,* 861–864.

Delis, D.C., Kramer, J.H., Kaplan, E., & Ober, B.A. (1994). *California Verbal Learning Test (CVLT).* San Antonio, TX: The Psychological Corp.

Korkman, M., Kirk, U., & Kemp, S., (1998). *NEPSY: A Developmental Neuropsychological Assessment.* San Antonio, TX: The Psychological Corp.

Meyers, J.E., & Meyers, K.R. (1995). *Rey Complex Figure Test (RCFT).* Lutz, FL: Psychological Assessment Resources (PAR).

Miller, L.J. (1988). *Miller Assessment for Preschoolers (MAP).* San Antonio, TX: The Psychological Corp.

Mutti, M., Sterling, H.M., & Spalding, N.V. (1978). *Quick Neurological Screening Test–Revised (QNST-R).* San Antonio, TX: The Psychological Corp.

Olson, H.C., & Burgess, D.M. (1997). Early intervention for children prenatally exposed to alcohol and other drugs. In M.J. Guralnick (Ed.), *The effectiveness of early intervention* (pp. 109–145). Baltimore: Paul H. Brookes Publishing Co.

Sparrow, S.S., Balla, D.A., & Cicchetti, D.V. (1984). *Vineland Adaptive Behavior Scales (VABS).* Circle Pines, MN: American Guidance Service.

Stratton, K., Howe, C., & Battaglia, F. (Eds.). (1996). *Fetal alcohol syndrome—Diagnosis, epidemiology, prevention and treatment.* Washington, DC: National Academy Press.

Streissguth, A.P., Barr, H.M., Kogan, J., & Bookstein, F. (1996). *Understanding the occurrence of secondary disabilities in clients with FAS and FAE: Final report to the Centers for Disease Control and Prevention.* Seattle: University of Washington Press.

Wechsler, D. (1991). *Wechsler Intelligence Scale for Children–Third Edition.* San Antonio, TX: The Psychological Corp.

Woodcock, R.W., & Johnson, M.B. (1989). *Woodcock-Johnson Tests of Cognitive Ability: Standard and Supplemental Batteries.* Allen, TX: DLM.

Chapter 16

A Child with
Prader-Willi Syndrome

Vanja A. Holm, Theresse Douglass,
Betty L. Lucas, Kathleen A. Washington,
Anne Hay, and Truman E. Coggins

This chapter's case study of a child with Prader-Willi syndrome (PWS) illustrates the classic clinical presentation of this disorder from birth. The infant had been inactive in the womb and was born floppy. During the first few days, the baby was lethargic with a weak cry. She also was a poor feeder who needed to be gavage fed early. Hypotonia (low muscle tone) slowly improved, but the child continued to present with poor weight gain, or failure to thrive (FTT), for several months. A picture emerges of a child with delayed development and excessive weight gain during the toddler years with accompanying behavior problems of overeating, food foraging, stubbornness, and excessive temper tantrums.

PWS exemplifies the difficulties presented to parents whose child has been diagnosed with a complex genetic disorder that has overwhelming implications for the future. What parents read about this disorder is frightening, and observing older children with the disorder and talking to their parents is not much comfort. The clinician's role is to put into perspective the information gleaned by the parents of young children with PWS and to emphasize the positive factors. The case study in this chapter also depicts how familial and cultural factors play an important role in adjusting to the stresses of parenting a child with a disability. The necessary support services available to help families of young children with PWS are emphasized. Finally, this case illustrates how an interdisciplinary team evaluates a child comprehensively to provide parents with a view of the child's strengths and weaknesses as well as a perspective for making realistic plans to meet the child's complex needs.

DIAGNOSIS OF PRADER-WILLI SYNDROME

Until 1981, the diagnosis of PWS was made on clinical features alone. At that time, a special chromosomal study was described that showed that a deletion of the proximal part of the long arm of chromosome 15 (called *15q deletion*) was the cause of the syndrome in 60%–70% of the cases. Later, it was found that chromosome 15 with the deletion was donated by the sperm and that one could get the same syndrome if both chromosome 15s came from the egg. This later circumstance, called *maternal disomy,* is the cause of about 30% of the cases of PWS. Both deletion and disomy cases can be detected by a test that shows an absence of paternal DNA in the crucial area of chromosome 15. This genetic abnormality occurs randomly in all races and is not inherited in families (Holm, 1996).

CASE BACKGROUND

Kim, a child of Chinese ancestry with PWS, had been known by the clinic professionals since she was first diagnosed with this condition at 12 months of age. A team consisting of clinicians from the disciplines of pediatrics, nutrition, and nursing has followed Kim since she was 14 months old. The full assessment discussed in this chapter was initiated when Kim's mother contacted the clinic with particular concerns when Kim was 4 years and 2 months old.

The information obtained in previous visits was reviewed by the pediatrician, who was the service coordinator for Kim's case. At this time, a full reevaluation seemed indicated and was planned to include representatives from the disciplines of pediatrics, nursing, nutrition, physical therapy, psychology, and speech-language pathology. As part of the reevaluation process, questionnaires regarding Kim's preschool education, motor development, and communicative behavior (see the Appendix at the end of this book) were sent to her school.

Chart Review

Review of Kim's clinical chart provided the following information. Kim had been the result of her then 34-year-old mother's second pregnancy, which lasted 39 weeks. Birth weight, length, and Apgar scores were within typical limits. The child's hospital stay was only 2 days, but she was readmitted at 4 days because of hypotonia and FTT. Sepsis was suspected, and she was treated with antibiotics until blood cultures showed no growth. She was gavage fed in the hospital and sent home on bottle feedings with special nipples having large holes. No etiological diagnosis was made at that time.

Because of the complicated early history and noted developmental delays, her pediatrician referred Kim to a high-risk infant follow-up (HRIF) clinic. At the evaluation at 12 months of age, Kim had a history of poor feeding and FTT. She also continued to have hypotonia, and she showed facial features of PWS. A tentative clinical diagnosis of PWS was subsequently confirmed by laboratory findings, and Kim was transferred to a clinical team with special expertise in the condition.

PWS is a genetic disorder for which the symptoms vary depending on age. The clinical picture in early childhood is described in this report. In later childhood, gross obesity and behavior problems in the form of temper tantrums and food preoccupation become significant. In adolescence, the obesity frequently becomes life threatening if not curtailed, and the behavior difficulties escalate to include lying about and stealing food, violent outbursts, and constant verbal perseverations. Even though mental retardation requiring limited support is typical, the adult with PWS usually needs to be in sheltered living situations for health reasons in order to control excessive, compulsive food intake (Cassidy, 1984).

In-Depth History

The team first saw Kim at 14 months of age. She had severe hypotonia and was lethargic but smiled responsively when approached. Her length was at the 25th percentile and weight for height was below the 5th percentile. Kim had been a poor feeder from birth, taking 20 minutes to ingest 2 ounces (oz) of formula in the early months. At 14 months of age, she was taking about 20 oz of iron-fortified formula per day in the bottle and small amounts of infant cereal and junior foods. It was recommended that Kim be offered solids three times a day to include more textured table foods. Other suggestions were to add oil and butter to foods and to offer more finger foods.

Kim's father was a professional engineer, and her mother was a homemaker. Her older brother was healthy. The mother's family lived in Taiwan and was described as having strong ties to traditional Chinese culture. The father's family lived in Canada and was said to have adopted a Western lifestyle. Kim's mother was not as proficient in English as her husband, but she still communicated well on her own.

In terms of supports, the pediatrician gently explained the implications of the diagnosis of PWS to the family. They were provided with information about the Prader-Willi Syndrome Association (PWSA), a national support group with a local chapter in the family's city of residence. Home-based physical therapy services recommended by the HRIF clinic were in place. The mother found public health nurse (PHN) visits, also initiated by the HRIF clinic, helpful as well.

The PHN had weighed Kim weekly. At a brief follow-up visit 2 months later, with nutrition and nursing, her weight for height was still below the 5th percentile. However, there had been a catch-up in her weight during the past 2 months. At this time, Kim ate three times a day, and her diet consisted mostly of table foods (e.g., vegetables, rice, chicken). The mother reported that Kim enjoyed finger feeding and was showing interest in using the spoon. Formula intake had decreased to 12–16 oz per day. Food records showed Kim's usual daily diet to contain about 750 calories. This or a slightly higher level of intake would be needed to continue the catch-up in growth. Recommendations focused on increasing the calories with solids as well as switching to cow's milk and offering Kim a cup daily.

Kim's mother said that she had been unable to speak to her family in Taiwan about her daughter's medical difficulties and the diagnosis, even though a close relative was a physician there. She felt that the attitude toward disabilities in her home country would be less understanding than what she had encountered in the United States and from her husband's family.

Reassessment at 18 months by pediatrics and nutrition was prompted by the parents' and therapist's concern that Kim seemed to be listing to one side when pulling to stand. When sitting, a spinal curvature was present that did not fully straighten when she was held in vertical suspension. Kim was referred to a pediatric scoliosis clinic. She was described as a quiet baby, but her parents reported that they occasionally heard her say "mama" and "dada" nonspecifically. In-home speech-language therapy had been added. Her weight for height had reached the 5th percentile. Kim's diet was similar, but she now sometimes used a spoon. She also had successfully switched from formula to milk. However, because her mother was unfamiliar with milk labels, Kim had been given 2% milk instead of the 4% milk that she needed. It was explained to the parents that although Kim needed whole milk at this time, later she would likely need to be given low-fat milk. PHN visits occurred biweekly during this period.

Three months later, the PHN reported by telephone that Kim's weight for height was at the 10th percentile, which was within typical limits. Kim enjoyed eating a variety of foods and almost never refused anything. Her parents were very pleased with her feeding progress and weight gain. The mother was looking for a job and had visited nearby developmental programs but wanted to find out about employment options before making a change from the home-based services.

Reevaluation at 26 months disclosed that Kim had been found to have mild right-sided scoliosis and was being closely followed in the specialty clinic. Her weight for height had reached the 25th percentile. Kim continued to eat from the family menu, which was of their culture (i.e., rice with meat and vegetables, noodle soups, fruit), but she also ate breads and cereals. Her mother reported that Kim loved McDonald's hamburgers and french fries, and she had this meal about once a week. Because the father usually worked late, Kim frequently ate a second dinner with him before going to bed. It was suggested that Kim instead be offered a small snack during the social time with her father. She now walked with assistance. The parents heard no words beside the still nonspecific "mama" and "dada." Kim attended a developmental program twice a week, where she was exposed to signing. The mother did not get a job but had learned to drive and was taking Kim to school. By this time, she had shared the diagnosis with her relatives in Taiwan and reported that they seemed to understand. The parents had been reading the PWSA newsletters but did not find them very relevant to their needs, as the information mostly dealt with the problems encountered by parents of older children. The PHN still made monthly visits.

At 2 years and 10 months of age, Kim was again evaluated by the team. Her scoliosis had improved. Receptive language and cognition had been measured at the 24-month level by her developmental program, but they reported her expressive language at the 12- to 14-month level. It had been decided that Kim would be transferred to the public preschool special education program at age 3. Her weight for height was at the 25th percentile. She ate a healthy Asian diet and was not seeking food but also never refused any foods. Food records showed Kim was taking in approximately 900 calories per day, about 10 calories per centimeter (cm). She had become stubborn and refused to have her teeth brushed. Cavities were noted, so she was referred for dental services. Kim's parents had noted that her right eye sometimes turned in, and her physician referred Kim to a pediatric ophthalmologist for regular check-ups. The parents were aware of her short stature and hypoplastic genitals, and the endocrinology of PWS was again discussed with them. They had yet to attend any PWSA meetings. At this time, the father was concerned that layoffs at his workplace could affect him. The father's family was said to love Kim dearly, visiting often. They did not seem to understand Kim's special nutrition needs, however, saying that she looked fine to them.

A reevaluation was carried out at 3 years and 6 months of age by the team members from pediatrics, nursing, and nutrition. The parents reported that Kim's scoliosis continued to improve by radiological measurements and that bracing never had been suggested. This information was confirmed in a letter from the orthopedic specialist. Her height continued to be below the 5th percentile, but her weight for height was at the 75 percentile. The lack of growth in height was a major factor in the change of her proportion. Although Kim ate the same foods at home, her mother had noticed that Kim would sometimes help herself to food that was left out. Education was provided regarding consistently keeping food out of Kim's sight. She was in a public special education preschool where she received a daily snack, but her mother was not sure of the kind or quantity. It was suggested that Kim's mother provide examples of portion sizes to the school staff. Her parents' main concern was Kim's delayed speech, but they were satisfied that the school program was filling her needs for help with language. They recognized that their daughter was stubborn. Behavioral aspects of the syndrome were discussed at some length. The parents thought that school personnel were familiar with the syndrome and the accompanying need to watch the weight of children with PWS. The mother was reminded of the upcoming national meeting of the PWSA to be held in her city in a few months. The PHN still made occasional visits.

The comprehensive interdisciplinary team evaluation that is the focus of this chapter was initiated when Kim was 4 years and 2 months old. At this time, the mother called the clinic with concerns about her daughter's short stature. Kim's mother was also very worried about her daughter's slowness in speaking, even though her understanding of language seemed quite good. Kim was no longer receiving direct physical therapy services, and her mother asked if these services would still be beneficial to Kim. In addition, the mother had attended the national conference of PWSA a few months earlier and, for the first time, observed many children and adults with this condition. She now wondered how Kim's development compared with other children with PWS and with other children her age. Kim was in special education preschool, but her mother questioned what the educational plan should be when Kim reached kindergarten.

PRELIMINARY AND PREASSESSMENT CONFERENCE

A summary of the team's experience with Kim and her family was shared with the larger group during a combined preliminary and preassessment conference. Specifically noted were the following: 1) the unequivocal medical diagnosis of PWS because of the 15q deletion; 2) FTT was present up to 21 months of age; 3) excessive weight gain had occurred by $3^1/2$ years of age; 4) expected developmental delays for children with PWS had been present since infancy; 5) appropriate intervention with home-based therapy followed by an infant program and a developmental preschool had been in place, but next year Kim would be eligible for kindergarten; 6) occasional foraging for food had just begun to be noticed by $3^1/2$ years of age; 7) her parents described Kim as "stubborn," but no behavior problems were obvious the last time she was seen; 8) the mother was a first-generation Chinese immigrant who had strong ties to her culture, and her family lived in Taiwan; 9) her father was a second-generation Chinese immigrant who had acclimated to American culture, and his family lived in Canada approximately 200 miles away; 10) the father's family did not understand the diagnosis; as a result, they questioned the treatment; 11) English was the family's second language; 12) the mother felt the home visits by the PHN were helpful; 13) little data existed about parenting style, parental unit resiliency, and cohesiveness; 14) Kim's parents had recently gained access to support via the PWSA; and 15) scoliosis, strabismus, and short stature needed medical monitoring, and continued medical interpretation and support might be indicated.

At the time of the preliminary planning for the full interdisciplinary assessment, Kim's parents reported no changes in the family circumstances. However, the parents relayed concerns about Kim's behavior. She was becoming more stubborn, was having more frequent tantrums at home, and had begun hitting her mother when angry. Information obtained from Kim's preschool indicated that she had been performing successfully in her developmental program. However, a school assessment 1 year earlier indicated that the child's cognitive skills were mildly delayed, and the school personnel said that Kim's language skills were more delayed than expected. Kim was reported to get along well with her peers, but she sometimes had tantrums at school when frustrated. The school also stated that she sometimes had tantrums when food was restricted. The school staff wanted input about an appropriate kindergarten placement for Kim, focusing on whether she should be in an inclusive kindergarten, and if she would need substantial support in that environment, or whether she should be placed in a self-contained special education class.

From the preliminary information, it was known that Kim's mother wondered if it was appropriate that her child no longer received physical therapy services. Records from the physical therapist at the preschool revealed that Kim was receiving physical therapy services using a consultative model. The therapist had a monthly consultation with Kim's classroom teacher to update eye–hand coordination and dressing activities. She also provided the teacher with suggestions for activities to be used during a daily gross motor time. The physical therapist saw Kim quarterly for evaluation of the child's individualized education program (IEP) and to update activities. The therapist was aware that Kim was being monitored for scoliosis and that the physical therapist at the hospital where follow-up occurred had given Kim's parents a home exercise program for the child.

Regarding other background material, no school report was obtained from the school speech-language therapist. However, the parents said that Kim was receiving such services. The nutritionist requested that the parents complete a 5- to 7-day food record, including food intake during preschool.

The pediatrician was selected as the service coordinator. The team discussed whether a social worker should participate. It was finally determined that the nurse and the psychologist would help this family negotiate community and professional resources and would deal with family coping and cultural issues. This decision was made because the nurse was involved in the case, and a social work referral could be made in the future if needed.

DISCIPLINE SUMMARIES AND RECOMMENDATIONS
A clinic schedule was arranged involving pediatric, nursing, nutritional, physical therapy, psychology, and speech-language pathology evaluations. Joint assessments were planned when possible to minimize the burden on Kim and her family. Kim and her parents visited the clinic once again at age 4 years and 6 months of age for this comprehensive team assessment.

Pediatrics

A review of Kim's medical history since her last visit revealed that she continued to be in good health with no recent illnesses. She had seen her ophthalmologist, but there were no longer concerns about strabismus. Kim's parents only saw her eye "wander" when she was tired. The scoliosis was no longer measurable on X-rays, and she had been discharged from orthopedic care. The parents' main medical concern was that Kim did not seem to be growing much. At the national PWSA conference, Kim's mother learned that sometimes daily growth hormone injections were used to treat short stature and wondered whether Kim was a candidate for this procedure. Other concerns raised by the parents were behavioral. Kim had become quite stubborn, and food foraging had become an issue at home, but not at school. Kim also had begun to display temper tantrums more regularly when parents refused to comply with her wishes.

The physical examination showed that Kim's height was below the 5th percentile, with a further deviation from it than on previous visits. Her weight was in the 25th percentile, and weight for height was above the 95th percentile. Distribution of cutaneous fat gave her a pear-shaped appearance with a relatively thin upper body and an increased accumulation of fat over the abdomen and upper thighs. Facial features disclosed her Chinese inheritance with superimposed PWS characteristics: a narrow diameter of the forehead, almond-shaped eyes, and downturned corners of the mouth with crusted saliva at the corners. The child's hands were small (at the 10th percentile) with a straight ulnar border (a lack of the normal bulge between the wrist and the little fingers), and her feet were also small (below the 5th percentile). Her immature female genitals were missing inner vaginal folds. Skin showed bruises on the lower extremities and evidence of skin picking on the hands and lower arms. The rest of the general physical examination was typical for her age; of note was that her previous eye deviation was no longer present, and her spine was straight. The neurological examination showed residual hypotonia but no other remarkable features. She quietly played by herself during the interview and did not resist the examination. Toward the end, she became restless and insisted that it was time for lunch; her language was only partly understood by the examiner.

The pediatrician's impression from Kim's medical history and physical examination was that the child showed a typical clinical picture of a child her age with PWS. Acute medical issues included growth retardation, mild overweight status, and developing behavior difficulties characteristically seen in children with PWS.

Recommendations

The pediatrician explained to Kim's parents that children with this syndrome bruise easily and that this bruising is not caused by any blood disorder. The skin picking was not a major concern at this time, but they had heard from other parents that it was difficult to stop. The parents were told that Kim's short stature was part of the endocrinological abnormalities often present in PWS and that this was the time to further explore whether treatment was indicated. The mother was again reminded of the need to continue to follow Kim's sexual development, as this aspect of endocrinological maturity often is atypical and might benefit from hormone treatment in the future. Recommendations for an endocrinological consultation, to evaluate possible growth hormone deficiency, were initiated by formal written referral request. Further recommendations were postponed until the interdisciplinary team meeting took place. The weight problem and behavioral issues would be further examined by other team members and discussed at the team conference.

Scoliosis is a common problem in PWS (approximately 85% of individuals with PWS are eventually affected). It sometimes occurs in infancy and then often, but not always, resolves as it did for Kim. Because it might return and become exacerbated by growth hormone treatment, the importance of follow-up was stressed. This could be done by Kim's physical therapist and her regular physician, but Kim's mother was also taught how to perform scoliosis checks on this visit.

Nursing

The nursing assessment plan was to observe the developmental pediatric history and physical examination and to follow with a brief interview. Certain issues of culture had to be kept in mind during interviewing. Because English is their second language, these parents were at risk for not understanding the clinicians' communications. It was also culturally appropriate for this mother not to question authority figures, even if she did not understand what was being communicated. For example, in this case the mother felt more relaxed with the nurse and was able to ask her to explain again the rationale and risks involved in growth hormone therapy previously discussed during the pediatric examination.

Parents of young children need to be educated about potential behavioral problems in PWS. This is best accomplished by reading appropriate material and meeting other parents of children with this disorder. Thus, the nurse complimented the parents for becoming active in the PWSA.

Kim's temper tantrums were mild at this time. When frustrated or denied something she wanted, Kim whined, stomped her feet, and banged objects. The parents were encouraged to ignore this behavior and, instead, to praise desired behaviors. They were told to try to anticipate situations in which Kim might lack the expressive skills to communicate her needs or in which impulse control was a concern. It was suggested that they help their daughter express her desires or divert her attention. Dealing with mild temper tantrums in this manner would reduce the chance of their becoming more serious.

Upon inquiry the parents identified different parenting thresholds for dealing with the behavior difficulties. Kim's mother felt that her efforts were sabotaged by the father. He did not check with her or ask Kim what her mother had already conveyed. Instead, he gave Kim what she wanted. The mother was angry that Kim's father could be the "nice guy," while she was left being the "mean" parent. Facilitating this conversation allowed Kim's father to become aware of the mother's anger and frustration regarding this issue. During this disagreement, it became clear that the parents had spent minimal energy nurturing their parental dyad. The complex needs of a child with PWS include expert management of often exceedingly difficult behaviors. A high level of communication within the marriage is a prerequisite for parents to handle this arduous task.

Support from the extended family is important to all parents of children with special needs as well. Kim's parents were encouraged to problem-solve with the paternal grandparents and to tell them effective ways to deal with Kim. At this point, Kim's father was also made aware of the pressures his parents placed on his wife and the need for him to take an active role in educating them.

Recommendations

As a result of this evaluation, two additional recommendations were made. First, the visiting PHN would be advised by the nurse of the need to support the parental unit, particularly in relation to Kim's behavior problems. Second, the team should consider inviting the grandparents to a future evaluation.

Nutrition

Although infants with PWS often experience FTT due to a weak suck, prevention and management of obesity is the primary nutritional concern from toddlerhood through adulthood. The unique aspects of the overweight issue in this syndrome include 1) hyperphagia—always wanting to eat; 2) short stature and, thus, reduced energy (calorie) needs; 3) less energy required for growth and activity compared to peers, even considering this short stature; 4) increasing food-seeking behaviors with age (e.g., sneaking, foraging, gorging); and 5) temper tantrums and other negative behaviors when food is restricted.

Most weight management efforts for children with typical development include modifying food selection and preparation, parent education regarding diet and behavior, and physical activity—but not restrictive diets. This general approach does not work in children with PWS. Rather, a specific caloric diet (using formulas based on calories per cm of height) needs to be determined for each child, depending on goals of slow weight gain, weight maintenance, or weight loss. Periodic adjustments must be made as the child grows or as goals are achieved. As food-seeking behaviors become evident, environmental controls need to be implemented, such as keeping food high and out of sight and locking cupboards, refrigerators, and freezers. Intervening for negative behavior and temper tantrums is critical to ensure that the diet is implemented. Education regarding the dietary and behavior management and using environmental controls is essential in all environments, including home, school, child care centers, and the homes of neighbors and relatives. A nutritionist or registered dietitian is a key source of support for children with PWS and their families (Holm & Pipes, 1976).

Interim Dietary Intake and Feeding Behavior

Both of Kim's parents accompanied her during the assessment and interview. A 5-day food record from within the previous 2 weeks indicated that Kim was consuming similar foods as in the past (e.g., rice with vegetables and meat, cereals). She regularly ate three meals at home, a morning snack at preschool (crackers, juice, or fruit), and an evening snack while her father ate dinner. Kim's mother tried to keep the portion sizes the same as in the past, but Kim often asked for more and, at times, had a minor temper tantrum when denied. The mother said that sometimes she ignores the tantrum, but at other times it is easier to give Kim more food. Although food is not left on the table or counters, the parents noticed in the preceding 6 months that Kim had started helping herself to food in the refrigerator or cupboards more often. Her parents usually stopped her but did not adjust her intake for the rest of the day.

The staff at Kim's school and her grandparents required more education regarding the unique needs for dietary management in children with PWS. They needed to understand that continuing to make exceptions could result in poor dietary control and increased behavior problems. The preschool snack had recently been a problem because Kim ate fast, asked for more, and frequently became upset when restricted. The staff told Kim's parents that when Kim threw tantrums, it was better for the group as a whole to give Kim a little more snack food. In addition, Kim's parents said that although they agreed on the need for controlling Kim's diet, the child's paternal grandparents thought it was rather harsh, especially as Kim was just plump. It was always frustrating visiting the grandparents because they would offer food to Kim despite the parents' request not to do so. The mother was hoping to accompany the father on an upcoming week-long business trip, and the grandparents had offered to take care of Kim. Now Kim's parents were wondering if they should go, even though they had not had more than a weekend alone together since Kim was born.

The food record was calculated to contain 1,075 calories per day, including estimates of two occasions involving extra food. This translated to 11.5 calories per cm of height. Other nutrients appeared to be well supplied, although Kim's iron intake was only 50% of the recommended dietary allowance (RDA). Kim's growth was confirmed as follows:

- Height: 93.5 cms (less than 5th percentile)
- Weight: 15.8 kilograms (kg) (25th percentile)
- Weight for height: greater than 95th percentile
- Body mass index: 18.2 (less than 95th percentile)

In the preceding 15 months, Kim had grown 4.5 cm in height and gained 2.8 kg, or about 6 pounds (lb). Although this weight gain (less than $^1/_2$ lb per month) would be within typical limits for preschool-age girls, her continued slow growth in height had resulted in significant overweight.

Kim's diet was basically low fat and quite nutritious; her parents were doing a good job. The extra calories appeared to be coming from second portions at home and school, as well as Kim's taking extra food. The total daily energy intake needed to be reduced in order to produce small weight loss over the next 6–9 months, allowing Kim's weight for height to fall between the 75th and 90th percentiles.

Recommendations

The nutritionist compiled a list of recommendations for Kim's parents. First, Kim's diet had to be adjusted to provide 10 calories per cm of height, or 935 calories per day. An exchange diet pattern was planned with the parents, incorporating usual eating patterns and typical foods and emphasizing portion sizes. The diet was planned to provide 900 calories per day, plus a weekly treat of 250 calories. Kim also needed to receive a daily children's chewable multivitamin containing iron.

It was necessary to monitor her height and weight and to plot these measurements monthly. If she started growth hormone treatment, weight might be lost too rapidly and the diet would need to be increased. Once weight for height was between the 75th and 90th percentiles, the calories could be adjusted for maintenance.

Problem solving was done with the parents regarding limiting Kim's access to food at home. They would keep problem foods in the pantry and put a lock on it. They were reluctant to lock the refrigerator but would consider it if physical monitoring did not work. Managing Kim's tantrums around food was also discussed, including the need for both parents to be consistent in following the diet pattern and offering other alternatives to requests for extra food. The parents welcomed the offer for the team to meet with current school staff. This meeting would provide education regarding the dietary management of children with PWS and consultation on behavior management.

As Kim might go into a full-day kindergarten program the next fall, the new school staff needed to be given information on her weight management program and the need for environmental monitoring. Objectives regarding Kim's lunch and snack, handling treats in the classroom, preventing food foraging, and dealing with negative behavior around food had to be included in the IEP. If Kim ever bought the school lunch instead of bringing one from home, the school lunch menu, by federal law, would need to be modified. A sample diet prescription for school lunch was given to the family. Food-related classroom activities would need to be closely monitored.

Finally, Kim's parents were encouraged to take their planned trip together. Written material would be given to the grandparents about prevention of obesity in PWS and the extreme consequences of obesity without diet control. Kim's parents would ask her grandparents to contact the nutritionist as necessary during their time of providing care for Kim. The mother would plan specific menus for Kim for the week of the parents' absence, and she indicated that the older brother would be able to help by reminding the grandparents of Kim's diet. Her parents were told that although some lapses may occur during that week, Kim could get back on the program when they returned. The time of the follow-up appointment, as well as what should be included, would be decided later, at the team conference.

Physical Therapy

The preliminary plan for the physical therapy assessment was to interview the family to clarify concerns about educational placement and therapy services; to determine the current status of orthopedic follow-up for scoliosis; to administer the Peabody Developmental Motor Scales (PDMS; Folio & Fewell, 1983); to establish developmental levels for gross and fine motor skills (the PDMS had been administered by the school therapist 9 months earlier, so this would be a good longitudinal measure and could be used to establish eligibility for school services); and to conduct clinical observations of muscle tone, automatic reactions, functional gait, balance, and posture.

Kim was accompanied to the evaluation by her mother, who remained in the room. Kim readily participated in the fine motor table activities and responded with smiles and hand claps to her accomplishments. Hand flapping was also observed when Kim was very excited about a presented activity. During the gross motor activities, some refusals occurred and Kim had more difficulty attending to the tasks. Kim's speech was inarticulate and her mother needed to clarify her daughter's communications. The therapist felt that the following test results were reliable indicators of Kim's motor abilities.

Neuromuscular Status/Clinical Observations

Muscle tone of the trunk was hypotonic. As measured by consistency and resistance to passive range of motion, tone in the upper and lower extremities was also hypotonic. Equilibrium reactions tested in sitting on a large therapy ball were immature, partly due to low trunk tone and poor trunk strength. Kim was giggly and appeared somewhat fatigued when protective extension reactions in her arms were tested. She often would not respond or was slow to respond; thus, protective extension reactions of the arms were present but inconsistent. No evidence of scoliosis was detected. Mild bilateral genu valgum (knock knees) was noted. When walking, Kim used excessive hip internal rotation and flexed her trunk forward. Kim ran with an awkward, flat-footed gait, with some knee circumduction noted.

Gross Motor Development

Peabody Gross Motor Scales were used, and the following results were obtained:

- Basal: 15–17 months
- Ceiling: 30–35 months
- Age equivalency: 22–24 months
- Standard deviation (SD): −2.05

During gross motor testing, Kim was cautious and very slowly navigated the stairway while holding on to the railing, preferring to mark time with her feet. She would not attempt jumping down from any of the steps. Broad jumping with two feet was accomplished without difficulty, but one-footed standing and hopping could not be done. Kim could not independently get to standing from sitting on the floor. W-sitting was a frequent position for Kim. Highest level ball skills included throwing a tennis ball and a rubber ball 3–4 feet and kicking them 3 feet. Kim was unsuccessful at catching.

It became apparent during gross motor testing that Kim had significant difficulty with functional motor tasks, such as getting to standing from sitting and stair climbing, that might limit her independence and ability to participate at her new school. It was decided to ask the physical therapist at Kim's new school to administer the School Function Assessment (SFA; Coster, Deeney, Haltiwanger, & Haley, 1998) in the fall. This assessment would provide valuable information about Kim's participation in various school-related activity environments, as well as indicate which school-related tasks might require adult assistance or adaptations or modifications. The test also assesses a child's resource requirements for performing cognitive and behavioral tasks (e.g., compliance with adult directives and school rules) specific to an educational environment.

Fine Motor Development
Peabody Fine Motor Scales showed the following scores:

- Basal: 36–41 months
- Ceiling: 60–71 months
- Age equivalency: 49–52 months
- SD: -1.28

Kim worked quickly and with determination on several of the fine motor activities. She consistently used her right hand for most tasks and demonstrated a tripod grasp with a pencil. Kim was able to copy simple shapes, including a circle and a square, while using a pencil. She had some difficulty manipulating the scissors but was able to cut out simple shapes, though not in the required time limit. Kim had the most difficulty with buttoning tasks; she could not properly manipulate even large buttons. Kim easily completed tasks such as stringing beads, stacking cubes, and copying cube designs.

Self-Care Skills
Kim's mother was interviewed regarding the child's self-care skills. She reported that Kim was able to take off her pants and underwear and could put on socks, although she sometimes refused to do so. In order to save time, her mother often dressed Kim, who could not yet manage any fasteners. On grooming tasks, Kim managed with moderate assistance. At mealtime, Kim was very neat and coordinated in the use of a fork and spoon. Kim's mother

reported that her daughter tended to play by herself and preferred to interact with adults rather than with other children. She liked to play grocery store, kitchen, and house (with her dolls); she also enjoyed music. She had recently shown interest in jumping on a trampoline.

In addition to her concern that Kim was no longer receiving one-to-one physical therapy services, Kim's mother indicated some confusion about the nature and purpose of the physical therapy services that Kim was presently receiving (i.e., consultative services). To support Kim's transition to kindergarten, it was decided that a discussion was needed with Kim's mother during which the intent of related services, such as physical therapy, under the law would be clarified. It was stressed that these services must be educationally relevant and provided with the purpose of assisting children to achieve optimal participation in and benefit from their educational programs. Thus, a consultative model is appropriate for many children, including Kim.

Recommendations

Upon completion of disciplinary assessment, the physical therapist developed the ensuing suggestions. In terms of school, Kim should continue to receive regular, consultative physical therapy services. Emphasis should be placed on working with the classroom teacher on fine motor skills as prerequisites for increasing independence in self-care and in preacademic tasks and play. Consultation with the adaptive physical education teacher regarding gross motor activities was also recommended. Furthermore, assessment, using the SFA to determine Kim's level of adaptive motor skills and resource requirements in a functional environment, was suggested the fall she started her new school.

Kim would benefit from a structured program to encourage greater independence in her dressing skills. School personnel could work with her parents to establish appropriate expectations and behavioral reinforcers for Kim. The parents could encourage Kim to try more self-care activities and choose garments within Kim's skill range (e.g., Velcro for shoes, large buttons for shirts).

At home, continued participation in gross motor activities, especially those centering around Kim's interests—such as moving and dancing to audiotapes with simple verbal directions and jumping on the trampoline—should be encouraged. Activity at the playground and community classes were appropriate choices as well. Enrollment in a swimming class for children with special needs was also recommended to strengthen back musculature and to promote overall conditioning. Resources in the local community would be provided to Kim's parents.

Psychology

The planned psychology assessment included general cognitive development, kindergarten readiness, adaptive functioning, and behavioral issues. Because Kim's prior testing indicated cognitive skills at the junction between the mildly

delayed and borderline ranges, her eligibility for school special education programs would be decided partially on the results of the testing. It was decided
to use the fourth edition of the Stanford-Binet Intelligence Scale for Children
(Stanford-Binet-IV; Thorndike, Hagen, & Sattler, 1986) to measure cognitive
functioning because that test is widely accepted by school districts and is normed
for a wide age span. The Stanford-Binet-IV was also used to assess Kim 1 year
earlier, so a current score would permit consideration of her progress in that
time. The Test of Early Reading Ability (TERA-2; Reid, Hresko, & Hammill,
1989) would be used to evaluate reading readiness, one of the factors to consider
in kindergarten readiness for the next year. The Vineland Adaptive Behavior
Scales (VABS; Sparrow, Balla, & Cicchetti, 1984) interview is typically used to
evaluate adaptive functioning. A clinical interview with the parents would be
used to address behavioral issues.

Kim was brought to the clinic by her mother. In the lobby, she responded
cheerfully to a greeting and willingly entered the testing room, accompanied
by her mother. Kim was able to separate from her mother without incident, so
she was tested alone while her mother observed from the adjacent room. During the formal testing, Kim was generally cooperative and showed good attention to the tasks. She was also very sociable and talked a great deal during the
evaluation. Some of her speech was difficult to understand and off topic. Kim
did not seem distressed when tasks became difficult for her, and she seemed to
be unaware of success or failure on individual items. Toward the end of the
session, she said more than once that she was hungry. After testing, Kim was
given toys to play with while her mother answered interview questions. Kim
played appropriately for approximately 20 minutes. She then came over to her
mother and asked about lunch several more times. It was a half hour earlier
than her usual lunchtime.

On the Stanford-Binet-IV, Kim achieved a test composite IQ score of 70,
at the 3rd percentile for her age. This composite score was derived from four
area scores:

- Verbal Reasoning: 62 (at the 1st percentile)
- Abstract/Visual Reasoning: 73 (at the 5th percentile)
- Quantitative Reasoning: 79 (at the 8th percentile)
- Short-Term Memory: 78 (at the 8th percentile)

Kim's memory and quantitative skills were relative strengths, while her verbal
skills were an area of weakness. She had a good understanding of counting and
comparing numbers. In addition, she showed very good visual short-term
memory, with borderline verbal memory.

Kim's adaptive functioning seen at home was measured by the VABS
through an interview given to her mother. Based on her mother's responses,
Kim received the following domain standard scores (and age equivalents):

- Communication Domain: 58 (2 years and 3 months)
- Daily Living Skills: 70 (3 years)
- Socialization Domain: 69 (2 years and 9 months)

These scores indicated that Kim's adaptive functioning as judged by her mother was developing below the range expected for her age. Of note, Kim's communication skills were lower than her other functional skills but compatible with the expressive language delays noted during testing. Her daily living (self-help) skills were also below the range expected. This may have been due in part to the fact that Kim's mother continued to perform most self-care tasks for her, such as dressing and bathing. This may reflect a cultural difference or result from limited motor skill on Kim's part.

The TERA-2 was given to assess Kim's prereading skills. She achieved a Reading Quotient of 64, at the 5th percentile for her age. Kim recognized familiar signs and logos and some letters of the alphabet. However, she did not have a good grasp of the alphabet or of sound–symbol correspondence. This suggested that Kim is not ready to begin learning to read.

Following formal testing, Kim's mother discussed current behavioral concerns. Kim had been showing increased stubbornness and tantrums, especially around food issues. The tantrums were somewhat more frequent when she was with her grandparents. Kim's mother was concerned that Kim was learning to manipulate others through these episodes. Some of the tantrum behavior was seen during her evaluations at the interdisciplinary clinic. So far, Kim's parents managed her tantrums by ignoring her or removing her to another room, and this was sometimes effective. Another behavior of concern was Kim's hitting others when frustrated. The parents had tried time-out for hitting, using a time-out chair in the kitchen. However, they had difficulty keeping Kim in that chair. Finally, Kim's mother mentioned that she and Kim's father did not always agree on discipline issues, and that this was causing some stress in the marriage.

In sum, Kim's cognitive and adaptive skills were developing below the range expected for her age, indicating a mild developmental delay. If her skills continued to develop at the same rate, she would eventually be classified as having mental retardation requiring limited support for the purposes of school programming. Kim had also begun to show the behaviors typical of children with PWS.

Recommendations

Kim continued to need special education support at school. Kim would be eligible for a full-day kindergarten program through her school district, and an ideal school situation for Kim would be one combining special education support with opportunities for integration with typically developing children. For example, Kim would be well served by a program that combines a half-day in a special education kindergarten with a half-day in a general kindergarten classroom. The exact format of Kim's kindergarten program would be decided by Kim's parents and her school district at their spring IEP meeting.

Kim would likely continue to require speech-language therapy to help her deal with relatively weak communication skills. Details regarding this matter would be discussed after consultation with the speech-language pathologist during the team meeting.

Kim's parents were encouraged to enroll her with the Division of Developmental Disabilities (DDD). This agency in the family's state provided support for individuals with developmental disabilities and their families, including behavior management specialists. Respite care for caregivers would also be available. In addition, by enrolling with this state agency, Kim's family would allow the state to predict more accurately the number of its citizens needing special services in the future.

Behavior management help was also available from private clinical psychologists. Kim's parents did not think that they needed outside help at this time. However, they were made aware that assistance was available if and when they needed extra help managing Kim's behavior at home. If they later decided to find a private clinician, the interdisciplinary clinic could provide a list of therapists having experience with children with developmental delays or even specifically PWS.

Speech-Language Pathology

Kim's mother had a primary concern about her daughter's slowness in speaking. Although it was not completely clear what Kim actually understood, her comprehension of language was reported to be stronger than her expressive language. Prior to the assessment, and with the help of an interpreter, Kim's mother completed the words and sentences section of the MacArthur Communicative Development Inventories (CDI; Fensen et al., 1993). Kim's expressive vocabulary of 250 words was near the 50th percentile for 21- to 22-month-old typically developing girls. Given Kim's age at testing, the magnitude of Kim's delay substantiated her mother's apprehension.

Standardized tests and nonstandardized measures were used to determine Kim's level of understanding. The Auditory Comprehension subscale of the Preschool Language Scale–3 (PLS-3; Zimmerman, Steiner, & Pond, 1992) was administered. Kim achieved a standard score of 69 (percentile rank = 2), which yielded an age equivalent of 3 years and 3 months. Her standard score on the Peabody Picture Vocabulary Test–Revised (Form L) was 75.

Kim's understanding of several early relational meanings was assessed with nonstandardized procedures. She understood several two-word relations that coded both probable (e.g., bounce ball) and improbable (e.g., kiss apple) events. However, she did not respond correctly when requested to perform improbable three-term semantic meanings. For example, when Kim was asked to "make the wagon push the boy," she picked up the male figure and had him push the wagon. This response suggested that Kim understood the words *boy*, *push*, and *wagon*, but she did not fully grasp language outside familiar contexts.

Kim continued to rely on nonverbal tactics (e.g., probable event strategy) to aid her in comprehending adult sentences.

An elicited production probe was used to assess Kim's understanding of *yes* or *no* and *wh-* questions (who, what, where, when, and why). The examiner posed a series of predetermined questions while reading the storybook *The Tale of Peter Rabbit*. Kim responded with semantically appropriate information to interrogatives consistent with an age of mastery between 2 and 3 years (e.g., *yes/no, where* questions) but had difficulty beyond that level (e.g., *how* and *when* questions).

Following the story, Kim and the clinician interacted socially for 20 minutes of low-structured play. Low-structured activities were designed around sets of thematically related toys. Kim made transitions between sets of toys with ease. Whenever and wherever possible, the clinician followed Kim's lead, attempting to expand or extend any spontaneous utterances.

Kim's rate of speaking was relatively low. On average, she produced approximately three utterances per minute. The average length of Kim's utterances was calculated to be 1.50 morphemes; a sentence length typically observed in 23-month-old children. Kim's longest utterance was four morphemes in length. Three different semantic relations were observed in this sample. Kim spontaneously combined the words *baby* and *bed* to form the two-word possessive relation *baby bed*. In addition, she produced two examples of an agent–action relation (i.e., *mommy sit, doggy run*) and several attributive–entity relations (e.g., *little book, happy doggy, more milk*). Kim did not use any grammatical morphemes (e.g., */ing/, /s/*) in this sample. All of Kim's single words and word combinations were spoken in English.

Kim was a socially engaging child. She participated in a variety of reciprocal activities with the examiner, had appropriate eye contact, and maintained joint attention. As a conversational partner, Kim was responsive, but not particularly assertive. She used her language for a variety of intentional communicative acts. She commented on objects and actions and requested information. Her responses to the examiner's queries for information were both adjacent and contingent. During one low-structured activity, Kim used the word *giger* while playing with a group of animals. The clinician was unable to decipher the meaning of *giger*. When Kim produced the word a second time, the clinician asked, "What did you say?" Kim put her hands near her face, formed her fingers into claws, repeated "giger," and then growled. The examiner then understood *giger* meant *tiger*.

In sum, Kim's performance profile presented an interesting pattern of delayed development. Her expressive language process was unquestionably delayed. She had a reduced vocabulary and was just beginning to combine a few words into simple sentences that code immediate events, ongoing actions, and salient objects or people. Although Kim had a clear desire to communicate, her vocal productions were few. The consequence of these delays was a sub-

stantial expressive impairment. Overall, Kim's level of expressive language
was near a 2-year-old's level. Kim gave the appearance of understanding much
of what was said; in reality, her comprehension was more consistent with that
of a 3-year-old child. This was a clinically meaningful delay that placed Kim
at considerable risk for academic problems and interpersonal difficulties.

Recommendations
The therapist determined that Kim should receive speech-language services to
foster both receptive and expressive language. Focused play activities and indirect language stimulation would be reasonable management strategies. If
Kim's expressive delays continued to persist, however, specific intervention
options would need to be discussed with Kim's mother and teachers.

TEAM CONFERENCE AND FINAL RECOMMENDATIONS
A conference with both parents was attended by the team members who had
evaluated Kim and her family. The team recognized that Kim's parents had
excellent basic knowledge of the diagnosis of PWS through their long-term
contact with the PWS clinic team and recent contact with the national parent
association. An effort was made throughout this conference to depict the findings of Kim's assessment in the framework of their understanding of PWS.

Physical Status
Kim's parents had observed marked short stature to be common in adults with
PWS. At the time of this conference, they had already arranged for an endocrinological appointment to have Kim assessed for growth hormone deficiency
and were eager to go ahead with treatment if indicated. Even though Kim's
early severe hypotonia had improved as expected, it was still present and explained the finding of her more severe delays in gross motor skills (testing at
the 22- to 24-month level) as compared with fine motor skills (at the 49- to 52-
month level). This is a common finding in preschool-age children with PWS.
The parents were told that growth hormone treatment usually improves muscle mass and gross motor skills. In view of this observation, the physical therapist emphasized the importance of practicing the suggested gross motor activities. Success on the playground would be likely, and this could enhance Kim's
self-confidence. As growth hormone treatment might increase the risk for a re-
occurrence of scoliosis, the therapist added a recommendation for the school
physical therapist to examine Kim's spine on a quarterly basis.

　　 Kim's weight gain had become excessive for the first time by the time of
this visit. The parents understood that their previous management of her diet,
which had been successful so far, now needed to become more vigilant. At
home, her mother had already incorporated the changes in the management
of Kim's diet that had been suggested by the nutritionist. Reading about and
observing other children with PWS had prepared these parents for the likelihood of a serious weight problem. They understood the need to prevent the

life-threatening obesity that is the outcome in untreated children. The biggest issue for them at the time of this assessment was how to impress upon others—grandparents, school personnel—that Kim's present "plumpness" was a fore-runner to a potential serious medical problem and that they needed every-body's cooperation to keep Kim's weight under control. They had tried to talk to the grandparents many times to no avail. Therefore, the team recommended that the grandparents be invited to the next reevaluation, which was set for 6 months and would include representatives from nursing, pediatrics, and nutrition. The plan for this visit would involve a discussion with Kim's grandparents regarding the medical seriousness of obesity in PWS. A pamphlet about PWS directed to educators was given to the mother to share with the school. The psychologist asked if low-calorie rewards could be used as reinforcers at school, and the nutritionist gave the mother a list of suitable items to share with Kim's teacher. The parents were reminded that, at their request, any team member would be happy to consult with school personnel about PWS by telephone or in person.

Developmental and Behavioral Status

The profile of Kim's cognitive development was reviewed according to the results obtained from the psychological and speech-language assessments. At 4 years and 6 months of age, she was functioning below age level in all areas, ranging from borderline to mildly delayed levels of development. Kim showed definite strength in quantitative reasoning (counting and numbers) and short-term memory and relative strength in visual reasoning, but weakness in verbal reasoning. The testing confirmed the mother's observation that Kim's understanding of language (at the 3-year level) was better than her expressive language (at the 2-year level); however, she was still delayed in both areas. The parents were told that this developmental profile is quite typical for preschool-age children with PWS. The assessment of Kim's adaptive functioning in the home reflected her measured skill levels in the communication domain (2 years and 3 months of age) but not in her daily living skills. Her performance level at home (3 years) did not reflect her fine motor skills as determined by the therapist (49–52 months). Kim's mother acknowledged that she probably prompted Kim more than necessary and would like to help Kim become more independent. Consequently, the therapist offered to share specific written suggestions with her. In view of the persistent discrepancy between receptive and expressive language, the speech-language therapist decided to develop a list of specific recommendations for activities to foster expressive language skills, which would be given to Kim's teacher and parents.

Kim was beginning to show some early behavior problems—such as stubbornness, tantrums when food had to be withheld, preoccupation with food, and sneaking of food—which, if allowed to escalate, would become significant problems in the future. The team spent some time discussing these PWS behavioral issues with Kim's parents with an emphasis on prevention. The parents confirmed that they needed to become more consistent with respect to handling food-related infractions and said that the discussions with the nurse had been helpful in this area. Continued nursing support was offered in the form of telephone consultation, and the clinic nurse would also contact the visiting PHN for assistance in this area. The psychologist reviewed her list of available community resources should Kim's parents feel they need more aid in this area later. The parents were told that the behavior difficulties experienced by families with children with PWS are a result of poorly understood psychological characteristics that are caused by the genetics of the disorder, not poor parenting. Most people try to become "super parents" to deal with their children having PWS, and seeking assistance in this process is usually advisable.

Educational and Social Issues

Kim was eligible to receive special education support because of her developmental delay. In the future, she would also be eligible for support through other suitable special education classifications until she turned 21 years old. The parents would have to plan her educational placement with the school from year to year. The next year's placement would be negotiated between the school and the parents in a few weeks; then, decisions would be made regarding remaining in a special education preschool, moving to regular kindergarten, or combining them as suggested by the team psychologist. The parents would take relevant reports (from physical therapy, psychology, and speech-language) to the IEP meeting, and team members in those disciplines offered to be available to assist them in this process if necessary.

Kim's family was well functioning and had considerable strengths. Extended family members living nearby were supportive, and they had connections to a unique culture with traditionally strong family ties. They had recently contacted the local and national PWS parent associations and had begun to receive support and information from these important resources. At this time, they also needed to learn of state services available to them for their daughter's disabilities through the DDD. Kim's parents had always been diligent in providing what was best for their daughter, seeking and acting on advice, using their own judgment. They were complimented for a job well done, and the team wished them good luck in the journey ahead.

CONCLUSION

PWS is a genetic disorder with complex clinical manifestations changing with age. The most serious disability—in the absence of intervention—is inevitable life-threatening obesity in older children. This chapter describes an interdisciplinary guidance program during the first years of life aimed at preventing this devastating health hazard. Nutritional, medical, and behavioral interventions are used to overcome the strong urge to overeat in PWS. The goals are an improved quality of life and an increased life span in people born with this challenging disorder.

REFERENCES

Cassidy, S.B. (1984). Prader-Willi syndrome. *Current Problems in Pediatrics, 14,* 1–55.

Coster, W., Deeney, T., Haltiwanger, J., & Haley, S. (1998). *School Function Assessment (SFA).* San Antonio, TX: The Psychological Corp.

Fensen, L., Dale, P., Reznick, J.S., Thal, D., Bates, E., Hartung, J., Pethick, S., & Reilly, J. (1993). *MacArthur Communicative Development Inventories (CDI).* San Diego, CA: Singular Publishing Group.

Folio, M.R., & Fewell, R. (1983). *Peabody Developmental Motor Scales and Activity Cards (PDMS).* Itasca, IL: The Riverside Publishing Co.

Holm, V.A. (1996). Prader-Willi syndrome. In A.J. Capute & P.J. Accardo (Eds.), *Developmental disabilities in infancy and childhood: Vol. II. The spectrum of developmental disabilities* (2nd ed., pp. 245–253). Baltimore: Paul H. Brookes Publishing Co.

Holm, V.A., & Pipes P.L. (1976). Food and children with Prader-Willi syndrome. *American Journal of Diseases of Children, 130,* 1063–1067.

Reid, D.K., Hresko, W.P., & Hammill, D.D. (1989). *Test of Early Reading Ability, Second Edition (TERA-2).* Austin, TX: PRO-ED.

Sparrow, S.S., Balla, D.A., & Cicchetti, D.V. (1984). *Vineland Adaptive Behavior Scales (VABS).* Circle Pines, MN: American Guidance Service.

Thorndike, R.L., Hagen, E.P., & Sattler, J.M. (1986). *Stanford-Binet Intelligence Scale for Children* (4th ed.). Itasca, IL: The Riverside Publishing Co.

Zimmerman, I., Steiner, V., & Pond, R. (1992). *Preschool Language Scale–3 (PLS-3).* San Antonio, TX: The Psychological Corp.

Chapter 17

A Child with
Fragile X Syndrome

Nuhad D. Dinno, Anne Hay,
William Eric Strong, Truman E. Coggins,
Susan Wendel, and Douglas S. Cook

Fragile X syndrome, identified as the most common cause of inherited mental retardation, is an X-linked recessive disorder, diagnosable by DNA molecular analysis. Carrier detection is possible, as well as prenatal diagnosis. It is estimated that 1 in 1,250 males and 1 in 2,000 females are affected. Eighty percent of males carrying the fragile X gene show mental retardation requiring intermittent to extensive support and hyperactive, aggressive, and autistic-like behaviors. Carrier females are less seriously affected. The most common physical findings are those of either atypically placed or somewhat prominent, large, or low-set ears with some underdevelopment of the helix. Other physical findings noted are a high-arched palate, a long face with a prominent forehead, and an increased distance between the eyes. Epicanthal folds (skinfolds on the inner corner of the eye) and ptosis (drooping eyelids) can occur as well. The next most common characteristic associated with fragile X in males is macroorchidism (large testes). It is seen more frequently in postpubertal boys.

351

Other findings include hyperextensibility of the joints, joint laxity with scoliosis, and pes planus (flat feet). Hypotonia (low muscle tone) is a common finding, and both fine and gross motor coordination are delayed. Failure to thrive
(FTT) is recognized in early infancy; however, this improves. Occasionally,
gastroesophageal reflux has been observed. Seizures also occur with some frequency in fragile X syndrome.

Behavior characteristics are striking. They include hyperactivity, autistic-
like behaviors, stereotypies, tics, and aggressive outbursts. Although children
with fragile X syndrome tend to have eye gaze avoidance, they do relate socially; nevertheless, they are anxious, easily overstimulated, and subsequently
avoidant in an autistic-like manner. Perseverative speech, hand biting, and occasionally characteristic calluses on the hands are noted with hand flapping and
poor eye contact. Shyness, social withdrawal, or other social oddities in relating
characterize many carrier females. Psychiatric problems include depression and
social anxiety (Reiss, Hagerman, Vinogradow, Abrams, & King, 1988).

Although the majority of individuals with fragile X syndrome have mental retardation, they demonstrate strength in vocabulary, memory, and visual-
perceptual tasks such that reading and spelling may be better than their overall
IQ scores would indicate. Weaknesses are seen in abstract reasoning, sequential
processing, and math. Speech and language are characterized by distinctive impairments in auditory memory, reception, and articulation. Other findings include presence of echolalia, verbal perseverations, and atypical intonation and
rhythm of speech. Speech is cluttered (American Academy of Pediatrics, Committee on Genetics, 1996).

This chapter's case study of a child with this inherited disorder demonstrates several issues and challenges frequently encountered by an interdisciplinary evaluation team. The medical, genetic, neurodevelopmental, and behavioral issues of a child with fragile X syndrome are complex and can overwhelm
the family. In the case illustrated in this chapter, the mother's understanding
of these issues and her ability to follow through with the team's recommendations are of concern. In part, her history of a learning disability and a recent
diagnosis of depression present major challenges to the team.

The team's knowledge and expertise in identifying local and community
supports is critical for any child with a developmental disability. As such, this
case also emphasizes the importance of communicating the needs of the child
and the family to other professionals and local community agencies for the coordination of services. In this instance, the child's teacher was extremely important in helping implement the educational and behavioral interventions
recommended. Finally, this case highlights the process of establishing communication among the family and the professionals and resources identified.

GENETICS OF FRAGILE X SYNDROME

Fragile X syndrome has been shown to be caused by an unstable CGG repeat
within the fragile X mental retardation-1, FMR(1), gene. The repeat is typically

polymorphic with 6 to 52 repeats, while affected males and females exhibit a massive expansion resulting in 200 to more than 1,000 repeats. Such expansions, called *full mutations,* are associated with atypical methylation of the FMR(1) gene, leading to transcriptional suppression. The resulting absence of the encoded protein FMRP, the RNA binding protein, is believed to result in the phenotype. Nonpenetrant male carriers and many female carriers exhibit premutation alleles of intermediate length (50 to 200 repeats), which are normally expressed. Male carriers transmit only unstable premutations while female premutation carriers can have carrier offspring with premutations or affected children with full mutations. The risk of having an affected child is directly related to the number of maternal repeats, with sequentially increasing probabilities of these alleles converting to full mutations as they are transmitted to subsequent generations. Advances have led to highly accurate lab diagnosis of both carrier and affected individuals as well as markedly improved prenatal diagnosis. As the premutation is transmitted vertically through a family, it tends to increase in size; therefore, greater numbers of affected children are observed in later generations, and greater numbers of carriers are seen in earlier generations.

Fragile X syndrome should be considered in any undiagnosed child with developmental delay or mental retardation. Because the mutation is so frequent and the phenotype is so subtle, particularly in young children, exclusion of fragile X syndrome on clinical grounds alone is not warranted. Once a child is identified as having fragile X syndrome, family members should be evaluated, as many could be at risk of having affected children. A woman at risk may wish to have her pregnancy monitored to determine prenatally whether the fetus has fragile X syndrome.

CASE BACKGROUND

James was a 5-year-old boy who had an established diagnosis of fragile X syndrome. He returned to the child development clinic because of mild ongoing developmental delays. Results of a previous assessment completed at 2 years of age showed physical findings as well as a developmental and behavior profile commonly seen in children with fragile X syndrome. He presented then with mild global developmental delays. Attention difficulties were also noted. Several recommendations were provided to the family, including a referral to an early intervention program. In addition, the parents were referred to a genetics clinic in their community for genetic counseling regarding the diagnosis of fragile X syndrome and its implications. An appointment was also scheduled for them through the interdisciplinary team clinic.

During the interim period, James attended a developmental preschool and received speech-language and occupational therapy services. The family also received services for behavior management through the Division of Developmental Disabilities (DDD). They did not follow through with recommended further genetic evaluation and consultation, even though an appointment was scheduled for them at the genetics clinic in their community.

The parents requested a reevaluation because of concerns about their son's aggressive behavior and hand biting. Moreover, the family felt that James's school was not providing him with programs usually provided to children who have fragile X syndrome. Additional concerns were an increased level of activity, attention problems, and poor social interactions. The child's parents also felt that James was not making as much progress as anticipated, and they questioned whether he would benefit from a sensory integration approach as part of his therapy. The mother again raised some questions about the genetic implications regarding fragile X syndrome as well.

PRELIMINARY AND PREASSESSMENT CONFERENCES

During the preliminary conference, information was gathered from James's previous clinic visit, preschool program education forms, and the occupational therapy and speech-language evaluation provided through his preschool program. Furthermore, James's medical history, provided by his primary care physician, and records from the Department of Social and Health Services' psychology consultation services were reviewed.

Based on the information provided, it was recommended at the preassessment conference that a reevaluation should include developmental representatives from the fields of pediatrics, occupational therapy, psychology, speech-language pathology, and social work. Because the family lived 200 miles away from the clinic, they were offered the opportunity of having the evaluation done over a period of 2 consecutive days. At the end of the second day, the team would then be able to meet with them and discuss findings and recommendations. It was also decided that having James's teacher at the parent conference would be crucial for implementing educational and behavioral needs. Permission was to be obtained from the parents to contact James's teacher.

DISCIPLINE SUMMARIES

Each team member participating in this case assessed James according to his or her discipline specialty. The findings from each field are described next.

Pediatrics

James was born at 41 weeks' gestation to an 18-year-old mother after her first viable pregnancy. The pregnancy was complicated by fever and flu symptoms during the seventh month. The mother took prenatal vitamins, reportedly smoked about five cigarettes a day, and drank some alcohol intermittently prior to learning that she was pregnant. Delivery was by cesarean section secondary to cephalopelvic disproportion. Birth weight was 7 pounds 4 ounces, length was 51 centimeters (cm), and head circumference 35 cm. Apgar scores were 8 and 9 at 1 and 5 minutes respectively. James remained in the nursery for 4 days with no reported neonatal complications. There were some initial feeding difficulties and a mild degree of FTT, both of which were resolved. James had had no problems since then, and his weight gain had been appropriate.

Developmental History

James's parents were concerned when he started rocking at 7 months old. However, no evaluations were performed at that time. James's early developmental milestones were delayed. At 2 years of age, he was referred to and received services from a birth-to-3 early intervention program. He also attended a child care center to provide interaction with typically developing children.

At the time of his initial referral to the interdisciplinary clinic at $2^{1}/_{2}$ years of age, there were concerns that James had features possibly associated with fetal alcohol syndrome. Yet upon further examination, it was determined that these features were not related to prenatal alcohol exposure. However, because of developmental delay and other suspicions, a chromosome analysis was performed; it reported a normal male karyotype (46,XY). DNA molecular analysis for fragile X syndrome was also done, and the results were consistent with the diagnosis of fragile X syndrome. The family was informed of this diagnosis and its genetic implications.

DNA molecular analysis was performed on James's mother, who was found to have a premutation status found in carriers of the gene for fragile X syndrome. At that time, it was recommended that James's family receive further genetic counseling and seek assessment for other maternal family members' genetic status. Consequently, an appointment was scheduled to attend a genetics clinic in their local community.

Educational History

At the time of assessment, James attended special education preschool services. He received speech-language and occupational therapy as part of his educational program. In addition, the school psychologist had been working on behavior management strategies in the classroom. James also attended a child care center after school because both of his parents worked. The child care provider had been experiencing difficulties with James's aggressive behavior and increased activity level.

Family History

James's mother was 23 years old at the time of her son's assessment and reportedly had a history of depression. In the past, she had been placed on medication but chose to discontinue it. The mother described herself as a slow learner, although she was tested at school and found to have typical intelligence. She said that she could be easily distracted and had a short attention span; she also reported having difficulties in school, especially in math. The biological father was unknown. The stepfather was 24 years old and in good health. He had no learning difficulties and was a high school graduate. Both parents worked outside of the home. James's stepfather worked in construction, and his mother was a medical records secretary. James had a half sister who was 18 months old and developing typically. She would, however, be undergoing testing for fragile X syndrome at the genetics clinic in the local community. In fact, several members of the mother's family were scheduled for fragile X syndrome testing at the genetics clinic. The maternal grandmother was reported to function "like a 13-year-old."

Past Medical History

Past medical history included frequent otitis media with three sets of pressure equalization tubes. His hearing had been assessed on several occasions and was found to be normal. A vision screening through the school was reported to be normal as well.

Physical Examination

On examination, James's height of 111 cm was at the 60th percentile, weight of 18.5 kilograms was at the 50th percentile, and head circumference of 50 cm was at the 50th percentile. Blood pressure was 92/50. He had a suggestion of downward-slanted eyes and a long face with a prominent chin. He had minimal epicanthal folds and a high forehead. He had hypertelorism (increased distance between the eyes), and the inner canthal distance (distance between the inner corners of the eyes) measured 3.2 cm, which was greater than the 75th percentile. Ears were slightly low set and prominent, and both helices were underdeveloped. Ear length was 5.5 cm on the left and 5.6 cm on the right, which was near the 25th percentile. He had a high-arched, narrow palate. He had a few calluses on the dorsum of both hands. The genitalia revealed a Tanner Stage 1 (prepubertal sexual development) with testicular volume of 2–3 cubic cm bilaterally. He had hyperextensibility at the wrists and hypermobility of all joints.

James had mild generalized hypotonia, and both fine and gross motor coordination were poor. Deep tendon reflexes were 2+ (considered a normal response). Cranial nerves were grossly intact. He was in constant motion and easily distractible throughout the examination. He mouthed objects frequently, and he showed decreased focus and attention. He had fairly good eye contact with parents and the examiner; however, he had a tendency to look sideways. He had a wide-based gait. James also had a tendency to perseverate over some words and was heard to use two- or three-word phrases with an explosive pattern in his speech.

Psychology

James was evaluated by the psychologist through standardized testing. On the Stanford-Binet Intelligence Scale for Children–Fourth Edition (Thorndike, Hagen, & Sattler, 1986), he achieved a Test Composite Score of 45, which was below the 1st percentile for his age. On the Vineland Adaptive Behavior Scales (VABS; Sparrow, Balla, & Cicchetti, 1984), he had a Communication standard score of 56, which was below the 1st percentile for both expressive and receptive language and showed an age equivalency of 3 years and 1 month. On the Socialization Domain, James had a standard score of 68, which was at the 1st percentile and equivalent to 3 years and 9 months of age.

A behavior assessment was also carried out. During free play, James was less agitated than during the standardized testing. Initially, his play was well organized; then it became more active and disorganized as the play time progressed. He talked to himself as he played, describing activities of animals, and he had a tendency to repeat statements many times. His hand flapping became more evident, and hand biting and aggressive behavior were observed as well.

James's mother completed two questionnaires to aid the assessment of her son's behavior: the Conners' Problem Solving Scale (Conners, 1989) and the Achenbach Child Behavior Checklist (CBCL; Achenbach & Edelbrook, 1986). Based on the mother's report, James's primary behavior problems were hyperactivity, aggression, and frequent hand biting. The information sent by James's school targeted his poor attention, high activity level, and unusual behaviors of hand flapping and hand biting. A videotape provided by the school showed significant disorganized, active behavior in the classroom that was often disruptive to the other students. The videotape also documented the teacher's efforts to modify James's behavior in the classroom.

Overall, James showed cognitive delays and many behavioral concerns that are typical of fragile X syndrome. His increasing attention difficulties and aggression were also consistent with children who have fragile X syndrome. It was the psychologist's conclusion that James also met criteria for the diagnosis of attention-deficit/hyperactivity disorder (ADHD).

Speech-Language Pathology

James's mother believed her son had made steady progress over the past 2 years. She felt he understood most everything that she said. Nonetheless, James's teachers and support personnel were concerned about his lack of meaningful progress. Thus, assessment was vital in resolving this discrepancy. A speech-language evaluation included standardized testing as well as clinical observations, and there was a nonstandardized assessment whereby data were collected and scrutinized while James displayed spontaneous language samples. A review of records revealed a recognizable pattern of performance consistent with what has been reported in the literature concerning fragile X syndrome.

The Preschool Language Scale–3 (PLS-3; Zimmerman, Steiner, & Pond, 1992) was utilized. Because this test was administered at James's previous clinic assessment, the results could be used to compare previous and present performance. The Communication and Symbolic Behavior Scales (CSBS; Wetherby & Prizant, 1993) were used to organize and categorize the findings. In addition, the child's mother completed the MacArthur Communicative Development Inventories (CDI; Fensen et al., 1993) to document the words James was using at home.

The results of the evaluation indicated that on standardized assessment James was demonstrating receptive and expressive speech and play behaviors exhibited by 2- to 3-year-old children developing typically. He obtained Receptive and Expressive Language standard scores of 58 and 59. When comparing his present assessment with the previous one, it appeared that James had made language gains. In a 24-month period, his receptive skills had increased by 11 months. The parent report and formal testing indicated a 5- to 8-month increase in expressive skills. James also demonstrated a limited number of communicative intents and had poor joint attention and inadequate turn-taking skills. These findings were not unlike data reported in the literature for children with fragile X syndrome, and the results were consistent with school reports and testing.

Occupational Therapy

Tools used for this evaluation included a child-administered standardized assessment, parent interview, and self-administered parent questionnaire. The therapist used the Peabody Developmental Motor Scales (PDMS; Folio & Fewell, 1983) to establish James's motor abilities and to document developmental progress. On the Gross Motor Scale, his performance was at the 3-year level, and performance on the Fine Motor Scale was at the 2-year level. This showed that James had made gradual progress in gross motor development, with less significant progress in the fine motor and object manipulation development, since his previous clinic visit.

Sensorimotor skills were tested by having the mother fill out a completed Sensory Profile (Dunn, 1994). Self-care skills were evaluated utilizing the Pediatric Evaluation of Disability Inventory (PEDI; Haley, Coster, Ludlow, Haltiwanger, & Andrellos, 1992). James demonstrated delays in independent self-care skills and social function, and he appeared to require an extensive amount of caregiver assistance compared with peers. His independent mobility was average for his age.

James exhibited atypical sensory processing, shown by hypersensitivity to touch and visual and auditory input, gravitational insecurity for movement in space, and difficulty regulating sensory information. As a result, James had emotional outbursts that were difficult for his family to manage. This sensory profile is frequently observed in children with fragile X syndrome (Scharfenaker et al., 1996; Stackhouse, 1994). In addition, during the evaluation, James exhibited a variety of stereotypic behaviors (e.g., hand biting and flapping) with increasing frequency during less structured aspects of the session.

The mother questioned whether her son should receive sensory integration therapy. The term *sensory integration* is used by occupational therapists in one of two ways. It describes a clinical frame of reference developed by Ayres (1972, 1979) for the treatment of people who present with disorders in sensory processing. Sensory integration may also be used to describe the human process of receiving, integrating, and responding to varied sensory information for the purpose of producing a functional and purposeful response or behavior. The use of sensory integration theory is an important and unique contribution of occupational therapy within the context of an interdisciplinary team.

The sensory integration frame of reference is built on neurobehavioral theory and Ayres' pragmatic belief that the brain's function of sensory processing, particularly the proximal senses (vestibular, tactile, and proprioceptive), serves as a foundation on which complex occupations (i.e., play and social skills) are scaffolded (Parham & Mailloux, 1996). Disturbances in sensory integration may result in a child's avoiding certain sensory experiences (e.g., refusing certain clothing textures, refusing to swing at the playground) or seeking excessive amounts of certain input (e.g., spinning, body rocking, touching and pressing up against furniture and walls). Parents and teachers may describe a child exhibiting behavior, social, or motor coordination problems, and it is the occupational therapist's role to investigate whether a sensory processing problem may underlie these problems.

There are several methods for evaluating a child's sensory processing. The Sensory Integration and Praxis Test (SIPT, Ayres, 1989) is the only standardized evaluation tool specific to the assessment of sensory integrative functions and requires certified training for administration. For those children who cannot be tested using standardized methods, other systems of assessment are utilized. One option is to observe the child clinically during play or other purposeful performance in a natural or clinical environment. A second alternative is the administration of a parent or teacher interview, using a sensory history questionnaire. As of the end of the 20th century, research is ongoing to develop standardized, reliable, and valid sensory questionnaires (Dunn, 1994; Dunn & Westman, 1997).

Therapeutic intervention for children with sensory integration difficulties entails a variety of sensory activities specifically selected and sequenced for the child's needs. The explanation of sensory integration intervention is complex and difficult to describe briefly. Wilbarger (1984) developed one mechanism for distilling this process, described as the *sensory diet*. The sensory diet utilizes the analogy of sensory input serving as nourishment to the brain. The right balance and combination of sensory input supports optimal levels of performance (Wilbarger, 1995; Williams & Shellenberger, 1992). The occupational therapist, in collaboration with the teacher and parents, may develop a sensory diet—which includes specific sensory experiences, consistent routines, and adaptations to the environment—to support the child's most optimal performance in the classroom or home.

Social Work
The social work interview was held with James's mother while his stepfather attended the psychology evaluation. The social worker had met with both parents at James's 2-year visit. When asked how life was going for her family, James's mother focused on concerns about the adequacy of the child's school

program, his activity level, and his aggressive behavior at home. A different set of issues emerged when she was asked what was most stressful for her and her husband. James's stepfather worked 60–70 hours each week, and the child's mother worked part time; the couple never felt they had time to spend with just each other. James's mother also noted that her depression had increased following her daughter's birth and that she was still on medication but not always using it.

The extended family's reluctance to have genetic screening emerged later in the interview, with James's mother saying that she had felt extremely embarrassed when she had been identified as a fragile X carrier. However, she had continued talking to the extended family about her son's condition. At this time, she was sure that they would agree to being tested for fragile X.

Throughout the interview James's mother was praised for the actions she had taken to determine her carrier status and to encourage her relatives to undergo fragile X testing as well. She was also given support regarding the difficulty of parenting a child with developmental disabilities and her struggles with depression.

To elicit the family's coping strategies, the social worker asked how each member dealt with stress. James's mother identified simply talking to her minister as being the most helpful. It appeared that the content of these discussions and her prayers was general and aimed at reassuring the mother. This is an example of passive or palliative coping. Adaptive coping was also part of the family's coping strategy, as the stepfather had started taking James on an outing each Saturday afternoon for 3–4 hours. This allowed James's mother and sister to spend time with family members. James's stepfather was said to be somewhat isolated from his extended family, but he talked weekly with several of his brothers who lived nearby. The mother's and stepfather's extended families would also occasionally get together for picnics, and both parents felt supported by that circumstance.

Overall, it appeared that the family used palliative coping more than adaptive coping. This idea was suggested by the fact that both the nuclear and the extended family focused on caring for individual family members. Although this was clearly helpful for the family's day-to-day coping, formal organizations that might increase resources over time were not identified, with the exception of their church. It seemed somewhat difficult for James's family to utilize formal services.

Tentative Recommendations

Tentative recommendations were discussed with James's mother to ascertain whether they were realistic for this family. A local organization that helped families develop individualized education programs (IEPs) was identified. Given James's continued aggression at home, it was anticipated that the family might want to use a state-funded home behavioral consultation team for families with children who have behavioral issues as well as developmental disabilities. In addition, James's mother was encouraged to make an appointment regarding her depression medication. It was suggested that the parents might want to initiate a 3- or 4-hour outing for themselves, without the involvement of children or chores, once or twice a month. (Having some time together, even occasionally, seems to help parents reduce their stress.) James's mother responded positively to these recommendations, which would be reviewed again at the parent conference. She also revealed that her minister had suggested that she present a seminar at her church about fragile X syndrome, and James's mother thought it was something that she could do if she had a little more information. Therefore, the social worker provided her with a pamphlet and an article about fragile X syndrome.

The enthusiasm James's mother showed for resources during this interview was much stronger that it had been during the two previous visits. She seemed ready to advocate for her child at home and at school as well as to begin seeking and using other potential resources. Her willingness to talk to her church members about James's condition was a great leap from feeling guilty about being a carrier. These changes were especially notable because parent advocacy is absolutely necessary for establishing supports for children with disabilities. In addition, parental involvement with service planning ensures that interventions are culturally appropriate and family centered.

INTEGRATION OF THE DISCIPLINARY INFORMATION AND RECOMMENDATIONS

The team members who evaluated James convened briefly before meeting with the parents to discuss their findings. Conclusions regarding the diagnosis and recommendations were drawn based on the results of the professionals involved. Several issues were taken into consideration, as James's developmental, educational, and behavioral requirements had to be addressed. It was also important to meet the parents' needs. Identifying support services for the family, such as a family resource person in the community, was crucial for the implementation of the team's suggestions.

The team—which included professionals from developmental pediatrics, psychology, speech-language pathology, occupational therapy, and social work—decided it was best that only the pediatrician and the social worker meet with the parents; the presence of all team members might be overwhelming to them.

James's teacher participated in the discussion at the parent conference. Her presence was critical because she would be helping the family actualize some of the team's recommendations in the future. Her attendance would also provide her with knowledge to clarify questions the family might have later. The parents were, of course, aware of James's diagnosis of fragile X syndrome. However, a general explanation of fragile X syndrome was again given to the parents. It was strongly emphasized that they should keep their appointment at their community genetics clinic to carry out further genetic testing of James's sister as well as other maternal family members.

The discussion then shifted to the findings regarding James's current level of intellectual functioning, language profile, and motor development. James had mental retardation requiring limited to intermittent support. His parents were informed that, in addition to having fragile X syndrome and the corresponding developmental delay, their son also had ADHD, which is commonly associated with fragile X syndrome. New behavior management strategies needed to be considered for dealing with James's ADHD diagnosis and meeting his developmental needs. Increased structure both at home and school was strongly recommended. Several suggestions were given as well as reading materials on ADHD and behavior management, and a list of community mental health resources was provided. A family resource coordinator was also suggested to identify appropriate mental health specialists for behavior management. The team representatives stated that regular, long-term work with a behavior specialist would be most beneficial for dealing with James's current, and possibly future, difficult behavior. That person could also communicate with the school to maintain continuity. James's teacher was aware of local professionals who could provide such services, so she would assist the parents in contacting these specialists. In addition, the possibility of trying medication for ADHD and aggressive behavior needed to be discussed with the primary care provider as an adjunct to behavior management interventions.

Continued speech-language therapy was also advised. James's speech-language goals were judged to be appropriate based on the information provided from his school. His speech-language pathologist needed to consult with James's mother and teacher to increase the likelihood that these objectives would be addressed in everyday situations to aid developing comprehension. James's teacher would communicate this recommendation to the school speech-language pathologist.

On another note, it was suggested that James receive ongoing occupational and physical therapy services through the public school system. From review of his IEP, it appeared that the occupational therapist at school was incorporating a sensory integrative approach in her work with James, which seemed appropriate. It was further recommended that this therapist work closely with James's classroom teacher to help organize, calm, and regulate the child's sensory and behavior responses. The possibility of a private-practice occupational therapist providing in-home consultation was discussed. This could assist James's parents in having their son perform some of the school activities and setting up a daily self-care routine for James. It could be done on a monthly basis as permitted by the family's finances.

Supportive services for families having a child with developmental disabilities were also addressed. The parents were again encouraged to contact the DDD to provide them with resources such as respite care or behavior management consultation. They were also encouraged to contact the National Fragile X Association to meet other parents having children with fragile X syndrome as well as to receive mailings regarding new developments in understanding fragile X syndrome. Another suggested resource was Parents Are Vital for Education (PAVE), which could aid them in advocating for James's educational needs. Furthermore, the parents were encouraged to spend time together, without their children, to reduce stress. Finally, follow-up was recommended within a year or two to determine James's developmental progress and needs. The family and James's teacher were encouraged to contact the clinic if they had questions or additional concerns.

REFERENCES

Achenbach, T.M., & Edelbrook, C.S. (1986). *Child Behavior Checklist and Youth Self-Report.* Burlington, VT: Author.

American Academy of Pediatrics, Committee on Genetics. (1996). Health supervision for children with fragile X syndrome. *Pediatrics, 98,* 297–300.

Ayres, A.J. (1972). *Sensory integration and learning disorders.* Los Angeles: Western Psychological Services.

Ayres, A.J. (1979). *Sensory integration and the child.* Los Angeles: Western Psychological Services.

Ayres, A.J. (1989). *Sensory Integration and Praxis Test (SIPT).* Los Angeles: Western Psychological Services.

Conners, C.K. (1989). *Conners' Rating Scales (CRS): Instruments for the assessment of childhood psychopathology.* North Tonawanda, NY: Multi-Health Systems.

Dunn, W. (1994). Performance of typical children on the Sensory Profile: An item analysis. *American Journal of Occupational Therapy, 48,* 967–964.

Dunn, W., & Westman, K. (1997). The Sensory Profile: The performance of a national sample of children without disabilities. *American Journal of Occupational Therapy, 51,* 25–34.

Fensen, L., Dale, P., Reznick, J.S., Thal, D., Bates, E., Hartung, J., Pethick, S., & Reilly, J. (1993). *MacArthur Communicative Development Inventories (CDI): User's guide and technical manual.* San Diego, CA: Singular Publishing Group.

Folio, M.R., & Fewell, R. (1983). *Peabody Developmental Motor Scales and Activity Cards (PDMS).* Itasca, IL: The Riverside Publishing Co.

Haley, S.M., Coster, W.J., Ludlow, L.H., Haltiwanger, J.T., & Andrellos, P.J. (1992). *Pediatric Evaluation of Disability Inventory (PEDI).* San Antonio, TX: Therapy Skill Builders.

Parham, D.L., & Mailloux, Z. (1996). Sensory integration. In J. Case-Smith, P.N. Pratt, & A.S. Allen (Eds.), *Occupational therapy for children* (pp. 307–353). St. Louis, MO: Mosby.

Reiss, A.L., Hagerman, R.J., Vinogradow, S., Abrams, M., & King, R.J. (1988). Psychiatric disability in female carriers of the fragile X chromosome. *Archives of General Psychiatry, 45,* 25–30.

Scharfenaker, S., O'Connor, R., Stackhouse, T., Braden, M., Hickman, L., & Gray, K. (1996). An integrated approach to intervention. In R. Jenssen & A. Cronister (Eds.), *Fragile X syndrome: Diagnosis, treatment, and research* (pp. 349–411). Baltimore: The Johns Hopkins University Press.

Sparrow, S.S., Balla, D.A., & Cicchetti, D.V. (1984). *Vineland Adaptive Behavior Scales (VABS).* Circle Pines, MN: American Guidance Service.

Stackhouse, T. (1994, March). Sensory integration concepts and fragile X syndrome. *American Occupational Therapy Association Sensory Integration Special Interest Section Newsletter, 17*(1), 2–6.

Thorndike, R.L., Hagen, E.P., & Sattler, J.M. (1986). *Stanford-Binet Intelligence Scale for Children* (4th ed.). Itasca, IL: The Riverside Publishing Co.

Wetherby, A., & Prizant, B. (1993). *Communication and Symbolic Behavior Scales (CSBS) manual: Normed edition.* Chicago: Applied Symbolix.

Wilbarger, P. (1984, September). Planning an adequate "sensory diet": Application of sensory processing theory during the first year of life. *ZERO TO THREE: National Center for Infants, Toddlers, and Families Bulletin, 5*(1), 7–12.

Wilbarger, P. (1995). The sensory diet: Activity programs based on sensory processing theory. *American Occupational Therapy Association Sensory Integration Special Interest Section Newsletter, 18*(2), 1–4.

Williams, M.S., & Shellenberger, S. (1992). *An introduction to "How does your engine run?": The alert program for self-regulation.* Albuquerque, NM: Therapy-Works.

Zimmerman, I., Steiner, V., & Pond, R. (1992). *Preschool Language Scale–3 (PLS-3).* San Antonio, TX.: The Psychological Corp.

Section IV

INTERNATIONAL PERSPECTIVES

Chapter 18

Interdisciplinary Assessment within Early Intervention in Russia

Elena Kozhevnikova

Efforts to develop methods of early intervention involving many disciplines in Russia began in the late 1980s, primarily as a reaction against the prevailing methods of medical interventions for children with disabilities in the former Soviet Union. From the start, however, there were many diffuse beliefs and unrealistic expectations of what could be achieved. In addition, creating a

The St. Petersburg Early Intervention Institute would not have been possible without the support of colleagues and friends from the United States, Sweden, Norway, the United Kingdom, and Finland. A special debt of gratitude is owed to Professor Bengt Borjeson from Stockholm, without whom this chapter could not have been written. Of course, my colleagues from the St. Petersburg Early Intervention Institute have been critical to the success of our program. Special thanks to N. Baranova, V. Balobanova, I. Chistovich, S. Dovbnya, I. Kalmikova, E. Klochkova, S. Kulikova, T. Morozova, V. Ryskina, and T. Vasilieva for their fine work and support.

professional resource of knowledge and a professional exchange together with colleagues within the United States and Europe was attempted. Unfortunately, at the same time, democratic Russia was confronting social and economic struggles—problems and difficulties that are more and more pronounced in Russia at the end of the 20th century.

As of 2000, it is not possible to give a reliable picture of the development of the field of knowledge of early intervention in Russia. The concept, as such, has gained recognition and does work as a positive force. In fact, several programs in Russia have started categorizing their work as early intervention, although most do not really understand the implications of this professional strategy. The Early Intervention Institute (EII) in St. Petersburg probably still is the only organization in Russia where a professional team tries to combine clinical assessments of children with disabilities with systematic intervention efforts. Applied research and evaluation of outcomes also contribute to the methods used.

A self-evident starting point for the work within the field of early intervention in Russia is the efforts to acquire knowledge and methods that have been developed in the Western world. For EII, which is the focus of this chapter, this has meant exciting meetings for staff with professionals from many disciplines, essentially meetings with different professional cultures. Being faced with the development of the professional work at EII, staff members have taken part in different university programs, international conferences, and seminars.

The experiences from this international exchange have, of course, been enriching but also paradoxical in a sense. From the start, there was from the Russian professionals' side an almost blind trust regarding the possibility of applying techniques developed in the Western world and translating them for use within the specific social situation that exists in Russia in 2000. The conclusion is that, on the one hand, the established Western knowledge on early intervention is indispensable for Russia. On the other hand, it is very difficult, if not impossible, to transfer these methods to Russian society. In a way that is sometimes very evident and almost invisible at other times, the work of early intervention is dependent on the specific conditions of the given social context. These invisible conditions become drastically obvious, however, when an attempt is made to implement the programs. This has been made clear by numerous restrictions that prevent professional application of the knowledge. On a personal level, these restrictions are experienced as extremely strong frustrations. At a professional level, one is in an absurd situation in which he or she has learned a great deal about the nature of conditions for which early intervention is effective, but the possibility of using this knowledge for the best of the society and for people is limited.

STARTING POINTS FOR THE DEVELOPMENT OF EARLY INTERVENTION IN RUSSIA

During President Gorbachev's *perestroika* and *glasnost*, Russians suddenly found much new—and, in many cases, shocking—information about their country.

At the same time, a feeling developed that something can be done, that professionals can change the situation. When the communist regimes of various countries fell in the early the 1990s, the Western world was confronted with dramatic pictures from the former socialist countries' treatment of—and, thus, the misery of—people with disabilities. Before this period, there were four categories of people that could be described as destructive by society: children with disabilities, children and youth with psychosocial problems, people with mental illnesses or mental retardation, and those who were criminal (antisocial). For the unhappy individuals who fell into these categories, the rule was that treatment was determined in a nonprofessional and arbitrary way and expressed a lack of concern for human suffering. All of this is an indelible disgrace for the former socialistic systems. Although the author has used past tense to describe these conditions, it remains a tragic fact that they are still prevalent at the end of the 20th century.

Extremely scarce resources may be one explanation. This obviously is the interpretation made by many supportive international organizations when they were confronted with the conditions of orphanages, institutions for young children, and mental hospitals and prisons in former communist countries. Convoys of trucks with clothes, food, and toys wheeled over the boundaries of the countries of Eastern Europe with the hope that these efforts could at least alleviate the acute maltreatment. After this first phase, it was hoped that the new economic system would take over, directing the emerging flood of resources to even the most neglected individuals within the population.

Essentially, this interpretation of misery as a result of lack of resources is very doubtful. Even institutions having terrible conditions cost a great deal to run. From the perspective of resources, extensive institutional care is economic madness. Therefore, one is forced to conclude that the treatment of individuals with disabilities in Russia was a logical consequence of the ideology of the social system that was responsible for maltreatment. The destructive treatment was a way to deal with the "unsuitable" individuals who, by their disabilities, were a "disgrace" for utopian socialistic society. Socialistic society strove for a lack of social classes; it would embrace all human beings. In reality, there was a very important restriction: "all" meant "all suitable." Those not able to correspond to this criterion were pushed out of society and treated in a way that practically eradicated any confrontation with society regarding disabilities. The walls of institutions were considered a protection for society, implying that one would not be disturbed by the misery of human beings in the midst of utopia.

Therefore, when the socialistic systems disintegrated there was hope everywhere that social intervention would be created to provide justice and offer adequate services for many people who had been eliminated from the fellowship of society. There was optimism that a decent life even for those with physical or mental impairments would be created and that they would have a place in the open, democratic society. During the 1990s, many in Russia had strong ambitions to go in this direction. Developing methods of early intervention is a case in point. Nonetheless, in the year 2000, there is a lack of re-sources, or, more often, the resources are in the wrong hands. There is not yet a willingness to fund those creating professional groups working with the "not suitable," and resources have not been established for families to make them capable of keeping a child with a disability within the family instead of institu-tionalizing him or her.

St. Petersburg is an exception. Early in the 1990s, its city council and city government were the most democratic in Russia. In 1992, these bodies de-cided to develop an early intervention program in the city. By 1999, the city government supported some social programs for children with disabilities, for homeless people, and for older adults. Its associations of parents of children with disabilities are the strongest in the country, and authorities listen to the opinions of parents. Czar Peter I built St. Petersburg as a window to Europe, and it is still the most "European" city in the country.

ATTITUDES IN RUSSIA
TOWARD PEOPLE WITH DISABILITIES

A definite obstacle when trying to implement service programs in general and early intervention programs in particular is the Russian population's prevalent distrust of people with disabilities. The former Soviet Union developed a rhetoric on the honor of work. As a result, a damaging attitude against people who received support without earning it also developed, even though these people should have been sustained by the theory of social policy. There were strong prejudices against those who might not have been able to exist without support and, thus, were entirely dependent on the system.

The psychological parallel was a contempt for the person with physical or mental impairments, a syndrome very characteristic of those societies having utopian ideology. In the Soviet Union, there were only healthy and happy in-dividuals, utopian human beings. The attitudes of the parents toward their children with disabilities reflected this double-edged intolerance. Many felt ashamed and condemned their children.

Institutional care for children with disabilities, therefore, had broad sup-port within the population, even among many family members. Developing methods of early intervention means fighting against these attitudes. In partic-ular, a program of early intervention has to be anchored in efforts that create a positive opinion among people for such measures. It is essential to make the program of early intervention legitimate among the people. Yet the desire to alter public opinion is not just an undertaking to promote better conditions for the program of early intervention. The ambition to change attitudes about people with disabilities in general is a goal in itself, a contribution to creating a broader system of social policy in which humanistic perspectives of the indi-vidual and individual differences are main themes.

PROFESSIONAL SOCIETIES'
UNDERSTANDING OF HUMAN BEINGS

It is not entirely fair to point at the negative attitudes of the Russian citizens about people with disabilities as the biggest difficulty for developing an early intervention system. At least as problematic, perhaps even more so, is resistance from professional societies. In Eastern European countries, a perspective exists that has led to the development of the discipline of *defectology*, which focuses on disabilities. This discipline encompasses many different disciplines within medicine as well as within the behavioral sciences. There are at least two philosophies within defectology that are contradictory to the program of early intervention. The first has to do with thought and theory regarding diagnostics. According to defectological science, diagnostics have a scientific purpose, or at least the diagnosis is scientifically grounded. In reality, the diagnostic systems are crowded with negative values and prejudices regarding people with disabilities; they do not look for potential, only for the person's impairments. When it comes to children with disabilities, defectology's intention is always to reach the final point of the diagnosis—the differentiation between those children who are able to learn and those children who are "uneducable." This final point of diagnosis is the starting point for the maltreatment of the majority of children in orphanages and other institutions. Those described as educable, however, are given rather intense education and training in different forms of special early childhood programs, schools, and so forth. In turn, countries where defectology is prominent have the tragicomic situation that efforts for the children with disabilities are directed toward those who have only very mild delays. For instance, there are many special logopedic preschools for children with articulation problems.

The other philosophy within the defectological perspective that is counterproductive to interdisciplinary early intervention is specialization. Every form of disability is believed to be a specific disability. Of course, the specific disability is a conceptual construction that lacks correspondence with the real nature of a child's disability. The neurological basis for many children with mental retardation is mostly diffuse, even when the cause of the disability is very specific, such as Down syndrome. Specialization within defectology is a response to professional demands for structuring the world and creating professional hierarchies, but this ambition lacks relevance for a real understanding of the needs of the child with a disability.

Accordingly, those philosophies developed within the frame of reference of defectology are a major threat to creating programs of early intervention. Early intervention is challenging the tradition of knowledge that was established within the Soviet system and in which there are still strong investments for keeping the hegemony of the defectological perspective (Strebeleva, 1998). Unfortunately, this view is antagonistic toward an interdisciplinary understanding of developmental disabilities and of human development in general.

IDEOLOGICAL PERSPECTIVES
FOR INTERDISCIPLINARY
ASSESSMENT WITHIN EARLY INTERVENTION

The program of early intervention at EII in St. Petersburg has to be understood from the previously discussed ideological perspective. EII's work must start from a fundamentally new way of understanding the child with a disability compared with the perspective related to the discipline of defectology. The child with a disability must be viewed from an interdisciplinary perspective, for diagnostic and assessment procedures as well as for the child's intervention program.

The interdisciplinary approach means that, out of *a priori* reasons, it is assumed that even a specific disability has general consequences for the person, and the experiences of the person with a disability are deeply personal. A hearing impairment is specific to the audiological system, but this observation must fit into a general understanding of the psychological and social needs of the child experiencing this disability and his or her parents. The specific disability is of decisive importance when it comes to the child's formation of self-concept, and this has far-reaching consequences for development.

Social perspective is absolutely necessary for understanding the child's needs. The child with a disability lives within a primary social context, the family, in which the responses of the parents and of the siblings are of major importance for the child's development and self-understanding. It is therefore axiomatic that every effort of early intervention must include family members.

The very concept of *disability* implies that there is a lack of "normal" capacity of the child. This view most often has negative implications for the design of services for the child. Those at EII have tried to develop an assessment of possibilities, to direct professional awareness to the field of strengths instead of describing the child's impairment. This is a difficult undertaking, however, and this chapter, to a large extent, tries to make the problems clear. Late 20th-century diagnostic instruments almost always have typical functioning as the criterion for judging the atypical functioning of a child with a disability. The professional routines for determining the child's potential are few and not well developed. This is not simple neglect; it is a matter of course that there is something more substantial if one is trying to describe a delay. That is, there is something to describe and measure. In contrast, potential is a symbolic construction; it is more of a way of thinking than of seeing something that is there to observe.

Nevertheless, this is not a checkmate situation. Those at EII think it is more or less impossible to measure the potential of the child as part of a diagnostic process before intervention starts. It is much more feasible to observe the child's strengths if the intervention program is used as an important way of understanding his or her capacity. In other words, EII has tried to create professional routines by which services to the child should at the same time constitute a continuous assessment, with the emphasis on the child's positive responses to the intervention.

This outlook implies a general and ideological conclusion: Diagnosis and assessment must be considered as hypotheses that should be revised according to the child's reactions to the intervention, and they also are consequences of critical discussion within the professional group. To be a professional in the field of early intervention, working with a child with a disability means that one is always, perhaps reluctantly, changing one's opinion.

Developing the Program

Will it be possible to put into use the interdisciplinary process approach? For the professional group at EII this is a difficult question, and some of the conditions established at EII in an effort to develop a program of early intervention are discussed in the following section.

The first strategy is to create a group of professional staff members who manifest an interdisciplinary knowledge. EII accepts 400–500 new families every year, who come to the institute via recommendations from a polyclinical unit of St. Petersburg, by referral from a hospital for children, or by the family's initiative. The age of the child always is between birth and 3 years. Regardless of the reason for referral, it is clear that these families represent a selective and positive sample due to the fact that the parents' ambition is to help their children and, in many cases, to avoid placing them in an institution. This is also a primary desire for the intervention program at EII—to prevent placing of a child outside of the family.

The diagnostic-assessment panorama is very extensive. The stated intent is to accept all families seeking help and, in those cases for which the task extends the professional competence of the group at EII, to assist the families in finding complementary support outside EII. Some of the children have severe disabilities, yet, the clinic often sees children with relatively mild delays that can be dealt with by rather simple supports. The professional group at EII consists of physicians, special education teachers, psychologists, speech-language pathologists, physiologists of vision and hearing, and speech scientists.

The programs at EII are extremely varied. The majority of families have 4–10 meetings with its staff members, but for other families, it means contact on a regular basis for more than a year. The staff members have a duty over and above clinical work to take part in a program of applied research, with emphasis on evaluating the results of the program of intervention.

EII has an obligation to foster interdisciplinary competence for its staff members. But what are the means for developing such a competence, and in what ways should it be put into play? A crucial step for establishing the interdisciplinary approach is to choose a qualified "gatekeeper," who works in a service coordinator role. This is a pediatrician; his or her responsibility is, in cooperation with the parents, to make a preliminary assessment of the needs of the child and the family and to make an initial intervention plan. Without such a qualified assessment available from the start, the child and the family will not receive the necessary supports. This first stage of assessment is both preliminary and decisive. It is preliminary in the sense that only tentative plans are made for the child and for the family but decisive in the sense that the parents are confronted with the different types of resources that can be offered by EII. For many parents who hope their children with disabilities can be healed, this is very provocative.

A second category of instruments for establishing an interdisciplinary approach regarding the child and family needs is detailed parent questionnaires. Every child is assessed by his or her parents, and this evaluation constitutes the primary basis for subsequent professional efforts. For Russian conditions, this represents a revolutionary professional procedure. It challenges ordinary and self-evident routines in a country where parental knowledge is seen as irrelevant and, therefore, completely neglected. Yet this is a very important element of early intervention. If work is based on the parents' judgments, it is easier to establish a cooperative relationship with the family. The logic is very simple: The initial process means that one starts with parental knowledge and then transforms it into an assessment and the need for further family cooperation to make the intervention process successful.

Still-Prevailing Traditions of Services for Children with Disabilities in Russia

The interdisciplinary approach of EII is a radical departure from prevailing professional tradition in Russia concerning the assessment and intervention of young children with disabilities. This tradition implies the following:

1. Implemented services have a strong emphasis on medical care. Only medical staff, physicians within different specialties, nurses, and so forth work with children younger than 3 years of age.
2. There are very few special education teachers, psychologists, speech-language pathologists, and other specialists working with children younger than 3 years of age. These kinds of professionals usually examine children older than 3 years of age, and then the specialists work only with children with minor disabilities.
3. Physical therapy and occupational therapy as specialties are nonexistent in Russia.
4. Speech-language pathologists do not work with early childhood communication.
5. The relationships among professionals are strictly hierarchical. Physicians make all decisions regarding the child's needs and who should work with him or her. The interplay with parents is exclusively directive. Mothers get instructions without understanding their meaning, even if they have a firm conviction that the child does not have the problem the physician assumes.

6. Delayed or impaired development is always considered a result of organic damage (if this damage cannot be verified, it still exists as a matter of course). The importance of the family situation and of the environment in general, as well as normal individual variations among children (e.g., "late starters"), is neglected.

7. There is no cooperation and no coordination among the different specialists. A physician and a teacher seldom discuss a child's problems together. The result is, of course, that their recommendations to the family often will be contradictory.

8. There are two types of institutions for young children with severe disabilities: orphanages and, if the child still is within the family, medical institutions for rehabilitation. Special preschools (e.g., for children with cerebral palsy or developmental delays) are very few in number for children older than 3 years of age. For children with multiple disabilities, the possibility of getting a placement at a special preschool is very limited.

Taken together, these conditions in Russia create numerous organizational problems regarding the professional work at EII. The family of a child with a disability has a learned fear of society and social officials. This fear also applies to other people, neighbors, relatives, and friends. Parents whose child has a disability are constantly confronted with requests to institutionalize the child or statements that the child will never learn, and it is better to give him or her away. There is no literature available for parents to get information about how to make simple supports for their children. Moreover, special aids for children with motor disabilities are almost nonexistent. Imported aids are impossible to buy because of the extremely high costs. Parents of children with disabilities do not get financial support, and there are no homes adjusted to the special needs of a child with a disability. These parents find themselves in an extremely difficult financial situation. The pension for the child is very small. There also is no established psychological support for the parents of a child with a disability. This is the reality with which the staff at EII have to live. These are the real conditions, but, of course, the intention is to work to alter them.

SCREENING AND ASSESSMENT

When the EII program in St. Petersburg was established, there were two ideological conditions for its work that were of decisive importance. The first was to accept, in principle, children with all types of disabilities: motor, sensory, cognitive, and psychosocial. The degree of difficulty or complexity of the disability would be of no relevance as to whether the child should be admitted. Yet there are selection mechanisms regardless of the professional efforts of EII. The staff often do not even meet the child with a very severe disability because of the attitudes of others. At medical units, parents are encouraged to refer that child to an orphanage. Even infants with Down syndrome are looked upon as incurable, and physicians recommend that parents send them to an orphanage directly from the maternity hospital. It is also more than probable that a child with a severe psychosocial background will not be seen by EII. These parents avoid contact with EII clinic professionals, whom they believe share society's view of their families. Especially among homes where there is heavy alcohol abuse, physical abuse, and so forth, the inclination to seek help and support is small. EII has tried, without great success, to develop strategies for connecting with hard-to-reach families.

The second condition for the work at EII is to make it possible to keep the child within the family. EII is not to be one more of those institutions that, in an open or a disguised fashion, encourages parents to abandon their children. Thus, a main goal of EII's professional efforts is to assist parents and help them take continuing responsibility for their children.

Staff at EII organize both screening procedures (i.e., a system to determine children's developmental delays or impairments) and intervention programs using interdisciplinary assessments at both stages of work. These routines must be accomplished so that 1) they contribute to the engagement of the parents as cooperative members of the team; 2) they help create a professional dialogue between different specialists; 3) they start from a nonhierarchical, collaborative philosophy among the specialists, in which the professional judgment that is most important depends on the problem in question; 4) interdisciplinary assessment, as a main purpose, is used to describe the child's potential and not his or her impairments; and 5) this assessment is open to new knowledge of the child gained during the sessions of treatment.

Screening Instruments

The main screening instruments used by EII are parent questionnaires, the Kent Infant Development (KID) Scale (Reuter & Bickett, 1985; Reuter & Reuter, 1990), and the Child Development Inventory (Ireton CDI; Ireton, 1992). Many screening instruments are characterized as "quick and dirty." The main asset of a good questionnaire is that it is inexpensive, not time consuming, and very useful. Psychometric qualities of the KID Scale and several of its national versions have been thoroughly investigated (Chistovich, Reuter, & Shapiro, 1997; Reuter & Wozniak, 1996) and shown to be valid and reliable. The same can be said about the MacArthur Communication Development Inventories (MacArthur CDI; Fensen et al., 1993; Fensen et al., 1994). Ireton's CDI also seems to have good reliability and validity (Ireton, 1997), although there are less data on the scale. Another point that is very important to EII is to work with families and to encourage the involvement of parents in the entire process. Questionnaires include the parents from the very beginning. An added advantage to using parent questionnaires is that families often then become more interested in their children's development.

The KID Scale is a caregiver-completed developmental assessment instrument appropriate for children who are chronologically or developmentally younger than 16 months of age. The KID Scale consists of 252 items that describe observable behaviors characteristic of an infant in the first 16 months of life. These items have been divided into five domains on the basis of their content: Cognitive, Motor, Language, Self-Help, and Social. Developmental ages, based on the full KID Scale, are used for the determination of overall developmental status. Age norms for the KID Scale have been developed and published in the United States, the Netherlands, Spain, Hungary, and Russia, and the assessment has been used in Germany and the Czech Republic as well. The Russian version of the KID Scale includes local St. Petersburg age norms, a user's manual (Chistovich, Reuter, & Shapiro, 1997), and a database computer program for scoring. The Russian normative sample is comparable in size and quality to the 2000 U.S. sample (about 700 children each).

The Ireton CDI is a later version of the Minnesota Child Development Inventory (Minnesota CDI; Ireton & Thwing, 1972). This 1992 update allows evaluation of the developmental age of children 1–6 years of age (15 months– 4 years of age in the Russian version) in six domains: Social, Self-Help, Gross Motor, Fine Motor, Expressive Language, and Language Comprehension. In the Russian version, some specific English language items have been substituted with appropriate Russian ones. In addition, 20 items particular to the Russian language were added for research purposes, but they are not included in the scale as of 2000. The Russian version of the Ireton CDI includes local St. Petersburg age norms (Chistovich & Shapiro, 1997) and a database scoring program.

Staff at EII devised the Word Comprehension Test with two aims: to get more objective data on word comprehension and to see if parents could and would do simple experiments with their children. The test includes 70 words of 6 classes: 20 commands, 15 locative words, 8 body parts, 6 colors, 5 quantitative words, and 16 qualitative words. Parents are given instructions in how to test comprehension. For example, a parent might put colored buttons before the child and say, "Give me the red one, now the blue one." After each trial, the button is put back, and parents are to mark the words the child uses. This test allows a gathering of extensive data on comprehension and production, although other subtests or supplementary scales are used to provide better estimates of language comprehension. Moreover, a translation of Actions and Gestures as part of the MacArthur CDI is also administered. It consists of First Communicative Gestures (12 items), Games and Routines (6 items), Actions with Objects (17 items), Pretending to Be a Parent (13 items), and Imitating Other Adult Actions (15 items). In Russia, there is not enough data in 2000 to develop local norms but, according to preliminary computations, the norms will be close to American ones. Thus, the American norms can be used for children 8–16 months of age. As of 2000, specialists at EII use this list informally to see what the child can do in these areas. Parents also are asked to record the words the child produces as well as his or her pronunciation of the word if it is not conventional. It is also requested that they list five examples of the longest phrases the child uses. The speech-language pathologists find these lists very informative. The data are used also for research purposes in EII and in the Child Language Department of the Pedagogical University.

Either at EII or the children's polyclinics, parents receive a test booklet and information and answer sheets. The test booklet contains instructions for filling out the information and answer sheets and a text of items. The information sheet is a form provided to record the child's name, gender, date of birth, and assessment date as well as the week of pregnancy during which the child was born, who completed the test, and some additional information about the child and his or her family. The caregiver marks responses on the answer sheet for each of the items in the test booklet.

Assessment by Gatekeeper

The pediatrician and one staff member with a specialized background (e.g., a psychologist, a speech-language pathologist) take part in the gatekeeper assessment. The aim of the evaluation is to decide if the child needs further assessment and a subsequent intervention program and, if so, to develop a working diagnosis and to decide to whom to refer the family. The information from the parents and the assessment tools is supplemented by visual and hearing screening and a pediatric examination. The process takes approximately 1 hour, and professional exchange among the professionals during this process, especially in the case of children with serious complications, is extensive.

In simple terms, the gatekeepers are opening the gates to two main groups of children: children who need early intervention, including those who have severe disabilities, and those who do not need early intervention but most likely do not receive proper medical treatment. In St. Petersburg in 2000, diagnosing children with encephalopathy has become extremely popular. There are some children's polyclinics where about 90% of children at 1 year of age have this diagnosis. They are receiving drugs, massage, electrotherapy, and other treatments. Certainly parents are very worried; they are coming to the EII to check if their children are developing typically and to ask about treatment. The gatekeepers try to calm parents by telling them that their children are indeed developing typically (as is true in most cases) and do not need special help. However, often this is not enough for parents, and the family is referred to a neurologist. There are also cases in which the child has some behavior problems and gatekeepers refer him or her to a neurologist and a psychologist, who together try to understand the situation. They often do months of follow-up in such cases.

Specific Assessments

Based on the working diagnosis of the gatekeepers, the child might be referred to different specialists at EII for an interdisciplinary assessment. Specialists include neurologists, physical therapists, special education teachers, speech-language pathologists, psychologists, audiologists, and physiologists of vision or ophthalmologists. The child may be referred to some other agency as well (e.g., a genetic center). All specialists working at EII can refer children to other specialists or other agencies, and very often staff have joint sessions. Usually, the child is seen in a single session or in sessions by interdisciplinary specialists. The specialists then meet and develop a plan for early intervention with the family. As discussed subsequently in this chapter, this is an important but preliminary step in the interdisciplinary early intervention process.

Audiology

Children who fail auditory screening and children with delays in language comprehension are referred to an audiologist. The audiologist tries also to test hearing in children with general developmental delays and in children with multiple disabilities. The audiologist uses standard methods of assessment: visual reinforcement audiometry (VRA) for children from 6 months to $1^{1}/_{2}$ years of age and conditioned play audiometry (CPA) for children from $1^{1}/_{2}$ to 3 years old. The method is chosen according to each child's developmental level, attention, and interests in play. The sounds are presented both in free field and through earphones and bone conductors. To make the procedure more interesting for the child, staff have started using moving sound for conditioning (stimuli that imitate movement from right to left and backward). As test stimuli, a standard set of pure tones (0.5, 1.0, 2.0, 4.0, 8.0 kilohertz) is used. Before starting audiological assessment, the child's orientation reaction to different sound stimuli (broadband and high-frequency noises of different intensity levels) is observed. Some types of speech audiometry are also used for testing children with speech comprehension delays. To be fitted for hearing aids, children are referred to specialized centers. By legislation, a hearing aid is recommended for children with hearing losses more than 55 decibels. Since 1996, it is possible to get individual earmolds and good quality foreign hearing aids in St. Petersburg. After the fitting, children return to the EII audiologist for testing. The audiologist not only tests hearing but also gives parents recommendations about auditory training.

Vision

Children who fail visual screening, have visual impairments according to medical records, have general developmental delays, and have multiple disabilities are referred to the physiologist of vision. To assess visual acuity, contrast sensitivity, and color vision, different tests from the LEA TEST SYSTEM (Hyvarinen et al., 1992) and BUST (Lindstead, 1988, 1997) are used. Informal tests are used to test field of vision and binocular fixation. To assess vision in children with multiple disabilities, observation of visual behavior is used. A set of materials from the Tomteboda Resource Centre in Sweden is extremely useful for these children (Jadne, Riesenfeld, & Wijk, 1996).

Although the clinic has modern tests and a rather strong group of physiologists of vision, this part of EII's work is not entirely satisfactory. The screening helps find children with very mild impairments and, in these cases, physiologists of vision can themselves recommend to parents ways to stimulate visual development. Yet in more serious cases, the children cannot be helped at EII; they are referred to city ophthalmologic services, where physicians often recommend that parents wait for treatment until the child is 3 years old.

Specialists working at EII with infants having vision impairments, with or without additional complications, use the vision assessment results for the development of an intervention program. It is very practical and efficient when all specialists participate in the assessment session or when they watch and discuss the video recording of that session together with parents and physiologists of vision.

Neurology and Physical Therapy

Children with general development delays, with delays in gross and fine motor development, with multiple disabilities, and without delays but with a neurological diagnosis are referred to a neurologist or a physical therapist. As of 2000, neurology and physical therapy are not divided into two separate specialties at EII. The clinic's physical therapists are actually child neurologists by education who received some knowledge of physical therapy. They are not dividing their functions with respect to neurology and physical therapy but, certainly with different children and in different situations, they are behaving mainly as neurologists or as physical therapists using methods of assessment obtained from two disciplines.

Neurological assessments used by neurologists in different countries are standard and, thus, quite similar. Working in the context of early intervention, the neurologist is trying to estimate the role of biological factors in the child's development. It is very important to have a physician on the team whose responsibility is to make or to define a medical diagnosis and to decide if some additional methods of assessment or medical treatments are needed. At EII, physicians work mainly as neurologists. However, they use not only standard neurological methods but also consider the KID Scale and the Ireton CDI results, as well as the results of assessments by other specialists.

For a child with motor disorders or with multiple disabilities, child neurologists are mainly playing the role of physical therapists. In this situation, the neurological assessment is always carried out by an assessment of the child's postural competence and movement abilities, which are added to aid in planning the intervention program. Different standard physical therapy scales are used for this purpose (Hare, 1993; Poutney, 1993).

Special Education

Assessment by the special education teacher is based on observation of the child and on discussions with the parent about the child's development and behavior. First, the teacher tries to understand how to establish contact with the child and to determine what is interesting for the child, his or her style of interaction with the surroundings, and the child's possibilities for solving different tasks. The assessment is done informally but, to a large extent, it is based on items from The Carolina Curriculum for Infants and Toddlers with Special Needs (Johnson-Martin, Jens, Attermeier, & Hacker, 1991) or the Portage Guide to Early Education (Shearer et al., 1976). The teacher tries to estimate the attention span of the child as well as the peculiarities of his or her contact and interaction with strangers (e.g., the teacher), parents, and peers (according to parents' report). During observations, the teacher notes the child's oral speech and gestures and tests speech comprehension and understanding, especially the child's ability to follow simple instructions. The teacher tries to estimate the level of the child's play, what kind of activities and toys are interesting for him or her, and the child's ability to imitate sounds and actions. The teacher is also interested in obtaining information about the child's self-help abilities. Usually, the special education teacher assesses children with multiple disabilities together with the neurologist.

Psychology

Children with delays in the social domain and children with socioemotional and behavior problems (in the gatekeeper's opinion) are referred to the psychologist. The psychologist tries to understand if a child's socioemotional development actually is atypical or if his or her behavior and parents' complaints are connected with peculiarities related to the child's age. The psychologist analyzes the history of the child's development, trying to find risk factors in psychological development such as disturbances in early infant–mother interaction, difficulties in breast feeding and weaning, early separation, and hospitalizations. The psychologist observes the child during the general assessment session with a special focus on the child's contact with the caregivers and the stranger (i.e., psychologist), interest in toys, and exploration activity level. The psychologist attempts to assess the extent to which parents understand their children's feelings and how parents' own issues (low self-esteem, anxiety, depression, disturbed relations in the family) influence their relationships with their children.

Of note, psychologists in Russia rarely see children with developmental delays, as parents of these children appear to try to avoid contact with psychologists. Perhaps it is because some of these families are rather closed, and the parents tend to explain their child's socioemotional behavior as a result of his or her delay or disorder. During the session with a child having serious delays, the psychologist tries to estimate the psychological needs of the child at the present moment using the same methods of observation and assessment as for children with milder delays.

At EII, joint assessments by the psychologist and the neurologist are used to define the roles of psychological and biological factors in the child's development. One of the serious difficulties for psychologists is a lack of formal assessment criteria. As of 2000, EII is adapting the Child Behavior Checklist (CBCL; Achenbach, 1992). However, high levels of subjectivity characterize EII's assessments.

Speech-Language Pathology

Children with delays in expressive language and language comprehension are referred to the speech-language pathologist. Both observations of the child and information from the family are used for assessment. The assessment usually consists of the following items:

1. Brief language anamneses (vocalizations, preverbal communication, babbling, first words) are monitored.
2. Expressive language (late babbling, vocabulary, prosody, imitation) is assessed. The vocabulary list gathered previously is used here. A vocabulary of more than 20–30 words, the beginning use of phrases, attempts at word modification, overgeneralizations, phonology, syllabic structure, stress, and phrase construction are also tested.
3. Language comprehension is evaluated by the Word Comprehension Test and by asking the family about the child's language comprehension in everyday life as well as if the child understands words without gestures. Staff also try to assess comprehension during the meeting, but this is often difficult because the child's reactions depend very strongly on his or her attention and general characteristics of communicative behavior.
4. Communication through gestures, mimicking, and communicative skills constitutes an additional component of the assessment. The Gestures List from the MacArthur CDI, observations of the child's communicative skills, and comparisons of the development of verbal and nonverbal communication are all used. Noting the parents' relationship with their child and their style of communication is another element. Many children can benefit from modification of language input or the parents' general style. The assessment has a rather intuitive character and is based on internal standards of typical development because, in Russia, there are no standardized measures of language acquisition or of early communication except the KID Scale and the Ireton CDI.

INTERDISCIPLINARY ASSESSMENT

Based on the assessments, various specialists integrate their information to develop a profile of developmental strengths for the child and to identify areas of concern. As many of the assessments by specialists occur together, ideas are shared on a routine basis. The overall purpose is to communicate the team's findings to the family and to develop a positive early intervention plan, if needed.

An underlying concept in this chapter is the intellectual effort to redefine the traditional Russian concept of diagnosis focused on impairments and to substitute in its place the concept of assessment, particularly interdisciplinary assessment, with its emphasis on describing a child's potential. This goal is of special importance for early intervention due to the destructive results of the diagnostic tradition as it has been developed within the discipline of defectology in Russia.

The strategy of the interdisciplinary assessment developed at EII can be summarized as follows:

1. The assessment of the child as well as the intervention should make use of the knowledge and engagement of the family. The parents are to be considered co-workers, and they must experience their share of successful work with the child.

2. The interdisciplinary assessment is built on an organization of knowledge exchange among professional colleagues during different phases of the work with the child and with the family. Yet knowledge exchange does not occur due to the goodwill of the colleagues. There is little time for this. This exchange has to be an organizational rule governing daily work.

3. The relationships among professionals representing different disciplines should be on equal bases. The psychologist and the special education teachers are not assistants to the physician; all experts have the same level of responsibility for the general program of early intervention. For every case in which the professional work will last for more than one or two consultations, there will be a team of experts, and one of its members will have main responsibility for the child. At EII, as a matter of course, there often is a primary person selected for the early intervention program who is a special education teacher or a psychologist (with one of the physicians as co-worker) on the team.

4. The professional work at EII is a major shift from the conventional diagnostic procedure toward using the interdisciplinary assessment as a starting point to understand the child's strengths and his or her capacity for development. With regard to the first three strategies, many of EII's ambitions are being fulfilled. Nonetheless, numerous problems still exist. At this fourth and crucial point, staff at EII find very significant difficulties. The main problem—one probably shared with colleagues in the field of early intervention everywhere—is that there is not a generally accepted way to describe the potential of the child that is analogous to a diagnosis of the child's impairment.

There are, of course, ways of avoiding this dilemma or at least minimizing its impact. One can define the assessment of the child as a continuous diagnosis to be made during the process of intervention. In such a case, there will be possibilities, starting with the preliminary diagnosis before intervention begins. It is important to follow the child's course of development and, at the same time, to try to understand the child's progress in relation to the intervention.

This is a way of working and a way of understanding the meaning of the concept of assessment that staff at EII plan to develop better. There is, however, a substantial risk of reducing the follow-along of the child's development to a routine of repeated assessments regarding the child's developmental level in different domains. Accordingly, EII staff are still bound to diagnostic thinking and its emphasis on the developmental disability of the child. The challenge, then, is to follow the child's development through a judgment of the flow of processes. In that way, there will be real possibilities of relating the development of the child to the efforts of the intervention. Yet such a goal means real professional collaboration and intensive efforts. Experts of diagnostic methods are more or less novices at describing processes of intervention. Thus, the colleagues at EII find themselves in an initial phase of professional development in this respect. Understanding interdisciplinary assessment as an ongoing study of the processes of development, in which the child is looked upon as an active participant, is truly a great challenge for the professionals at EII.

REDEFINITION OF THE CONCEPT OF ASSESSMENT

Is it possible to work with the child with a disability without using his or her disability as a guiding principle for the program of intervention? Staff at EII have asked this question and have also attempted to formulate some preliminary answers. The starting point of this thinking is an almost inevitable restriction of virtually all programs directed toward early intervention. To a certain extent, the efforts of developing the child's potential will always be directed toward eliminating or mitigating the effects of a child's given disability.

The goal of intervention will thus be limited and related to the judgment of the disability. This is true even when one tries to use the interdisciplinary assessment of the child's strengths to describe the intervention in terms of conventional processes. In an effort to bring about a fundamental rethinking, professionals at EII have tried to adopt some theoretical perspectives that are being developed foremost in the United States, where the starting point of the study of the child is the conviction that the child learns the world by creating and recreating "theories" (see Gopnik & Meltzoff, 1997). By adopting this formula, EII states the following general rules regarding the child perspective of the interdisciplinary assessment: 1) the child's cognitive development means that the child, through relating to the external world, is in a systematic way developing, deepening, testing, formulating, and reformulating his or her theories of the world; 2) it is at least partially possible to follow and to understand these developing schemata by detailed observations and descriptions of social and linguistic occurrences when the child is an active partner; and 3) this ongoing description of the creation of the world is the raw material for the assessment of the child's structural cognitive capacity and potential.

Adding to these basic assumptions, there are supplementary assumptions regarding the assessment of the child. One example is the belief that the child with a disability, as well as the child with typical development, is engaged in the same but modified task of structuring his or her understanding of the world in terms of theories and meanings. Another supplementary assumption, more of a working hypothesis, is that understanding theory construction on the child's side does not in any way exclude different kinds of expertise among the professional staff members. Knowledge is needed from the physical therapist, the psychologist, and the special education teacher, and each has a high degree of relevance when interpreting the theoretical work of the child. Therefore, the professionals at EII are devoted to using the interdisciplinary expertise of the staff members to establish an understanding of the child's strategies, thereby further developing and redefining his or her cognitive structures. This is an undertaking in which it is taken for granted that it is necessary to observe this development within a context of communication and social exchange. The theoretical work of the child can be interpreted only within a social frame of reference.

CONCLUSION

This chapter demonstrates the optimism felt in Russia at the end of the 20th century regarding interdisciplinary early intervention. It begins by describing external difficulties in relation to EII's program of early intervention—particularly the rigid diagnostic understanding of the child, directed to his or her impairment, and the low priority in Russia given to intervention programs for children with disabilities. But the real difficulties are those that are shared with the professional community within the field of early intervention. In what ways should professionals define the concept of interdisciplinary assessment, and in what ways should a program of early intervention be implemented in order to fulfill professional standards? Those working in this field experience these problems with their colleagues all over the world. A lot can be learned from each other, and this is a very hopeful prospect!

REFERENCES

Achenbach, T.M. (1992). *Manual for the Child Behavior Checklist/2–3 and 1992 Profile.* Burlington: University of Vermont Department of Psychiatry.

Chistovich, I., Reuter, J., & Shapiro, J. (1997). *Manual on assessing infant development on the basis of Russian version of KID Scale.* St. Petersburg, Russia: St. Petersburg Early Intervention Institute Publications.

Chistovich, I., & Shapiro, J. (1997). Russian norms for Child Development Inventory. In H. Ireton, (Ed.), *Child Development Inventories in education and health care* (pp.124–126). Minneapolis, MN: Behavior Science Systems.

Fensen, L., Dale, P., Reznick, J.S., Bates, E., Thal, D.J., & Pethick, S.J. (1994). Variability in early communicative development. *Monographs of the Society for Research in Child Development, 59*(5, Serial No. 242).

Fensen, L., Dale, P., Reznick, J.S., Thal, D., Bates, E., Hartung, J., Pethick, S., & Reilly J. (1993). *MacArthur Communicative Development Inventories: User's guide and technical manual.* San Diego, CA: Singular Publishing Group.

Gopnik, A., & Meltzoff, A. (1997). *Words, thoughts and theories.* Cambridge, MA: The MIT Press.

Hare, N. (1993). The Physical Ability Scale. In *Physical Ability Scale and variants. Hare Association for Physical Ability* (pp. 7–26). Bulwell, United Kingdom: Wm. J. Butler & Co.

Hyvarinen, L., Colenbrander, A., Arditi, A., Land, M.A., Seidman, K., Kopidlansky, E., & Greening, C. (1992). *The LH Symbol Tests. A system for vision testing in children.* New York: Lighthouse Low Vision Products.

Ireton, H. (1992). *Child Development Inventory manual.* Minneapolis, MN: Behavior Science Systems.

Ireton, H. (Ed.). (1997). *Child Development Inventories in education and health care.* Minneapolis, MN: Behavior Science Systems.

Ireton, H., & Thwing, E. (1972). *Manual for the Minnesota Child Development Inventory.* Minneapolis, MN: Behavior Science Systems.

Jadne, K., Riesenfeld, A., & Wijk, C. (1996). *The Visual Screening Kit.* Laromedel, Sweden: SIH.

Johnson-Martin, N.M., Jens, K.G., Attermeier, S.M., & Hacker, B.J. (1991). *The Carolina Curriculum for Infants and Toddlers with Special Needs* (2nd ed.). Baltimore: Paul H. Brookes Publishing Co.

Lindstead, E. (1988). *Manual BUST–D, A Vision Test for Young Children and/or Handicapped Children/Adults.* Stockholm: Elysin.

Lindstead, E. (1997). *How well does a child see? A guide on vision and vision assessment in children.* Stockholm: Elysin.

Poutney, T. (1993). The clinical application of ability levels. In *Physical Ability Scale and variants. Hare Association for Physical Ability* (pp. 43–50). Bulwell, United Kingdom: Wm. J. Butler & Co.

Reuter, J., & Reuter, L. (1990). *Addendum to the second edition of the KID Scale manual.* Kent, OH: Kent Developmental Metrics.

Reuter, J.M., & Bickett, L. (1985). *The Kent Infant Development Scale manual* (2nd ed.). Kent, OH: Kent Developmental Metrics.

Reuter, J.M., & Woznniak, J.R. (1996). *The Kent Infant Development (KID) Scale user's guide & technical manual* (3rd ed.). Kent, OH: Kent Developmental Metrics.

Shearer, D.E., Billingsley, J., Frohman, A., Hilliard, J., Johnson, F., & Shearer, M. (1976). *Portage Guide to Early Education.* Portage, WI: Cooperative Educational Service Agency No. 5.

Strebeleva, E. (1998). Creation in Russia of the unified system of early detection and early correction of deviations in the development of children. In *Proceedings of the conference Problems of Special Psychology and Psychodiagnostics of Deviated Development* (pp. 116–119). Moscow: Institute of Education Publications.

Chapter 19

Interdisciplinary Assessment of Individuals with Disabilities in Italy

A New Model in Rome

Giorgio Albertini and Salvatore Rubino

The primary purpose of the Child, Adult, Aging Development Center Silvana Paolini Angelucci in Rome, Italy, is the evaluation of children, young adults, and older adults with developmental disabilities. As part of the Casa di Cura San Raffaele, the center employs an interdisciplinary, comprehensive, and longitudinal approach, having a close collaboration with the families and the communities served. This chapter provides a brief description of the model used at the Child, Adult, Aging Development Center Silvana Paolini Angelucci and the principles that guide its staff's practice of interdisciplinary assessment. The model applies to individuals with disabilities and their families throughout the life span but is especially relevant to young children who may be receiving their first comprehensive evaluation and their families.

THE MODEL

A main problem in the field of developmental disabilities in Italy is not simply obtaining a diagnosis, as that is guaranteed to come from medical centers, but receiving a thoughtful assessment and evaluation of the developmental characteristics of individuals with disabilities. This comprehensive assessment is essential in order to identify needs for the different phases of children's growth and development, thereby putting into effect the most current intervention strategies in the familiar contexts of the individual's home, school, and leisure time (Abroms & Sheiner, 1980). For the families, it means activating the resources that allow them to organize and maximize the impact of these intervention strategies.

Most theories formulated in the 1990s about brain development are well integrated with environmental factors. The plasticity of development in the early years in particular is a guiding principle. Similarly, educational and rehabilitative strategies are based on the concept of the area of potential development and on cognitive theories linking brain structure and function. Principles of developmental psychology involving dynamic interactions for promoting growth and development suggest the importance of a forward-looking assessment process and its connections to intervention strategies.

The activities originally carried out at the Casa di Cura San Raffaele are in many ways a replication of the English-American model, using assessment protocols and therapeutic methods supported by the majority of the scientific literature on developmental disabilities. By establishing interdisciplinary and longitudinal foci, a rich collaboration with families is created. This is equally true for those who temporarily reside at the center as inpatients. The goal is to allow—as quickly as possible—assessment, intervention orientation, and a return to one's community. This requires not only close communication with families but also transferring information to the school and to local agencies for intervention and leisure.

Children and families come to the center following a pediatric evaluation or a pediatric neurological evaluation. The physician then makes a schedule for clinical and medical consultations as well as for developmental evaluations. Specialists generally include physical therapists, speech-language pathologists, psychologists, and child neurologists. Families attend the center for 1 or 2 days, depending on the complexity of the evaluation. In more complex cases, families may attend the center longer. At the end of all the consultations, a staff meeting is conducted to discuss educational and rehabilitative activities. The family then meets with the center's director and with the professional whose discipline is most applicable for that child and his or her family. For some families, a period of intensive treatment at the center is a possible outcome of this process. Therefore, the center must host children and parents in an environment that is absolutely different from the traditional hospital environment, including play areas beyond those used for therapy. The next section discusses how the center was literally constructed and, more specifically, its structural features.

Structural Features

After an analysis of the project's characteristics, with a special emphasis on cultural issues and consideration of the difficulties the children have with clinical environments, the architect, Paolo Macoratti, translated the principles of the center staff into an architectural language. A deliberate choice was made to break with the dominant approach in which space is allocated primarily through the rational distribution of functions, equipment, and resources, all in the name of efficiency and mechanical use of technology. If that approach was followed, the structure produced would have aseptic, linear, and anonymous spaces, as well as no sociocultural references to the outside world.

The idea of thinking differently in the design of the center was reinforced by visiting the Children's Hospital of Boston and the Children's Hospital of Philadelphia, both in the United States. As a consequence, the idea to design a new structure arose, organizing functional spaces and rendering them more permeable, using new materials, and employing color schemes with therapeutic goals. The center was conceived according to the idea of how a house functions. It was divided into three levels. In a house, the entrance, hall, and living and dining rooms are usually situated on the ground floor; in the center, these spaces are the reception hall, a multifunctional area with play activities, and the canteen. The night area (hospital beds and bathrooms) is situated on the second floor to host children and their parents in their own private rooms, and the area reserved for work (the center's evaluation and treatment rooms and the specialists' offices) is situated in the basement. Images, scenes, colors, lights, and three-dimensional trees are all presented as an exterior within an interior in order to insert into the environment natural models such as earth, sky, and water. The space is also marked with roads, squares, parking areas, and corners. As structural characteristics orient educational and rehabilitative purposes, it is helpful for children, parents, and professionals to be in an environment that expresses the broad educational and integrated perspective of the center's model. Creativity, dynamic interaction with the environment, the individual's originality, and relationships among all people involved are some of the center's key features.

THE PROGRAM

The Child, Adult, Aging Development Center Silvana Paolini Angelucci is dedicated to children and adults, incorporating what the international literature calls a *life-span perspective*. The main element of the assessment process is the concept of developmental change over time through a dynamic process. This demands an interdisciplinary, comprehensive, and longitudinal approach designed to locate the individual's needs and strengths in relation to the context and to his or her developmental phase.

In particular, the center focuses on children with developmental delays, mental retardation, learning disabilities, motor impairments, and behavior disorders. In its diagnostic process, attempts are made to identify possible causes, including preconceptional or conceptional factors or prenatal, perinatal, or postnatal events (Crocker & Rubin, 1989; Pueshel, 1986). Environmental factors can also play a role in determining different kinds of neurodevelopmental disabilities. Although identifying a diagnosis and a possible etiology is important, so is the process of obtaining a developmental profile and determining an intervention program.

One of the center's intervention projects addresses early intervention for children with Down syndrome or cerebral palsy (Puccini & Perfetti, 1987). Another specific program is directed toward adolescents and adults with Down syndrome or cerebral palsy. In order to put these programs into effect, center staff use the latest technical instruments housed in the clinic, including computed tomography; magnetic resonance imaging (MRI); and other MRI and radiological, neurophysiological, and echographic supports (Barnes, 1992). Ophthalmological and audiological laboratories as well as a state-of-the-art movement analysis laboratory for the qualitative and quantitative analysis of movements provide information for designing interventions. Specialists who make important contributions to these intervention programs are neurologists with expertise in developmental disabilities, pediatricians, cardiologists, ophthalmologists, otorhinolaryngologists, audiologists, orthopedists, bioengineers, neuropsychiatrists, psychologists, developmental therapists, educators, social workers, and computer scientists. Using all of these components together, a comprehensive assessment and intervention plan is created.

In view of the comprehensiveness and complexity of this program, a service coordinator is critical. This person, usually the center director, is responsible for organizing the assessment phase, the intervention plan, and the intervention itself, as well as encouraging cooperation among the different specialists. Priorities are ascertained and specialists strive to complement one another.

CONCLUSION

Interdisciplinary clinical assessment of individuals with disabilities must be adapted to cultural factors across countries. One such example from Italy is presented in this chapter. Cultural and philosophical issues have guided the establishment of the discussed interdisciplinary model; its process and organization; and even the structural features of the Child, Adult, Aging Development Center Silvana Paolini Angelucci itself.

REFERENCES

Abroms, I.F., & Sheiner, A.P. (1980). *The practical management of the developmentally disabled child.* St. Louis, MO: Mosby.

Barnes, P.D. (1992). Imaging of the central nervous system in pediatrics and adolescence. *Pediatric Clinics of North America, 39*(4),743–776.

Pueshel, M. (1986). A center for the study of children with developmental disabilities. *Journal of Pediatric Neurosciences, 4,* 305–312.

Puccini, P., & Perfetti, C. (1987). *Rehabilitation of children with cerebral palsy.* Rome: Marrapese.

Rubin, L., & Crocker, A.C. (Eds.). (1989). *Developmental disabilities: Delivery of medical care for children and adults.* Philadelphia: Lea & Febiger.

Chapter 20

Assessment Philosophies and Practices in Sweden

Eva Björck-Åkesson, Mats Granlund,
and Rune J. Simeonsson

The growth of early childhood intervention programs and the importance of early intervention is expanding across nations. In Europe there is a growing interest in early childhood intervention as manifested by EURLYAID, an organization that aims at developing common European Union policy and legislation regarding early intervention. In 1993, a manifesto by EURLYAID declared a single vision for member states to provide the best possible aid to children with disabilities in the respective countries, based on the United Nations Convention of the Rights of the Child (De Moor, Van Waesberghe, Hosman, Jaeken, & Miedema, 1993). The manifesto was inspired by the Education of the Handicapped Act Amendments of 1986 (PL 99-457) in the United States and stated that children with disabilities are entitled to multidisciplinary assessment and intervention and to an individualized family service plan (IFSP). According to EURLYAID, early intervention is intended for all children who have developmental disabilities, who are at risk for developmental delay, or who are identified as being at risk on the basis of a diagnosed prenatal condition (De Moor, Van Waesberghe, Hosman, Jaeken, & Miedma, 1993). Intervention encompasses identification, training, and guidance as well as all forms of child-oriented training activities and parent-oriented guidance activities that are implemented to address the developmental condition directly and immediately. The focus for intervention encompasses the child and the family in the larger context.

The Child Assessment Manifesto by EURLYAID (1997) asserted that the purpose of assessment is to incorporate information needs in a broad way: "to identify children at risk; to define and document such a child's health, functional, psychological, and/or social condition; to define and document parent's and family's expectations, needs, concerns, and/or competencies; and to define and document outcomes of intervention" (p. 1). Both the child and the environment are viewed as part of the assessment, and the perspective is both developmental and functional, involving those in the assessment process who are part of the child's immediate environment.

Assessment is characterized as a process with several phases: 1) defining the concerns to be addressed and deciding how to assess them; 2) implementing assessment procedures (testing, observations, interviews); 3) interpreting results; 4) sharing information and using this material to analyze problems or to describe them further; 5) utilizing these descriptions as the basis for setting goals; and 6) following up on the assessment to answer the question "What additional information is needed?" (EURLYAID, 1997). In addition, assessment is part of a greater problem-solving process that starts with the identification of the family's primary concerns. Assessment planning is then based on these priorities. After implementing the assessment procedures and interpreting the results, the known facts may be used to define, prioritize, and explain the concerns to a greater degree.

Differences may exist, however, between theory and practice in early childhood intervention. The general assumptions underlying early childhood intervention are similar across European countries. Each country's culture, traditions, and laws influence the organization of early intervention services and how children and families are treated. Thus, there are differences in the nature of assessment and how it is conducted. In Scandinavia, *habilitation* is used for services provided to children and youth with disabilities and their families (Bille & Olow, 1992; Björck-Åkesson & Granlund, 1997; Jansson, 1996; von Tetzchner & Schiorbeck, 1992). The services are aimed at improving functioning, communication, and quality of life for children with developmental disabilities and their families. This reflects an emerging trend toward a holistic and functional perspective of the child's habilitation as well as an emphasis on the neuropsychological aspects of child development.

This chapter reviews in further detail assessment philosophies and intervention practices in Sweden, where the interdisciplinary approach is increasingly being adopted. To this end, the chapter is organized into four sections. First, a framework for the nature of assessment and the values behind evaluation and intervention are discussed. The function of assessment for clinical professionals, families, and children as well as the roles of professionals and parents are considered. Second, the context of early intervention in Sweden at the end of the 20th century is reviewed. Third, assessment practices and issues in Sweden during this time period are described. The International Classification of Impairments, Disabilities, and Handicaps (ICIDH) by the World Health Organization (WHO, 1980) and the draft of the ICIDH–2 (WHO, 1999) serve as a conceptual foundation for review of assessment tools. In this structure, assessment ranges from a *developmental perspective*, with impairment and disability as the main interests, to a *functional perspective*, which is ecologically oriented and emphasizes a child's daily activities in his or her environment. Finally, implications for the future direction of early childhood intervention in Sweden are proposed.

FRAMEWORK FOR ASSESSMENT IN EARLY INTERVENTION

Guralnick (1997) made a distinction between first- and second-generation research on the effectiveness of early intervention. In first-generation research, the focus was on the child and the methods used to assess and intervene at the level of the child's impairment and disability. In second-generation research, the focus expanded to address important issues in the day-to-day functioning of the child and family, including clinicians, educators, and other interventionists. This has broadened the scope of the discussion about assessment and intervention. Second-generation research frames assessment as an analysis of situations rather than the derivation of developmental diagnoses. As a result, the application of change and systems theory becomes central instead of categorical labeling. The transition to a second-generation assessment approach implies a concentration on the interrelationships between developmental and functional perspectives including the child, the environment, and the transactions between child and environment. Thus, fundamental questions asked when using this approach are "Why and how is assessment conducted?" and "What is the function of assessment in the intervention process?"

Family Intervention and Assessment

Within a systems-theoretical perspective, the primary purpose of intervention is to support children with disabilities in their development and to promote the quality of life for these children and their families. When child development is seen as a transactional process (Sameroff & Fiese, 1990), developmental ou comes are a function of the continuous dynamic interactions of the child with the overall environment, mediated by experiences provided by the family and the child's immediate environment. As a result, the focus for assessment may be the child, the family, the caregiving environment, or the interactions among these components.

The intervention process encompasses elements of initial screening, focused assessment, follow-up assessment, goal setting and designing methods, implementing intervention, and evaluating the effectiveness of intervention (Bailey &

Simeonsson, 1988). In this process, families participate in transactions with professionals. For this reason, the impact of intervention may begin as early as the initial screening, and both expected and unexpected outcomes of intervention will follow from each element added to the process. Sometimes the initial parts of an assessment may be the only intervention needed, such as when evaluation provides information that helps parents better understand their children.

At least seven purposes for assessment can be identified: 1) screening, 2) diagnosis, 3) classification or eligibility determination, 4) projection of goals, 5) intervention planning, 6) program monitoring, and 7) evaluation of outcomes. The first four of these purposes are typically bound to the child whereas the latter three may be of wider scope (e.g., including the environment). With a second-generation research perspective, there are other purposes: mutual learning, finding the nodal points at which intervention is meeting changing needs in everyday life, listing realistic goals for the child or family, and evaluating the results in child and family life. The goals of intervention may differ in relation to the focus of intervention, such as optimal development of the child or decreased family needs. Consequently, assessment may have different foci. Examples of these different foci include the child's development in various domains, the family as a developmental environment, the family as a system in emotional turmoil, the family as a resource for training, and the family members as decision makers. These domains presuppose different roles for the family in the assessment process (Björck-Åkesson, Carlhed, & Granlund, 1998). By definition, addressing family needs and decisions is superimposed on other purposes. With this perspective, assessment methods necessarily differ in terms of the problem addressed and the desired goal. Table 20.1 summarizes the elements of the family-centered assessment approach regarding the objective of intervention, the goal and type of intervention, information aggregation (the assessment itself), and family roles in the assessment process. The next section discusses the family elements themselves in greater detail.

Family as Environment
The child's primary environment is a source of stimulation and support that influences his or her ongoing behavior. The creation of a meaningful and sustainable environment is a central task for most families. When addressing the family as the environment for the child, intervention and assessment can take one of two forms. One is aimed at the construction and maintenance of daily routines that provide developmentally sensitive interactions (*proximal processes*) to promote the development and functioning of the child with a disability. The other focus is integrating specific interventions into the family environment. In this context, the family members act as information providers regarding the child's developmental level and progress.

Family Coping
The birth of a child with a disability is often a source of distress for members of the family (Bailey & Simeonsson, 1988; Lagerheim, 1988). Following the ini-

Table 20.1.   Family focus in intervention and assessment

Focus	Goal/ objective	Intervention	Focus of assessment	Role of family in assessment
The family as environment for the child with a disability	The child with a disability interacts optimally with people within the immediate setting and has a "rich environment"	Supervision and interaction coaching Parents given advice, adapted toys, etc. Integrate specific interventions into the family environment	Child development, interaction patterns, home environment, family adaptations, family resources	Providers of information about the child and the family structure and routines, recipients of services for the child
Family coping	Family has a typical family life cycle and accepts the child (e.g., copes with feelings)	Crisis therapy, respite care, redefinition of behavior of the child with a disability	Interview about family life, survey of family needs and coping strategies	Provide therapeutic support and services
Family as trainers	Optimal child development within specific area	Teach training program, supervise parents	Assess child's specific skills and progress Assess parent's skills and progress in training	Acquire skills and knowledge as students, serve as trainers and facilitators for child
Family needs	Decrease in perceived family needs	Fulfill needs at different levels: child, mother, father, siblings, extended family	Identify and prioritize needs	Recipients of services and guidance, collaborators
Family as decision makers	Family is actively involved in and perceives control over intervention process	Provide opportunities for involvement and control, teach problem-solving strategies	Problems in everyday life, child behavior, social and physical environments	Function as collaborators, decision makers, coordinators

tial turmoil, a grieving process occurs. This process may be extended, and different families and individuals within families usually cope in relatively competent ways. Over time, most families and individual family members develop coping mechanisms that support them when crises are experienced. The need for crisis intervention may therefore decrease as the child advances in age. Some interventions, however, have a crisis focus and are aimed at helping family members through crisis periods. Another aim is to help family members develop strategies for coping with recurring crisis periods. This type of intervention is meant to redefine the behavior of the child with a disability and, thereby, also change the way that family members respond to and interact with the child. A crisis focus implies that the professional is an "expert" and families are simply patients or clients receiving services. In reality, assessment in this context is geared toward parents' perceptions of their children and life situations. It is mainly informal and is based on a professional's interpretations of parents' behavior and verbal reports.

Family as Trainers

Family involvement in the assessment and intervention process has evolved from intervention programs in which parents merely implemented training methods designed by professionals. When family members are assigned training roles, the professional's task is to provide the rationale for training skills to family members, to help them apply the learned skills for working with the child with a disability, and to give feedback to family members. Such programs are in many instances based on a developmental perspective (i.e., the family environment is used for learning skills in a predetermined developmental sequence). Assessment in this context includes a child's specific areas of development and progress and can also involve information about the skills of the parents as trainers.

Family Needs

In the process of adapting to circumstances, families often identify possible solutions to problems they experience. This is seen as *expressing needs*. Needs can be related to the functioning of the whole family or of a specific member, most frequently the child with a disability (Bailey & Simeonsson, 1988; Roll-Pettersson, 1997; Roll-Pettersson, Granlund, & Steénson, 1999). Professionals working in early intervention must recognize and help address higher priority family needs before negotiating solutions to problems of lower priority. For families, concerns related to the child with a disability may not always be first priority; sometimes it may be necessary to solve other problems before attending to concerns related to the child. Professionals as well as families need to be skilled at defining problems in terms of the difference between how something is and how it should be.

Family as Decision Makers

It is important to involve the family members in decisions to the extent that they desire. Professionals should provide services in a fashion that gives family members opportunities to decide on assessment, goals, and methods for intervention. In this process of gaining mutual knowledge about the child, family members may act as collaborators and providers of information as well as decision makers. The family is thus involved in the assessment as an equal partner providing specific information that is valuable for the intervention process.

EARLY INTERVENTION CONTEXT IN SWEDEN

In Sweden, *early childhood intervention* is broadly defined as intervention practices for children with developmental disabilities from birth to 7 years of age (when children start compulsory school). All children in Sweden grow up within a family system; less than 1% of children younger than the age of 16 live in institutions. The social insurance system grants that one parent is entitled to stay home with the child during the child's first year of life with 80% wages and then for 90 more days with a lower payment. Thereafter, most children attend community-based child care services while their parents work part or full time. The support system for early childhood intervention for children with disabilities is organized on three levels: the community level, the county council level, and the national level. The law stresses the community's basic responsibility for all children, and the community provides fundamental services for all children and their families. Services from the community include social welfare and child care. Health care is implemented at well-baby clinics and child welfare centers, which provide preventive services to all children from birth until entering school. Services are provided by pediatricians; nurses; and, on some occasions, child psychologists, speech-language pathologists, and social workers.

The professionals at the child welfare center are responsible for identifying children at risk for developmental disabilities. Special assessment instruments are used by pediatric nurses to screen for developmental risk or disability in all children until the child starts school. Representative assessment measures are the Boel Test at 9 months of age (Stensland-Junker, 1975), a speech-language screening at age 3, and screenings of psychomotor and language development as well as hearing and vision tests at the age of 4. Pediatricians or general health physicians also examine children at specific ages during early childhood. The routines vary among different counties in the country. Parents may contact the child welfare center at any time when they have questions or problems or need advice. When a disability is indicated, further assessment and intervention are provided after referral to medical services or a habilitation center. In addition, services are offered to children with disabilities and their families according to the Support and Service Act (LSS, SFS:1993: 387) and the Health and Medical Services Act of 1982 (HSL, SFS:1982:763). The county council has the main responsibility for child health care and medical care as well as additional advice and support for children with disabilities and their families. At the national level, young children with visual or hearing impairments are attended to by the Institute for Handicap Issues in Schools. Special preschool educators give services to those children and their families in early childhood before they start school.

As mentioned previously, the concept *habilitation,* which is used to provide special services to children with disabilities and their families, partly overlaps the concept *early childhood intervention.* In Sweden, there are differences in the legal right to services depending on the type and degree of disability. Regional habilitation centers are responsible for serving the majority of the children with disabilities and their families; children with only a visual or hearing impairment are excluded. Services include medical treatment, physical therapy, occupational therapy, special education consultation, speech-language therapy, and psychological and social consultation. At these habilitation centers, professionals are organized in multidisciplinary or interdisciplinary teams. Common for all service providers at habilitation centers is that the intervention process starts with an assessment focusing on the diagnosis of a disability. The system for service provision is undergoing change, and services vary in their organization in different parts of Sweden.

Children determined to be at risk for developmental delays because of social and environmental factors are not included in the group initially served at the habilitation centers. These children and their families may receive continued support from the child health care organization and from child psychiatric clinics. When a disability is suspected after initial screening, these organizations refer the child to the habilitation center for further assessment. The remainder of this chapter addresses the assessment and intervention processes conducted at the habilitation centers.

ASSESSMENT PRACTICES AND ISSUES IN SWEDEN

Assessment in Sweden has traditionally been conducted from a developmental perspective. The child's optimal performance in specific domains of development has been emphasized by professionals using profession-specific instruments based on "normal" development in children (Björck-Åkesson, 1992, 1993; Björck-Åkesson, Brodin, & Fälth, 1997; Björck-Åkesson & Granlund, 1997; Högberg, 1996). Norm-referenced assessment instruments have been used that relate the development of the child with a disability to that of a typically developing child. Informal interviews and observations are often part of child assessment. Maximal levels of performance and complexity are often emphasized in assessment regardless of method for assessment. Assessment results usually describe the child's best performance and are based on the concept of *milestones*, which are common markers in a child's development.

Within a functional perspective (Björck-Åkesson et al., 1997; Björck-Åkesson & Granlund, 1997; Calculator, 1990; Granlund, 1993), everyday functioning and the social context of development serve as the focus for assessment. Scales and behavior measures are used in functional assessment with systematic observations often made of the child's interaction with the social environment. Structured interviews with parents aim to identify a child's needs, strengths, and weaknesses and the resources and limitations of the social and physical environment. The uniqueness of each child is emphasized, and individual differences are noted. The outcome of functional assessment is a description of everyday functioning with a focus on context competence and the goal of generalization over contexts. Frequency of behavior and functional problems manifested by the child are assessed in the environment. Biological or medical variables may be added to clarify impairments of body function or structure. Table 20.2 summarizes the developmental and functional approaches to assessment.

The elaboration of a functional perspective in assessment has drawn on the conceptual and taxonomic approach of WHO's ICIDH (1980). The ICIDH is among WHO's classifications of health and was designed to provide international terms for classifying the consequences of disease or injury. In addition to providing standard terminology regarding disability that is suitable

Table 20.2.   Characteristics of developmental and functional perspectives on assessment

Characteristic	Developmental perspective	Functional perspective
Relation to International Classification of Impairments, Disabilities, and Handicaps (ICIDH)	Addresses dimensions of disability/activity	Addresses dimensions of handicap, participation, environment
Focus of assessment	Optimal performance Specific domains Knowledge and skills of the child	Everyday functioning of the child in the family context Proximal processes Social domains Family assessment
Assessment instruments	Norm-referenced Criterion-referenced Interviews about child Observation of child Profession-specific	Functional scales Behavioral measures Interaction scales Structured interview about child and family/environment Observation of child in different contexts/environments Adaptation scales Coping scales Family needs scales
Criteria	Typical development	Individual development Child and family in social context Quality of life
Outcome	Maximal/optimal level Specific domains Complexity Best performance	Context competence Everyday functioning Frequency Most common behavior Adaptations
Goals	Milestones	Acquisition of competencies needed Empowerment

Based on Björck-Åkesson (1992).

for international use, a major contribution of ICIDH is the definition of three separate and distinct dimensions of consequences of disease or injury. Thus, the ICIDH defines *impairments* in terms of atypical structures or functions of the body, *disabilities* in terms of lacking or reduced abilities, and *handicap* in terms of disadvantage in social and societal roles. These distinctions provide a useful means for differentiating the focus and nature of assessment as well as giving direction for potential intervention efforts. For example, in the assessment of a young child with cerebral palsy, atypical limb functioning is defined as an impairment, problems of locomotion as a disability, and reduced physical independence and mobility as a handicap. Interventions can be documented in terms of one or more dimensions that serve as the focus for habilitative efforts.

In light of concerns about conceptual and technical features of the 1980 version of the ICIDH, a revision effort has been underway since 1994 to prepare the ICIDH–2. Among the concerns is a serious lack of coverage of childhood disability in the 1980 ICIDH, which should be addressed in the revision (Simeonsson, Lollar, Hollowell, & Adams, in press). Key features of the revised ICIDH include an expanded conception of *disability*, recognition of the centrality of the person's interaction with his or her environment, and neutral terms for dimensions of human functioning. The ICIDH–2 will thus provide guidelines for documenting disability in relation to three dimensions: body function and structure variations, activity limitations, and participation restrictions. In addition, classification of the environment will give opportunities for documenting each individual's context. The value of the ICIDH and the ICIDH–2 is that they provide a common nomenclature on aspects of disability and can serve as a reference for defining the focus and scope of assessment tools.

In many parts of Sweden, individualized service plans (ISPs) are based on the Quebec revision of ICIDH (Larsson & Nilsson, 1999; Sjögren, 1996), which builds on a functional perspective. In assessment based on this ISP model, a broad analysis of the family's and the child's situation is made to identify situational restrictions in different areas of everyday life. The collaborative problem-solving model (Björck-Åkesson, Granlund, & Olsson, 1996) is another functional approach for intervention that is frequently used. In this model, assessment is emphasized as a means for formulating and explaining concerns the child experiences in everyday life. The difference between the two models is that the ISP model is more formal, with assessment of specific domains, whereas the second model uses collaborative problem solving to address intervention.

Assessment Instruments

A survey was conducted of assessment instruments used by professionals in habilitation centers in 4 of 24 counties in Sweden and at a center for children with hearing impairments and cognitive disabilities (Granlund & Björck-Åkesson, 1999). A major aim of the data collection was to gain insight into assessment approaches in Sweden. The information was collected by students in a master's level course in early childhood intervention and family support. They also were working in habilitation centers as professionals from the following disciplines: special education, psychology, speech-language pathology, occupational therapy, and physical therapy. The students gathered data through interviews and review of documents from all professional categories (except pediatrics) in the five habilitation centers involved to determine how evaluation was conducted in their respective centers. The focus of assessment (as delineated in Table 20.2), the origin of material used, and the process of assessment were analyzed. Survey results revealed that each professional group tended to use tests and instruments specific to its field. In addition, a developmental perspective appeared to be the dominant approach. The survey also revealed a trend toward incorporating assessment instruments having a functional perspective, with professionals working together in an interdisciplinary fashion. When assessment was carried out by a team of professionals, the procedure tended to be informal. Natural observations or video observations were used as well as informal interviews. In addition, interdisciplinary play observations were conducted, in which professionals worked together utilizing play-based assessments.

The survey results also revealed that there are few formal instruments of Swedish origin for early childhood assessment and intervention. Many of the formal assessment instruments used originate from other European countries or the United States and then are translated into Swedish and adapted to Swedish conditions. For instance, Swedish psychologists use a British measure—Griffith's Developmental Scales—to evaluate children from birth to 2 years of age and from 2 to 8 years of age (Nordberg, 1997; Nordberg & Alin-Åkerman, 1983). Another example is the Pediatric Evaluation of Disability Inventory (PEDI), an American assessment tool translated and adapted to Swedish conditions (Nordmark & Orban, 1999). The PEDI is a multidisciplinary assessment instrument used by physical therapists, occupational therapists, speech-language pathologists, and other professionals on the habilitation team. It measures development and function in the areas of independence, movement, and social ability for children ages 6 months to 7 years and 6 months old. Motor-Perceptual Development (Holle, Bönnelycke, Kemp, & Mortensen, 1990) is a standardized observational schedule for assessing the motor-perceptual development of children from birth to 7 years of age and is used mainly by special educators. This particular measure is Danish in origin and has been translated into Swedish.

Manuals and material for tests of intelligence are often in English with test protocols in Swedish. These tools are administered by certified psychologists. The revised and expanded version (2 to 21 years old) of the Leiter International Performance Scale–Revised (Leiter-R; Roid & Miller, 1997) is available in an American edition, but a Swedish version is forthcoming. The revised Wechsler Preschool and Primary Scale of Intelligence (Wechsler, 1989), for children 3 to 7 years old, has been standardized on a Swedish sample with a Swedish manual and test protocols. The Snijders-Oomen Nonverbal Intelligence Scale (Snijders & Snijders-Oomen, 1994) is used for assessment of nonverbal intelligence in children (2 to 7 years old) with language impairments, such as those with hearing impairments. For assessing language development in children from 1 year and 3 months to 7 years of age, speech-language pathologists use an original English revision of the Reynell Developmental Language Scales–III (Reynell, 1974). The Illinois Test of Psycholinguistic Abilities (ITPA) was standardized on a Swedish sample (Holmgren, 1984) and is used by psychologists and speech-language pathologists to assess psycholinguistic ability in children from 4 years and 6 months to 9 years and 11 months of age.

For motor development and function, physical therapists use a Swedish translation of the Movement ABC (Henderson & Sugden, 1996) and the original American version of the Bruininks-Oseretsky Test of Motor Proficiency (Bruininks, 1978). A number of new tests for neuropsychological assessment were introduced in Sweden during the late 1990s. The Neuropsychological Investigation for Children (NEPSY; Korkman, Kirk, & Kemp, 1998) is based on the Soviet psychologist Luria's work on the neuropsychological assessment of adults. A version for 3- to 12-year-olds is under development, based on an earlier standardization for 4- to 7-year-old children (Korkman, 1990).

Family needs are most often assessed with informal interviews. There is a significant need for new instruments that may be used by different professionals in this area. Examples of instruments used are a Swedish version of The Family Needs Survey (Bailey & Simeonsson, 1988) and a translation of the theory of ecocultural assessment (Bernheimer, Gallimore, & Weisner, 1990; Gallimore, Weisner, Bernheimer, Guthrie, & Nihira, 1993; Granlund, Sandell-Andersson, & Björck-Åkesson, 1998), which was introduced in Sweden and in the Swedish-speaking part of Finland during the late 1990s.

Role of Professionals in Assessment

The previously discussed survey of assessment practices in Sweden (Granlund & Björck-Åkesson, 1999) also revealed that most assessment activities were discipline specific and performed by individual professionals. An explanation for this may be the tendency to emphasize the child's impairment or disability in assessment. Most instruments used for this purpose are standardized and norm-referenced. As they are typically not theory based, they do not lend themselves to a collaborative approach for interdisciplinary assessment. The impact of habilitation services on family accommodations was examined in a pilot study of the habilitation records for 15 children with disabilities (Granlund et al., 1998). The results revealed that most intervention goals were discipline-specific and that family information, services, and intervention were fragmented. The approach was more interdisciplinary when the intervention team had established routines for the IFSP process, and goals were defined in terms of minimizing the consequences of the child's disabilities.

Developmental Issues

Bjerre's 1998 survey of habilitation in Sweden described aspects of assessment and diagnostics in early childhood intervention. The following methods for evaluation were highlighted: arena, play-based, and family assessments; assessments of child–parent interaction, social support, and environment; and the *portfolio method* (i.e., using a sampling of the child's work or products over time). Nevertheless, in practice it appears that these methods are not the ones most frequently used. All of these techniques are based on a functional approach to assessment, but in everyday practice, traditional assessment methods based on a developmental or disability perspective still seemed to be employed.

The developmental perspective to assessment holds that the family is a "rich" environment for the child with a disability, and specific interventions are designed for that environment. Family members are not involved in assessment and tend to take roles as recipients of assessment information. The developmental approach in Sweden's habilitation process is shifting, however, toward a family and social context-oriented approach (Bjerre, 1998; Björck-Åkesson & Granlund, 1997; Högberg, 1996; Jansson, 1996). Assumptions about recommended practices are changing in relation to increased parent involvement and functional intervention. A team is often created around each child, offering support and services in the family context. The team may involve professionals both from local and regional service providers and the parents. An example of this is the ISP team in which professionals and parents work together setting goals for the child and implementing child-centered intervention. The concepts of participation and empowerment are emphasized when a family's role in the child's habilitation is stressed. Although quality in habilitation is difficult to characterize, Swedish literature has highlighted the following factors for definition: 1) equal rights to services for all children and families, 2) continuous quality assurance in relation to general standards, 3) an interdisciplinary character of services, 4) family involvement in the intervention process, 5) continuous and long-lasting contacts, 6) decreasing the handicap in the child's immediate environment and daily activities, and 7) implementation of ISPs (Bjerre, 1998; Bjerre, Ferngren, Lagerkvist, & Witt Engerström, 1999).

An important part of the assessment process in this perspective is how decisions are made about what to assess, how assessment should be conducted, and who should be involved in the assessment. It seems that evaluations of environmental components and family needs are commonly informal and sometimes made without explicit parental consent. The option of a broader formal assessment, in which environmental components are involved, is a fairly new approach in Sweden. The desire to conduct such evaluations constitutes wishful thinking, as instruments for such assessment are particularly uncommon in non–English-speaking countries.

Family Involvement Issues

Every phase in the assessment process must have a clear beginning and end, a process that can be represented by an intervention cycle (Simeonsson et al.,

1996). In formal assessment, the beginning and end of the information collection stage are clearly marked. This allows families to have a more active learning experience; it also helps them to compare the actual assessment with expectations and, thus, to ask questions throughout the data collection phase. As a result, it becomes easier for the parents to discuss and question the conclusions reached from assessment. For example, when a sample of Swedish parents were asked if they had gained knowledge about their children through collaborating with professionals, they were more positive if professionals worked in a traditional manner with formal test instruments (Granlund, Steénson, & Björck-Åkesson, 1999). In informal assessment, it is difficult for parents and other members in the child's immediate environment to determine if assessment is actually completed. Therefore, it becomes harder for parents to ask questions about the evaluation or to draw conclusions about its results. This phenomenon is especially pronounced in assessment on family issues that are almost exclusively informal.

If and when parents participate in the assessment process, the probability that they can learn about their children and themselves increases. It also improves their chances of judging the appropriateness of the assessment instruments used. Nonetheless, the form and content of these tools set the limits for the manner in which parents and others involved in the child's care can participate in collecting and interpreting assessment information. The way in which the concern is defined does affect the collaboration between parents and professionals in the intervention cycle. If it is identified in terms of impairment, standardized or criterion-referenced tests are used and the evaluation takes the form of experts measuring a child's responses to preset test items under set conditions. In many instances, parents tend to be passive recipients of information collected by professionals. A consequence of this situation is that professionals also select the goals and methods of intervention.

The tendency to identify the impairment or disability as the focus for intervention decreases with the age of the child. Many interventions for infants are based on assessment with a developmental foundation and have a prospective rationale. That is, professionals give advice based on what is considered the recommended practice associated with a diagnosis (e.g., Down syndrome) rather than the specific problems of an infant's interaction with the environment. As children grow older, their exposure to settings outside of the home increases the number of situations in which they experience handicapping consequences of their disabilities. Parents are the experts in identifying these circumstances. Therefore, when their children are older, parents are more active in the first phase of the intervention cycle (problem identification). Parents also tend to be more involved in the intervention cycle when ISPs based on the ICIDH model are used (concentrating on the consequences of the disabilities that place the individual at a disadvantage) as opposed to when intervention is implemented in a traditional manner (Larsson & Nilsson, 1999).

IMPLICATIONS AND CONCLUSION

The framework of first-generation and second-generation perspectives in early childhood intervention can be applied to services for children with disabilities in Sweden. There has been a shift from a developmental model, emphasizing impairment and disability, toward a functional model, stressing family participation and the child's functioning within his or her daily social context. This shift has challenged the traditional approach to assessment and intervention that emphasized diagnosing and treating the child's impairment and disability. With the 21st century approaching, there is a need for new assessment instruments in Sweden to complement existing measures. The newer methods include evaluating family and community needs and resources and the child's interaction with his or her immediate environment. This approach requires that the family and other caregivers collaborate and thus demands that professionals be competent in problem solving. Three dimensions can be identified as essential to this emerging approach in early childhood intervention: an interdisciplinary approach, parent–professional collaboration, and the outcome evaluations of both.

Interdisciplinary Approach

This change redefines the roles of professionals and families in the assessment and intervention process. Interdisciplinary collaboration among professionals and between professionals and parents is necessary to ensure that children and families receive individualized support adapted to their special needs. It requires analysis of problems in environmental contexts of everyday life by those involved and the application of transactional theory and systems theory. This change in paradigm from a disability-oriented to a systems-oriented perspective may cause conflicts among professionals about recommended practices and the scope of the professional role. Not everyone agrees with a social-oriented, family view. Greater acceptance and implementation of an interdisciplinary approach require more discipline-specific training in occupational therapy, pediatric medicine, physical therapy, and special education. In addition, knowledge about children with disabilities and their families, communication and collaborative problem solving, working in teams and with consultation, and intervention processes as a whole are needed.

Professionals approach new demands in different ways. One technique is to incorporate a family-oriented perspective, broadening the field of professionalism. Another is to concentrate on a particular professional field, for example, by highlighting specific training methods or new tools for diagnostics. This is evident when looking at perceived needs of in-service training (Brithon & Karlsson, 1998). There is, for instance, a growing interest in neuropsychological assessment in Scandinavia. A number of instruments for neuropsychological assessment have been developed or translated mainly from English during the 1990s. A future perspective is that both aspects—developing good practices for working with the child in the family context and for improving methods to obtain valid and reliable information about the child's specific impairment or disability—are important. Instead of treating discrepancies among different assessment outcomes as failures, multiple sources and measures can be used to strengthen the validity of the evaluation. From various tools and their accompanying results, hypotheses about the child's development can be derived that may be transformed into intervention strategies. Ideally, the assessment outcome should be a synthesis based on collaborative work and various types of information. Assessment of children with disabilities may be depicted as a puzzle, with different pieces revealing themselves continuously. Therefore, assessment must be an ongoing process that considers the child in the context of the primary caregiving environment.

The emerging approach to assessment and intervention in Sweden is consistent with Guralnick's (1997) view of second-generation research. Stenhammar and Ulfhielm (1998) reported that parents judge habilitation to be of good quality when support is given in such a way that parents participate in decisions. This means that parents should influence the process of assessment and intervention, gain information and knowledge, and perceive a clear relationship between the concern expressed and the intervention. The involvement of the family in the intervention process may, however, take different forms. Studies of family involvement (Björck-Åkesson & Granlund, 1995; Carlhed, 1998; Stenhammar & Ulfhielm, 1998) show that parents want to be more involved in decisions about assessment in general, evaluation procedures, and intervention. Professionals have also expressed the fact that they want more family involvement in assessment and intervention (Björck-Åkesson & Granlund, 1995; Carlhed, 1998). Limitations in the system for service provision may account for the fact that families are not as involved to the degree they desire and also for the ways professionals and parents relate to each other. Family-centered services are mainly discussed in relation to the service provision process in Sweden. The outcomes of these services at the family level have not been discussed to the same extent. These and related issues have implications, such as outcome evaluation and the nature of collaboration between parents and professionals, that can be identified for the continued development of assessment practices in Sweden.

Parent–Professional Collaboration

Collaboration between parents and professionals in the assessment and intervention process has been discussed extensively in Sweden (Bjerre, 1998; Björck-Åkesson, 1992, 1993; Björck-Åkesson & Granlund, 1995; Carlhed, 1998; Högberg, 1996; Larsson & Nilsson, 1999; Stenhammar & Ulfhielm, 1998). Tentatively, three dimensions of family involvement can be identified: activity, information exchange and knowledge gain, and relations/security (Björck-Åkesson et al., 1998). More attention, however, needs to be given to defining the roles and forms of the family and professionals in the collaborative process.

Table 20.3.   A model for collaborative problem solving

Problem description in terms of the child
"Adam does not attend to his mother."

Problem explanation in terms of the child and the social and physical environment
"Adam has a hearing impairment in his left ear." (impairment)
"Adam does not hear well enough." (disability)
"Adam's mother does not have good strategies to get and maintain Adam's attention."
(handicap)
"The room is too noisy." (handicap)
"Other children are noisy." (handicap)
"Adam is too far from his mother." (handicap)

Goals in terms of the child
"Adam attends to his mother."

Methods in terms of the child and the social and physical environment
"Adam receives a hearing aid." (impairment)
"Adam receives training in positioning so that he can use his hearing aid." (disability)
"Adam's mother learns effective strategies to get and maintain Adam's attention."
(handicap)
"Changes are made in the room to make it less noisy."
(handicap)
"The other children learn to be less noisy." (handicap)
"Adam is close to the teacher." (handicap)

Implementation of intervention
A detailed description is given of how, when, and by whom the chosen methods are
carried out within a time frame.

Outcome evaluation
Goal attainment, in terms of what the child does when the goal is reached, is scaled.

A model for collaborative problem solving based on systems theory (Björck-Åkesson et al., 1996) has been implemented in a number of habilitation centers. In this model, the roles of parents and professionals are highlighted. Assessment is regarded as a learning process for both parents and professionals. Basic to the model is the idea that problems are expressed as they are seen in everyday life and that multiple explanations for the concerns are addressed in the assessment. These explanations are sought at different levels corresponding to the ICIDH model in terms of the child, the social and physical environment, and the interaction between the child and the environment. This means that a number of assessment instruments, both formal and informal, are needed to obtain a clear picture of the child's and family's needs for support. The core of the model is that the different levels yield methods of intervention that are chosen collaboratively by the family and professionals. After implementing the intervention, outcomes can be evaluated with the goal-attainment procedure. The basic components of the model are presented in Table 20.3.

In this model of collaboration, parents and professionals have different roles (see Table 20.4). The parents are experts on problem formulation because they can best describe the structures, routines, and activities of their

Table 20.4.   Roles of parents and professionals in collaborative problem solving regarding assessment and intervention

Parents	Professionals
Experts on problem formulation	Experts on guiding parents to express problems
Experts on their everyday life and explanations to problems that may be connected to life history, roles, structures, routines, and activities	Experts on explanations of problems related to diagnoses, test results, developmental stages, and functions
Experts on their lifestyle and needs (i.e., prioritizing needs)	Experts on helping parents express and prioritize needs to make informed decisions
Experts on expressing goals	Experts on guiding parents to express goals
Experts on how to integrate methods into everyday life	Experts on designing methods and on integrating specific methods into everyday life
Experts on deciding goal attainment in everyday life terms	Experts on determining goal attainment in discipline-specific areas

everyday lives with their children. The professionals are experts in helping parents to express concerns. Regarding explanations, the parents are most qualified to provide those that are related to the behavior of the child and their own lives. Professionals are experts in guiding the parents to express valid explanations regarding diagnoses and information related to the child's impairment or disability. The parents are most capable of prioritizing problems, but they may need assistance from professionals in this process. The parents are also experts on the goals for their child and, of course, the goals are closely related to the prioritization of concerns. The professionals are experts on assessment, from which they can derive explanations for parents. These explanations, in turn, may serve as the basis for designing interventions. Nevertheless, the parents can best determine how to integrate methods into their everyday life. Finally, parents and professionals need to evaluate outcomes of intervention together. The use of goal-attainment scaling has been shown to be an effective technique for evaluating outcomes and enhancing the connection between problems and goals.

The preceding model details a collaborative problem-solving process that has clear roles for parents and professionals. It also emphasizes assessment in the intervention process. With this approach, a dual perspective may be reached, incorporating both developmental and functional approaches. Assessment is based on an analysis of problem situations by those involved in the intervention process and draws on each participant's special expertise. It is regarded as a mutual learning process that has gaining knowledge as the unifying dimension. The potential of problem explanation is used so that the competence of both families and clinicians is equally regarded. Assessment becomes a process in which families and professionals learn from each other about the child and the social context in which the child lives. This process in turn reflects a mutual undertaking based on solving problems experienced in everyday life, a desirable goal for early intervention with children and families in Sweden and elsewhere.

REFERENCES

Bailey, D.B., & Simeonsson, R.J. (1988). *Family assessment in early intervention*. New York: Merrill.

Bernheimer, L., Gallimore, R., & Weisner, T. (1990). Ecocultural theory as a context for the individual family service plan. *Journal of Early Intervention, 14*, 219–233.

Bille, B., & Olow, I. (Eds.). (1992). *Habilitation of children with physical disabilities*. Stockholm: Almqvist & Wiksell.

Bjerre, I. (1998). Good quality in child- and youth-habilitation. In *Evaluation of habilitation and rehabilitation* (Swedish National Board of Health and Welfare Report No. 1998-19-8). Stockholm: Socialstyrelsen.

Bjerre, I., Ferngren, H., Lagerkvist, B., & Witt Engerström, I. (1999). New possibilities to measure the quality of habilitation. *Läkartidningen, 96(15)*, 1833–1836.

Björck-Åkesson, E. (1992). Communicative interaction between non-speaking young children with physical disability and parents—a longitudinal study. *Göteborg Studies in Educational Sciences, 90*. Göteborg, Sweden: Acta Universitatis Gothoburgensis.

Björck-Åkesson, E. (1993). *Communicative interaction between young nonspeaking children with physical disabilities and their parents* (Handicap Research Group Report No. 13). Jönköping, Sweden: Högskolan i Jönköping.

Björck-Åkesson, E., Brodin, J., & Fälth, I.-B. (1997). *Intervention-Interaction-Communication: A model for family-oriented early intervention*. Rockneby, Sweden: WRP Förlag.

Björck-Åkesson, E., Carlhed, C., & Granlund, M. (1998, October). The impact of early intervention on the family system. In *Equal opportunities and quality of life for families with a young disabled child*. Presented at the fourth European symposium of EURLYAID, Butgenbach, Belgium.

Björck-Åkesson, E., & Granlund, M. (1995). Family involvement in assessment and intervention: Perceptions of professionals and parents in Sweden. *Exceptional Children, 61*, 520–535.

Björck-Åkesson, E., & Granlund, M. (1997). Changing perspectives in early intervention for children with disabilities in Sweden. *Infants and Young Children, 9*, 56–68.

Björck-Åkesson, E., Granlund, M., & Olsson, C. (1996). Collaborative problem solving in communication intervention. In S. von Tetzchner & M.H. Jensen (Eds.), *Augmentative and alternative communication: European perspectives* (pp. 324–341). London: Whurr Publishers.

Brithon, M., & Karlsson, M. (1998). *Attitudes to and expectations on in-service training: Interviews and inquiries to professionals in habilitation*. Västerås, Sweden: Mälardalen University.

Bruininks, R.H. (1978). *Bruininks-Oseretsky Test of Motor Proficiency*. Stockholm: Psykologiförlaget.

Calculator, S. (1990). Evaluating the efficacy of AAC intervention for children with severe disabilities. In J. Brodin & E. Björck-Åkesson (Eds.), *Methodological issues in research in augmentative and alternative communication: Proceedings from the first ISAAC Research Symposium in Augmentative and Alternative Communication* (pp. 22–35). Stockholm: ISAAC and Handikappinstitutet.

Carlhed, C. (1998). *Everyone wants good habilitation services.* . . . (From the Opuscula report series No. 37). Västerås, Sweden: Mälardalen University.

De Moor, J.M.H., Van Waesberghe, B.T.M., Hosman, J.B.L., Jaeken, D., & Miedema, S. (1993). Early intervention for children with developmental disabilities: Manifesto of the EURLYAID working party. *International Journal of Rehabilitation Research, 16,* 23–31.

Education of the Handicapped Act Amendments of 1986, PL 99-457, 20 U.S.C. §§ 1400 *et seq.*

EURLYAID Working Party. (1997). Child assessment manifesto. *Early intervention for children with developmental disabilities.* St. Vith, Belgium: Alefpa/Europe.

Gallimore, R., Weisner, T., Bernheimer, L., Guthrie, D., & Nihira, K. (1993). Family responses to young children with developmental delays: Accommodation activity in ecological and cultural context. *American Journal on Mental Retardation, 98,* 185–206.

Granlund, M. (1993). Communicative competence in persons with profound mental retardation. *Acta Universitatis Upsaliensis, Studia Psychologica Clinica Upsaliensia, 3.* Stockholm: Almqvist & Wiksell International.

Granlund, M., & Björck-Åkesson, E. (1999). *Survey of assessment instruments used at five habilitation centers.* Unpublished report. Västerås, Sweden: Mälardalen University.

Granlund, M., Sandell-Andersson, C., & Björck-Åkesson, E. (1998). *Eco cultural interviews—A pilot study.* Unpublished report. Västerås, Mälardalen University, Sweden.

Granlund, M., & Steénson, A.-L. (1999). *Classroom teachers and consultants working together.* In M. Granlund (Ed.), *Students with multiple disabilities in the special school: Effects and efficacy of education* (pp. 181–214). Stockholm: Stiftelsen ALA.

Granlund, M., Steénson, A.-L., & Björck-Åkesson, E. (1999). Management through inservice training. In M. Granlund (Ed.), *Students with multiple disabilities in the special school: Effects and efficacy of education* (pp. 383–472). Stockholm: Stiftelsen ALA.

Guralnick, M.J. (1997). Second-generation research in the field of early intervention. In M.J. Guralnick (Ed.), *The effectiveness of early intervention* (pp. 3–20). Baltimore: Paul H. Brookes Publishing Co.

Health and Medical Services Act of 1982 (HSL, SFS: 1982:763). Sweden.

Henderson, S.E., & Sugden, D.A. (1996). *Movement ABC. Manual.* Stockholm: Psykologiförlaget.

Högberg, B. (1996). *The handicapped child in the adult world.* Stockholm: Pedagogiska Institutionen, Stockholms Universitet.

Holle, B., Bönnelycke, K., Kemp, E., & Mortensen, L.T. (1990). *Motor-Perceptual Development.* Stockholm: Psykologiförlaget.

Holmgren, B. (1987). *Illinois Test of Psycholinguistic Abilities (ITPA).* Stockholm: Psykologiförlaget.

Jansson, U. (1996). Early intervention in Sweden. In M. Brambring, H. Rauh, & A. Beelmann (Eds.), *Early childhood intervention: Theory, evaluation, and practice* (pp. 72–91). Berlin, Germany: Walter de Gruyter.

Korkman, M. (1990). *NEPSY Manual.* Stockholm: Psykologiförlaget.

Korkman, M., Kirk, U., & Kemp, S. (1998). *NEPSY: A Developmental Neuropsychological Assessment.* San Antonio, TX: The Psychological Corp.

Lagerheim, B. (1988). *To develop with a handicap.* Stockholm: Nordstedts.

Larsson, M., & Nilsson, M. (1999). Individualized service programs: A working method for family centered habilitation. *Socialmedicinsk Tidskrift, 1,* 13–20.

Nordberg, L. (1997). *Griffith data.* Stockholm: Psykologiförlaget.

Nordberg, L., & Alin-Åkerman, B. (1983). *Standardization of Griffith's Developmental Scales for the ages two to eight years.* Stockholm: Psykologiförlaget.

Nordmark, E., & Orban, K. (1999). *Pediatric Evaluation of Disability Inventory (PEDI)– Swedish version.* Stockholm: Psykologiförlaget.

Reynell, J. (1974). *Reynell Developmental Language Scales–III (Manual).* Windsor, England: NFER Publishing Company.

Roid, G.H., & Miller, L.J. (1997). *Leiter International Performance Scale–Revised (Leiter-R).* Wood Dale, IL: Stoelting Co.

Roll-Pettersson, L. (1997). *Parents of children with disabilities tell about their emotional experiences.* Stockholm: Stiftelsen ALA.

Roll-Pettersson, L., Granlund, M., & Steénson, A.-L. (1999). Perceptions of needs for advice and support in families and teachers of children in the special school. In M. Granlund (Ed.), *Students with multiple disabilities in the special school: Effects and efficacy of education* (pp. 105–180). Stockholm: Stiftelsen ALA.

Sameroff, A.J., & Fiese, B.H. (1990). Transactional regulation and early intervention. In S.J. Meisels & J.P. Shonkoff (Eds.), *Handbook of early childhood intervention* (pp. 119–149). Cambridge, United Kingdom: Cambridge University Press.

Simeonsson, R., Huntington, G., McMillen, J.S., Haugh-Dodds, A., Halperin, D., Zipper, I.N., & Leskinen, M.M. (1996). Services for young children and their families: Evaluating the intervention cycle. *Infants and Young Children, 9,* 31–42.

Simeonsson, R.J., Lollar, D., Hollowell, J., & Adams, M. (in press). Revision of the International Classification of Impairments, Disabilities, and Handicaps: Developmental issues. *Journal of Clinical Epidemiology.*

Sjögren, O. (1996). *Individualized Service Plans.* Unpublished report, Nacka, Sweden.

Snijders, J. Th., & Snijders Oomen, N. (1994). *Snijders-Oomen Nonverbal Intelligence Scale.* Stockholm: Psykologiförlaget.

Stenhammar, A.-M., & Ulfhielm, K. (1998). How can we get what we want? In *Evaluation of habilitation and rehabilitation* (Swedish National Board of Health and Welfare Report No. 1998-2). Stockholm: Socialstyrelsen.

Stensland-Junker, K. (1975). *The young human being.* Stockholm: Naturoch Kultur.

Support and Service Act (LSS, SFS:1993:387). Sweden.

von Tetzchner, S., & Schiorbeck, H. (1992). *Habilitation: Interdisciplinary work with persons with congenital or early acquired disabilities.* Oslo, Norway: Ad Notam Gyldendal.

Wechsler, D. (1989). *Wechsler Preschool and Primary Scale of Intelligence–Revised.* San Antonio: The Psychological Corp.

World Health Organization (WHO). (1980). *International Classification of Impairments, Disabilities, and Handicaps (ICIDH).* Geneva, Switzerland: Author.

World Health Organization (WHO). (1999). *ICIDH–2 Beta 2 Draft Introduction.* Geneva, Switzerland: Author.

APPENDIX

Questionnaires for Parents

Parent Questionnaire
Feeding Clinic Parent Questionnaire
Child and Family Services Parent Questionnaire

Questionnaires for Professionals

Developmental Center/Preschool Questionnaire
Communicative Behavior Questionnaire
Social Work Family Assessment
Motor Development Questionnaire
Education Questionnaire
Occupational and Physical Therapy Services Survey

PKU Clinic

Checklist for Families New to the PKU Clinic
Management Guidelines for PKU

PARENT QUESTIONNAIRE

Date completed _____

Dear Parent or Guardian:

The following questionnaire is intended to provide information about your child and family so that we can better understand your concerns and needs. Your answers will be regarded as confidential information and will be used by the team evaluating your child at this center. This information will be shared with others only if you have given us written consent. If you need more space to answer the questions completely, please feel free to attach extra sheets of paper. If you have any questions regarding answering questionnaire items, please contact the program coordinator. Thank you.

Child Development Program Staff

Identification

Child's name _____ Birth date _____
Address _____ City/State _____ Zip _____
Parents _____
Person completing form _____ Telephone number _____
Relationship to child _____
Who referred you to us? _____
Has this child ever been evaluated at this clinic before? _____
Describe any specific events that led to this application: _____
_____

Community Resources Currently Used

Child's physician _____ Telephone number _____
Address _____
List other community services (e.g., specialty physicians, counselors, therapists, caseworkers, public health nurses, support groups):

Name	Agency	Telephone number

Developed at the Center on Human Development and Disability, University of Washington, Seattle
Interdisciplinary Clinical Assessment of Young Children with Developmental Disabilities
© 2000 by Paul H. Brookes Publishing Co., Baltimore

Educational Information

Name of child's current school _____ District _____
Address _____ Telephone number _____
Teacher _____ Program type (e.g., developmental preschool) _____

Describe any difficulties your child currently is experiencing in his/ her school or child care program: _____

_____

_____

List services your child is receiving through the school district or an early intervention program:

Service	Therapist's name	Telephone number
Physical therapy		
Occupational therapy		
Speech-language therapy		
Other		

Have you discussed your concerns about your child with anybody in the school? If so, with whom? _____

_____

_____

List previous school programs attended by this child:

Name and address	Program type	Grade	Date

List the names of people from the community or your child's educational program who should be invited to case or parent conferences:

_____

_____

_____

Developed at the Center on Human Development and Disability, University of Washington, Seattle
Interdisciplinary Clinical Assessment of Young Children with Developmental Disabilities
© 2000 by Paul H. Brookes Publishing Co., Baltimore

Areas of Concern

	Check if applicable	Comments
Physical health	☐	
Hearing	☐	
Vision	☐	
Weight (overweight or underweight)	☐	
Diet and/or feeding	☐	
Sleeping	☐	
Elimination	☐	
Coordination and/or motor skills	☐	
Development of self-help skills	☐	
Speech-language	☐	
School achievement or learning	☐	
Behavior	☐	
Discipline	☐	
Emotional adjustment	☐	
Other	☐	

Family

A. Complete as much of the following information as possible regarding the child's *biological family.*

Birth Mother

Name _____ Birth date _____
Occupation _____ Gross monthly income _____
Current position _____ Work telephone number _____
Last grade completed in school _____ Marital status _____
How long have you lived with current partner? _____
Are there any physical, learning, or emotional concerns of which we should be aware? _____
_____

Birth Father

Name _____ Birth date _____
Occupation _____ Gross monthly income _____
Current position _____ Work telephone number _____

Developed at the Center on Human Development and Disability, University of Washington, Seattle
Interdisciplinary Clinical Assessment of Young Children with Developmental Disabilities
© 2000 by Paul H. Brookes Publishing Co., Baltimore

Last grade completed in school _____ Marital status _____
How long have you lived with current partner? _____
Are there any physical, learning, or emotional concerns of which we should be aware? _____

List all the child's biological siblings (full and half):

Name	Birth date	Relationship	Place of residence

Are there any concerns with the child's siblings of which we should be aware? _____
_____
_____
_____

B.   If the child is living with *anyone other than his or her biological family*, provide the following information for the individual(s) who are primary caregivers.

Person #1

How are you related to this child? (Circle) adoptive parent, foster parent, stepparent, other (explain) _____
How long has the child lived with you? _____
Name _____ Birth date _____
Occupation _____ Gross monthly income _____
Last grade completed in school _____ Marital status _____
Telephone number _____
Are there any physical, learning, or emotional concerns of which we should be aware? _____
_____

Person #2

How are you related to this child? (Circle) adoptive parent, foster parent, stepparent, other (explain) _____
How long has the child lived with you? _____
Name _____ Birth date _____
Occupation _____ Gross monthly income _____

Developed at the Center on Human Development and Disability, University of Washington, Seattle
Interdisciplinary Clinical Assessment of Young Children with Developmental Disabilities
© 2000 by Paul H. Brookes Publishing Co., Baltimore

Last grade completed in school _____ Marital status _____
Telephone number _____
Are there any physical, learning, or emotional concerns of which
we should be aware? _____

_____

To be completed whether child lives with his or her biological parent(s)
or not—list all other people living in the household with the child:

Name	Birth date	Relationship to this child

Medical History

Information regarding pregnancy, labor, delivery, and family history
should be provided only as it relates to the child's biological parents.

How much weight did mother gain during this pregnancy? _____

What kind of medication or shots did the mother receive during
pregnancy?

Medication	Month of pregnancy taken

Did the mother experience any of the following conditions during
the pregnancy?

Condition	Check if applicable	Month of pregnancy
Fever		
"Flu"		
Skin rash		
Spotting or bleeding		
Toxemia of pregnancy (swelling of hands and feet, high blood pressure, dizzy spells, headaches)		

Developed at the Center on Human Development and Disability, University of Washington, Seattle
Interdisciplinary Clinical Assessment of Young Children with Developmental Disabilities
© 2000 by Paul H. Brookes Publishing Co., Baltimore

Was the unborn child exposed to any of the following during the pregnancy?

Item	Check if applicable	Month of pregnancy
X-ray procedures		
Tobacco smoke		
Alcohol		
Drugs (specify below)		

Specific drugs: _____

Was there anything unusual about the child's delivery? _____

Explain: _____

_____

_____

_____

Birth Measurements: Weight _____ Length _____

Head circumference _____

Did the baby cry immediately? Yes ___ No ___ Don't know ___

Any difficulties with the baby immediately after birth? _____

If yes, describe: _____

_____

_____

_____

Apgar scores _____ Child's place of birth _____

If born in a hospital, list name and address: _____

Physician in attendance _____ How many

days did the baby stay in the hospital? _____

Any difficulties during the baby's first month at home? _____

If yes, describe: _____

_____

_____

Has the child had any other medical problems that might be related to your present concerns about him/her? _____

Describe: _____

_____

_____

_____

Developed at the Center on Human Development and Disability, University of Washington, Seattle
Interdisciplinary Clinical Assessment of Young Children with Developmental Disabilities
© 2000 by Paul H. Brookes Publishing Co., Baltimore

List all pregnancies of the biological mother (including miscarriages) in order of occurrence:

Year	Length of pregnancy (weeks)	Birth weight (pounds/ ounces)	Check if difficulties		Status of children	
			during pregnancy	at birth	Is the child living, healthy, and developing typically?	If not, explain

Check any conditions present in the child's biological family:

Condition	Mother	Mother's family	Father	Father's family
Birth defects				
Mental retardation				
Learning disabilities				
Mental or emotional disorder				
Allergies				
Epilepsy				
Vision or hearing disorder				
Diabetes				
Inherited/genetic disorder				
Other health problems				

How would you describe your child's current health status? _____

_____

_____

_____

Developed at the Center on Human Development and Disability, University of Washington, Seattle
Interdisciplinary Clinical Assessment of Young Children with Developmental Disabilities
© 2000 by Paul H. Brookes Publishing Co., Baltimore

Describe current treatment of listed condition(s): _____

_____

_____

Which physicians/health care providers are primarily responsible
for treatment of the above conditions? _____

_____

_____

Developmental History
At approximately what age did your child do the following:

	Age (in months)
Smile	
Sit alone	
Walk alone	
Say first two to three clear words	
Put two or three words together to make a sentence	
Become toilet trained for daytime hours	
Stay dry at night	

List specific concerns you have about your child's development
and when they started: _____

_____

_____

What do you hope to get from this evaluation? _____

_____

_____

_____

_____

_____

_____

_____

_____

Thank you for your time and information.

Developed at the Center on Human Development and Disability, University of Washington, Seattle
Interdisciplinary Clinical Assessment of Young Children with Developmental Disabilities
© 2000 by Paul H. Brookes Publishing Co., Baltimore

FEEDING CLINIC PARENT QUESTIONNAIRE

Date completed _____

Dear Parent or Guardian:

The following questionnaire is intended to provide information about your child so that we can better understand your concerns and needs. Your answers will be regarded as confidential information and will be used by the team evaluating your child at this center. This information will be shared with others only if you have given us written consent. If you need more space to answer the questions completely, please feel free to attach extra sheets of paper. If you have any questions regarding answering items on the questionnaire, please contact the program coordinator. Thank you.

Identification

Child's name _____ Birth date _____

Address _____ City/State _____ Zip _____

Mother's name _____

Home/work telephone numbers _____

Father's name _____

Home/work telephone numbers _____

Person completing form _____

Relationship to child _____

Who referred you to us? _____

Has this child ever been evaluated at this clinic before? _____

Medical Information

Medical diagnosis (if any) _____

Current medical problems _____

_____

List any medications your child is taking: _____

Child's birth weight _____ Birth length _____
Head circumference _____

Developed at the Center on Human Development and Disability, University of Washington, Seattle
Interdisciplinary Clinical Assessment of Young Children with Developmental Disabilities
© 2000 by Paul H. Brookes Publishing Co., Baltimore

Length of pregnancy (weeks) _____ Problems during
pregnancy _____
How long was your child hospitalized after birth? _____
List any significant problems at that time: _____
_____

How would you describe your child's current overall developmental level?
_____ Delayed _____ At age level _____ Advanced _____ Not sure
Comments: _____

Feeding Information

This section focuses on feeding and nutrition. As the parent or primary caregiver, your input and insights are extremely important. Feeding is a major part of parenting, and you know your child better than anyone else. We consider you to be a part of our feeding clinic team and value your comments, questions, and insights.

Please briefly list specific *concerns or questions you would like addressed during this evaluation process* or what you hope comes out of this evaluation: _____
_____
_____
_____
_____

Please check the areas of concern regarding your child.
Star (*) the item(s) of **greatest concern**.

Underweight	_____	Overstuffs mouth	_____
Overweight	_____	Hypersensitivity around	
Reflux or vomiting	_____	mouth	_____
Constipation or diarrhea	_____	Messy eater	_____
Accepts limited variety		Poor positioning while	
of foods	_____	feeding	_____
Needs special diet	_____	Excessive time for eating	_____
Poor appetite	_____	Throws food	_____
Weak suck	_____	Refuses to eat	_____
Chewing or swallowing		Throws tantrums	_____
difficulties	_____	Easily distracted during	
Gagging or choking	_____	feedings	_____
Unskilled at using utensils	_____	Prefers fingers to utensils	_____

Developed at the Center on Human Development and Disability, University of Washington, Seattle
Interdisciplinary Clinical Assessment of Young Children with Developmental Disabilities
© 2000 by Paul H. Brookes Publishing Co., Baltimore

Does not give clear   Unpredictable mealtime
   hunger cues   ____   behavior   ____
Unable to feed self   ____   Other _____

Has your child ever been fed in a method other than orally (e.g., gastrostomy, nasogastric tube)? _____

If yes, please specify type: _____

Does your child have any food restrictions (e.g., due to allergies or cultural or religious beliefs)? _____

_____

_____

What types of food does your child eat?
     ____ Liquids only   ____ Baby foods
     ____ Soft table foods   ____ Regular table foods

Can your child self-feed? ____ Yes ____ No   If yes, indicate the manner of feeding:
     ____ Holds bottle   ____ Uses fork
     ____ Drinks from cup   ____ Uses spoon
     ____ Finger feeds

What is going well with feeding?_____

What have you or others tried in the past to improve the feeding problem? _____

Describe the results: _____

Current Educational and Community Resources

	Name and address	Telephone
Child's physician		
Current school		
Teacher		
Physical therapist		
Occupational therapist		
Speech-language therapist		
Nutritionist/dietitian		

Developed at the Center on Human Development and Disability, University of Washington, Seattle
Interdisciplinary Clinical Assessment of Young Children with Developmental Disabilities
© 2000 by Paul H. Brookes Publishing Co., Baltimore

Public health nurse _____ _____

Other (e.g., caseworker) _____ _____
_____

List others living in the same household with the child:

Name	Relationship to child	Age (if child)
_____	_____	_____
_____	_____	_____
_____	_____	_____
_____	_____	_____
_____	_____	_____

List other caregivers who regularly feed your child:

Name	Relationship to child
_____	_____
_____	_____
_____	_____

Other comments you would like to share with us:

Thank you for your time and information.

Developed at the Center on Human Development and Disability, University of Washington, Seattle
Interdisciplinary Clinical Assessment of Young Children with Developmental Disabilities
© 2000 by Paul H. Brookes Publishing Co., Baltimore

CHILD AND FAMILY SERVICES
PARENT QUESTIONNAIRE

Child's name _____ Date completed _____

Birth date _____

County/State providing services _____

Name/relationship of person completing form _____

This child is currently receiving	**Circle answer**	
Supplemental Security Income (SSI: Medicaid)	YES	NO
If yes, Financial & Medical	YES	NO
Medical Only	YES	NO
Supportive services from the		
Division of Developmental Disabilities (DDD)	YES	NO
Division of Children and Family Services (DCFS)	YES	NO
If yes, please check type(s): Foster Care ____		
Adoption ____ CPS ____		
Therapy/counseling	YES	NO
If yes, please check type(s):		
Speech-language ____ OT/PT ____		
Behavioral ____ Mental health ____ Other ____		
Health care from a pediatrician or primary care physician	YES	NO
Visits from the public health nurse	YES	NO
If younger than 3 years old, birth-to-3 services	YES	NO
Developmental preschool services	YES	NO
Special education services	YES	NO
If yes, is there an individualized education program (IEP) in place?	YES	NO

Developed at the Center on Human Development and Disability, University of Washington, Seattle
Interdisciplinary Clinical Assessment of Young Children with Developmental Disabilities
© 2000 by Paul H. Brookes Publishing Co., Baltimore

The family is currently receiving

Temporary Aid to Needy Families (Welfare)	YES	NO
Women, Infants, and Children (WIC)	YES	NO
Respite care	YES	NO

If yes, how many hours a month? ____

Who pays for this? _____

Counseling	YES	NO
Do you participate in any support group(s)?	YES	NO

Is there any assistance you'd like that you aren't

receiving now?	YES	NO

If yes, please describe:

Thank you for your time and information.

Developed at the Center on Human Development and Disability, University of Washington, Seattle
Interdisciplinary Clinical Assessment of Young Children with Developmental Disabilities
© 2000 by Paul H. Brookes Publishing Co., Baltimore

DEVELOPMENTAL CENTER/
PRESCHOOL QUESTIONNAIRE

To the teacher of _____ Date completed _____

The Child Development Program has been contacted regarding services for this child. Our clinic is interdisciplinary; therefore, this child will be seen by a variety of professionals during the evaluation. Because we want our clinical services to be as effective and efficient as possible, we would like our work to complement and reinforce school and community efforts. Your prompt return of this completed form will permit us to schedule the assessment without delay. In addition, please send test records and recent IFSP/IEP information if available.

1. **Basic Information**

    Person completing form _____ Telephone _____
    A. School name _____ District _____
        Address _____
    B. Classroom:
        Number of students _____ Age range _____
        Cognitive level of students _____
        Physical level of students _____
        Number of adults: Teachers ___ Aides ___ Volunteers ___
    C. What do you see as the child's strengths? _____
        _____

2. **Individual Performance Record**

    Do you have concerns in the following areas? If so, describe:
    A. Balance, learning gross motor skills, or physical activity level _____
        _____
        _____

    B. Fine motor movements, such as tremors, overreaching, weakness, or awkward finger coordination _____
        _____
        _____

Developed at the Center on Human Development and Disability, University of Washington, Seattle
Interdisciplinary Clinical Assessment of Young Children with Developmental Disabilities
© 2000 by Paul H. Brookes Publishing Co., Baltimore

C. Speech-language development _____
_____

_____

D. Cognitive and preacademic skills _____
_____

_____

E. Attending behavior _____
_____

F. Peer interaction skills _____
_____

G. Aggressive behavior _____
_____

H. Social behavior, personality areas _____
_____

_____

I. Health/hygiene _____
_____

J. Family issues _____
_____

3. Are there specific questions we can try to answer in our evaluation of this child? _____
_____

4. We would like input from school personnel. Who is available to participate in a staff and/or parent conference for this child to facilitate the implementation of recommendations?

Name	Telephone number

Thank you for your time and information.

Developed at the Center on Human Development and Disability, University of Washington, Seattle
Interdisciplinary Clinical Assessment of Young Children with Developmental Disabilities
© 2000 by Paul H. Brookes Publishing Co., Baltimore

COMMUNICATIVE BEHAVIOR QUESTIONNAIRE

(to be completed by the child's
communication disorders specialist)

Child's name _____ Date completed _____

Person completing form _____ Telephone number _____

School/clinic _____ Address _____

1. Please estimate this child's approximate level of functioning:

    Receptive
    language _____
    (expressed in age—
    year and months)

    Expressive
    language _____
    (expressed in age—
    year and months)

    Speech
    intelligibility _____
    (expressed as %)

2. What are your specific concerns about the child?

    _____

    _____

    _____

3. What are the current objectives of intervention?

    _____

    _____

    _____

4. What changes in communicative behavior have occurred in the past 6 months?

    _____

    _____

    _____

5. What procedures have been effective for the child?

    _____

    _____

    _____

    _____

    _____

Developed at the Center on Human Development and Disability, University of Washington, Seattle
Interdisciplinary Clinical Assessment of Young Children with Developmental Disabilities
© 2000 by Paul H. Brookes Publishing Co., Baltimore

6. Do the child's parents participate in the intervention program?
   Yes ＿＿ No ＿＿ If yes, how?

   _____

   _____

   _____

7. Do you have concerns about hearing?   Yes ＿＿ No ＿＿
   If yes, please note if the following apply:
   Recurrent middle-ear infections   Yes ＿＿ No ＿＿
   Child wears a hearing aid   Yes ＿＿ No ＿＿
   Documented hearing loss   Yes ＿＿ No ＿＿
   If yes, specify nature of loss: _____

   _____

8. What information would you like to obtain from an assessment
   at the Child Development Program?

   _____

   _____

   _____

   _____

   _____

   _____

   _____

Thank you for your time and information.

Developed at the Center on Human Development and Disability, University of Washington, Seattle
Interdisciplinary Clinical Assessment of Young Children with Developmental Disabilities
© 2000 by Paul H. Brookes Publishing Co., Baltimore

SOCIAL WORK FAMILY ASSESSMENT
(to be completed by the social worker as
a guide to the family interview)

Information for this form is taken from questionnaires sent to parents, school personnel, medical providers, and other professionals.

Today's date _____ Child's name _____
Address _____ Telephone _____
Birth date _____ Pediatrician's name _____ Hospital ID # ____
Child referred by _____ Reason _____

Names of family members	Relationship	Age	Marital status (m/s/d/w)	Other
_____	_____	___	_____	_____
_____	_____	___	_____	_____
_____	_____	___	_____	_____
_____	_____	___	_____	_____
_____	_____	___	_____	_____
_____	_____	___	_____	_____

Prior concerns _____
_____

Current concerns _____
_____

Emotional support (e.g., family, friends, religious, professional)
_____
_____

Issues at home _____
_____

Issues at school _____
_____

School name _____ Teacher _____

Developed at the Center on Human Development and Disability, University of Washington, Seattle
Interdisciplinary Clinical Assessment of Young Children with Developmental Disabilities
© 2000 by Paul H. Brookes Publishing Co., Baltimore

432

Issues in the community _____
_____
_____
_____
_____
_____

Current and past community services (e.g., respite care, family support, Division of Developmental Disabilities) _____
_____
_____
_____
_____
_____

Potential family concerns

	Yes	No
Alcohol abuse	____	____
Drug abuse	____	____
Depression	____	____
Mental health disorders	____	____
Finances	____	____
Domestic violence	____	____
Other	____	____

Needs identified by the family _____
_____
_____
_____
_____
_____

Suggestions _____
_____
_____
_____
_____
_____
_____

Developed at the Center on Human Development and Disability, University of Washington, Seattle
Interdisciplinary Clinical Assessment of Young Children with Developmental Disabilities
© 2000 by Paul H. Brookes Publishing Co., Baltimore

MOTOR DEVELOPMENT QUESTIONNAIRE
(to be completed by the therapist and/or teacher)

Child's name _____ Date completed _____

Person completing the form _____ Telephone _____

1. Are you concerned about this child's

    Fine motor development? Yes ____ No ____

    Concerns: _____

    Gross motor development? Yes ____ No ____

    Concerns: _____

    Perceptual development? Yes ____ No ____

    Concerns: _____

2. Please describe the physical and occupational therapy services
    this child has received (e.g., individual, group, consultation):

Description	Date started	Date completed	Frequency

3. Does the child need an assessment by this clinic's OT?

    Yes ____ No ____

    PT? Yes ____ No ____

    If yes, what specific questions or concerns should be addressed?

    _____

    _____

    _____

    PLEASE ANSWER THE FOLLOWING QUESTIONS ONLY IF
    CHILD IS INVOLVED IN THERAPY.

4. Major emphasis of therapy intervention (including therapy goals):

    _____

    _____

    _____

Developed at the Center on Human Development and Disability, University of Washington, Seattle
Interdisciplinary Clinical Assessment of Young Children with Developmental Disabilities
© 2000 by Paul H. Brookes Publishing Co., Baltimore

5. When did you most recently meet with the child's teacher?

    _____

    When did you most recently meet with the child's parents?

    _____

    How often do you meet with the teacher? _____
    Parents? _____
6. Have you suggested a home program? Yes ____ No ____
    If yes, what are your recommendations? _____

    _____

    _____

    _____

    _____

7. How well do you think the home program is carried out?

    _____

    _____

    _____

    _____

Thank you for your time and information.

Developed at the Center on Human Development and Disability, University of Washington, Seattle
Interdisciplinary Clinical Assessment of Young Children with Developmental Disabilities
© 2000 by Paul H. Brookes Publishing Co., Baltimore

EDUCATION QUESTIONNAIRE

To the teacher of _____ Date completed _____

The Child Development Program has been contacted regarding service for this child. Our clinic is interdisciplinary; therefore, this child will be seen by a variety of professionals during the evaluation. Because we want our clinical services to be as effective and efficient as possible, we would like our work to complement and reinforce school and community efforts. Your prompt return of this completed form will permit us to schedule the evaluation without delay. In addition, please send test records and recent IFSP/IEP if available.

1. **Basic information**

   Person completing form _____ Telephone _____

   A. School name _____ District _____
      Address _____

   B. Please describe the child's current educational program:
      Grade __ General class? __ Special education class? __
      Self-contained? ___ Open concept? _____
      Combined grades? _____
      Number of students _____ Number of teachers _____
      Number of aides _____ Number of volunteers _____
      Has the child's classroom instruction been mostly
      group? _____ Individual? _____

   C. List the extra resources currently provided for the child
      (e.g., reading, speech-language therapy) and the average
      number of hours per week provided as well as the instruction format (e.g., one to one, or small group):

      _____

      _____

2. **Individual performance record**

   To provide us with specific information relative to the child's functioning, please complete the following:

   A. What do you see as this child's strengths? _____

      _____

   B. Please list the child's specific problems: _____

      _____

      _____

Developed at the Center on Human Development and Disability, University of Washington, Seattle
Interdisciplinary Clinical Assessment of Young Children with Developmental Disabilities
© 2000 by Paul H. Brookes Publishing Co., Baltimore

C. Briefly characterize this child's relationship with
Peers _____
Teachers and adults _____

D. Does this child have a behavior problem in the classroom? Yes ____ No ____
If answer is yes, describe the nature of the problem and
interventions tried: _____
_____

3. When did you most recently meet with the child's parents?
_____

4. Do you have specific concerns or questions about the family?
Yes ____ No ____
If yes, please describe: _____
_____

5. Please indicate what evaluations or treatments have already
been provided by the school, and attach testing reports. Also,
please indicate if school testing is planned in the next year.

6. We would like input from school personnel. Who will be
available to participate in a staff and/or parent conference for
this child to facilitate implementation of recommendations?

Name	Telephone

Thank you for your time and information.

Developed at the Center on Human Development and Disability, University of Washington, Seattle
Interdisciplinary Clinical Assessment of Young Children with Developmental Disabilities
© 2000 by Paul H. Brookes Publishing Co., Baltimore

OCCUPATIONAL AND
PHYSICAL THERAPY SERVICES SURVEY
(to be completed by
the child's teacher and/or therapist)

In order to provide the most appropriate and comprehensive assessments, the occupational and physical therapy staff at the clinic would like information on each child prior to his or her visit. We value your input regarding your concerns, therapy services, and assessment results.

Child's name _____ Date completed _____

Person completing form _____ Telephone _____

Relationship to the child _____ Name of agency/school _____

1. Do you have concerns in the following areas? If so, describe:
   Fine motor development _____

   Gross motor development _____

   Perceptual development _____

   Oral motor skills _____

   Self-help skills _____

   Play skills _____

2. Describe the physical and occupational therapy services this child has received:

Type of therapy	Indi-vidual	Group	Consul-tation to teacher	Date started	Date ended	Fre-quency
Occupational therapy						
Physical therapy						
Other (specify)						

Developed at the Center on Human Development and Disability, University of Washington, Seattle
Interdisciplinary Clinical Assessment of Young Children with Developmental Disabilities
© 2000 by Paul H. Brookes Publishing Co., Baltimore

3. Provide information regarding most recent assessment(s):

Assessment tool	Date of testing	Age at testing	Standard score	Standard deviation score	Age equiva- lency

4. Describe the emphasis of current therapy intervention (includ- ing therapy goals): _____
   _____
   _____
   _____

5. Do you recommend that this child be evaluated at the inter- disciplinary clinic by _____
   An occupational therapist? ____ Yes ____ No
   A physical therapist? ____ Yes ____ No
   If yes, what specific questions or concerns should be ad- dressed? _____
   _____
   _____
   _____
   _____
   _____
   _____
   _____

Thank you for your time and information.

Developed at the Center on Human Development and Disability, University of Washington, Seattle
Interdisciplinary Clinical Assessment of Young Children with Developmental Disabilities
© 2000 by Paul H. Brookes Publishing Co., Baltimore

CHECKLIST FOR FAMILIES NEW TO THE PKU CLINIC
(to be completed by the nutritionist case manager)

1. **Basic information**
   Child's name _____ Birth date _____ Sex: ___ M ___F
   Mother's name _____ Birth date _____
   Father's name _____ Birth date _____
   Address _____ City/State _____ Zip _____
   Home telephone number _____
   Child's pediatrician _____ Telephone _____
   Address _____

2. **Diagnostic checklist**
   Birth weight: ___g or ___ lb ___ oz
   Gestational age: ___ weeks
   Birth order: _____
   Infant being fed _____ breast milk _____ proprietary formula

Diagnostic studies

Date collected	Sample (Guthrie/ quantitative)	Age	Date reported	Phenylalanine (mg %)	Tyrosine (mg %)

Biopterin studies

Date blood and urine collected for biopterin _____
Date results received _____

Treatment

Date phenylalanine-free formula introduced _____

Developed at the Center on Human Development and Disability, University of Washington, Seattle
Interdisciplinary Clinical Assessment of Young Children with Developmental Disabilities
© 2000 by Paul H. Brookes Publishing Co., Baltimore

3. Initial teaching guidelines

Date the following materials provided to the family _____

____ Family Care Notebook
____ New Parents' Guide to PKU
____ PKU Management Guidelines
____ Living with PKU
____ National PKU News sample copy and order form

Teaching topics at first visits:

Date _____   Date _____

A. PKU	C. Management of PKU
___ Genetics	___ Blood phenylala-nine levels of 2–6 mg %
___ Metabolic pathways	___ Phenylalanine-free formula is mainstay
B. Prospects for children with PKU	___ Milk is supple-mented
___ Preventing mental retardation	___ Low-protein fruits and vegetables
___ Typical growth and development with early and consistent treatment	___ Low-protein breads and cereals
___ Lifetime treatment	___ Avoiding Nutrasweet
	___ Dealing with childhood illnesses

Family home visit offered? _____

Home visit accepted? _____

Developed at the Center on Human Development and Disability, University of Washington, Seattle
Interdisciplinary Clinical Assessment of Young Children with Developmental Disabilities
© 2000 by Paul H. Brookes Publishing Co., Baltimore

MANAGEMENT GUIDELINES FOR PKU

Serum Phenylalanine Levels

Without early diagnosis and appropriate treatment, phenylketonuria (PKU) leads to mental retardation. Cognitive impairments can be prevented with good management. Serum phenylalanine levels of 2–10 mg% are safe and acceptable, but levels of 2–6 mg% are ideal and especially important for infants and young children. The current standard of care in the United States is to maintain these safe levels throughout life. No one with PKU should ever be "taken off diet."

Once newborn children are under satisfactory management, a monthly serum phenylalanine ("phe") level is recommended, which is drawn at the monthly clinic. If that level is out of the recommended range, a mid-month follow-up level is requested.

Food Patterns

Children with PKU must eliminate high-protein foods from their diet (meat, fish, dairy products, eggs, poultry) and restrict their intake of moderate-protein foods (potatoes, grains). As children grow older, they need to increase their intake of low-protein foods (certain fruits and vegetables, low-protein breads and low-protein pasta products) to maintain appropriate energy (calorie) intake and to prevent hunger. Adequate formula intake plus low-protein foods provide protein, phenylalanine, and tyrosine at the required levels as well as energy to support growth and all essential nutrients.

Formula

All formula is prescribed by a physician and monitored by a nutritionist. Infants and children who receive a consistent daily intake of a phenylalanine-free formula/medical food (roughly 85% of their protein needs and 90% of their energy needs) have the most stable and appropriate serum phenylalanine levels. The clinic policy is "formula first." Parents are taught that formula is given before other foods, both to meet nutritional needs and to satisfy appetite. Formula is necessary to maintain low blood phe levels that support long-term compliance and lead to the child's future completion of school, employment, and independence.

Developed at the Center on Human Development and Disability, University of Washington, Seattle
Interdisciplinary Clinical Assessment of Young Children with Developmental Disabilities
© 2000 by Paul H. Brookes Publishing Co., Baltimore

Nutrition Education

Teaching children to manage their diets by themselves is an important aspect of the program, starting with "yes/no foods" and moving on to "how much." At the monthly clinics, nutrition education activities are provided for each age group to aid children in learning about their diets.

Two concepts are reinforced by this clinic, the first being that parents are the teachers. Materials and ideas with which parents can continue to teach their children about the diet at home are provided. The importance of consistency and appropriate development of food habits is emphasized. The second concept is that of health. Children with well-managed PKU are typically developing, healthy children. Every possible attempt is made to treat them as such and not as if they have a disease. All aspects of the child—diet, physical fitness, self-esteem, and self-worth—are considered. The consistent food patterns and routines established by parents in early childhood are essential for dietary compliance when children are older and more independent.

Illness

It is important to treat usual childhood illnesses aggressively to prevent tissue catabolism and consequent elevated blood phenylalanine levels. During an illness or infection, it is important to maintain the formula intake as much as possible. The continuation of formula prevents the breakdown of muscle protein that increases the level of phenylalanine in blood. However, if a child refuses to drink formula, whatever clear liquid the primary care physician recommends is appropriate. Parents need to contact the primary care physician for management of the illness before calling the PKU clinic staff.

Lifetime Diet

The current standard of care is a low-phenylalanine diet, including formula/medical food, for life. The PKU Collaborative Study documented long-term dietary intervention as the only method to achieve optimal cognitive ability. When children are taken off the low-phenylalanine diet and their blood phenylalanine levels increase, their IQ scores or achievement test scores drop. Cranial magnetic resonance imaging (MRI) studies have documented that abnormalities consistent with breakdown of neural tissue of the brain, and the

Developed at the Center on Human Development and Disability, University of Washington, Seattle
Interdisciplinary Clinical Assessment of Young Children with Developmental Disabilities
© 2000 by Paul H. Brookes Publishing Co., Baltimore

severity of these changes, correlate with high blood phenylalanine levels. Central to long-term compliance is regular monitoring of progress: Monthly (or more frequent) monitoring of serum phe levels and food records is important in noting "benchmarks of progress" for people with PKU.

Clinic Format

There is a 2-day clinic cycle each month, which is the third Wednesday and the following Thursday. You will receive an appointment time for your child and meet with your child's age-appropriate nutrition education and parent group. Instead of giving children individual appointments, children and their parents are seen in groups based on age. Children meet with the nutritionist to work on a nutrition education project while parents meet in a separate group to discuss issues related to raising a child with PKU. After group time, families meet individually with the pediatrician, the nutritionist, and the social worker.

This group format was chosen for several reasons. First, it is a reliable and efficient way to educate children and parents and to keep them up to date on recent developments in PKU management. In addition, parents can support each other, and children benefit immeasurably from knowing other children with PKU.

Families are strongly urged to attend the monthly clinic. For families who live too far away to attend monthly clinics, a monthly serum phenylalanine level and a 3-day food record is required. Experience has shown that this monthly feedback is essential for maintaining good serum phenylalanine levels.

Maternal PKU

There is a special dilemma for females with PKU. It is difficult for a woman with PKU to have a typically developing child. Even when serum phenylalanine levels are kept low, there may be some damage to the fetus. The higher the serum phenylalanine level, the poorer the fetal outcome. Infants of mothers with PKU exhibit microcephaly, mental retardation, and growth retardation. Due to this adverse outcome, women with PKU are encouraged to consider all the risks of pregnancy carefully; other alternatives, such as adoption, are recommended. This matter is discussed early with the family so that the consequences are well understood and appropriate decisions can be made.

Developed at the Center on Human Development and Disability, University of Washington, Seattle
Interdisciplinary Clinical Assessment of Young Children with Developmental Disabilities
© 2000 by Paul H. Brookes Publishing Co., Baltimore

Index

Page numbers followed by "f" indicate figures; those followed by "t" indicate tables.

Expressive language, *see* Language and
  communicative development
  assessment
Expressive One-Word Picture
  Vocabulary Test, 46*t*
External case manager, *see* Service
  coordinator role
Extremities assessment
  for fragile X syndrome, 352
  as part of neurodevelopmental
    assessment, 73, 75
Eyes, assessment, *see* Vision

Facial features, appraisal of, 74, 75, 82
  for fragile X syndrome, 351
Failure to thrive (FTT), 120*t*, 327, 329,
    332, 336, 352
Familiarity with child and family, 162
Families at high risk
  premature infant, case study, 226–235
  treatment of phenylketonuria (PKU),
    case study, 276–277
Family
  daily life and routines, nursing
    assessment of, 94
  empowerment as result of social work
    assessment, 203–205
  occupational therapy assessment of
    priorities, 147
  Swedish views of role, 395*t*, 396
  see also headings starting with Parent
Family environment, *see* Environment
  of child
Family history
  autism and, case study, 297–298
  fragile X syndrome and, case study,
    355–356
  as part of neurodevelopmental
    assessment, 69
  speech-language assessment and, case
    study, 53*f*–54*f*, 55
  see also Information gathering as part
    of assessment
Family involvement
  in nutrition assessment, 107
  in physical therapy assessment, 173
  in psychological assessment, 186,
    197–198
  social work role in assessment,
    201–203, 204*t*

views on in Sweden, 403–404
  family-oriented perspective, 405
  trends, 406
  see also Parent–child relationship
Family Needs Survey, use in Sweden, 402
Family relationship with child, *see*
  Parent–child relationship
Family relationship with professionals, *see*
  Family involvement; Parent–
  professional relationship
Family services, *see* Individualized family
  service plans (IFSPs); Special
  Supplemental Nutrition Program
  for Women, Infants, and
  Children (WIC)
Family strengths, *see* Strengths of family
Family-centered care, summary
  of, 204*t*
FAS, *see* Fetal alcohol syndrome
Fat, *see* Growth parameters; Nutrition
  assessment; Obesity
Father, *see headings starting with Family
  or Parent*
Fear of social workers, effect of, 210
Feeding clinic
  Down syndrome, case study role,
    252, 254
  parent questionnaire, 252, 422–425
Feeding development and skills,
  119–120, 121*t*
Feeding difficulties
  case study of child with, 95–98
  premature infant, 228, 229,
    231–232, 246–247
  Down syndrome, case study, 252,
    254–256, 265
  interdisciplinary teams forming special
    groups to handle, 4
  occupational therapy assessment
    and, 131
  screening for, 120
  see also Nutrition assessment; Prader-
    Willi syndrome (PWS)
Fetal alcohol syndrome (FAS), 71, 71*t*
  age of child for assessment for, 324
  assessment process for, 309–310
  case study of child with, 310–326
    Attention-deficit/hyperactivity
      disorder (ADHD) diagnosis and,
      312, 319
    adoption of child, 312

see also Neurodevelopmental
assessment
Neuromuscular components of
movement, 158
Neuropsychological assessment, use in
Sweden, 402, 405
Newborns, *see* Infants
NICUs, *see* Neonatal intensive care units
Nonstandardized tests
in psychological assessment, 189, 191
in speech-language assessment, 45–47
Norm-referenced tests
occupational therapy assessment
using, 134, 139
physical therapy assessment using, 163
speech-language assessment using, 45
Sweden, use of, 398
North American Nursing Diagnosis
Association (NANDA), 86, 88
Nursing assessment, 85–103
assessment phase, 88–89
behavior in varied settings in data
collection, 92
case studies of decision making, 95–98
recommendations, 97–98
child and family strengths, importance
of assessing, 94–95
collaborative relationship with child,
family, and community, 86, 100
contexts of data collected, 92
cultural context and services provided,
101
diagnosis, 86–87, 93
diagnostic decision making, 89–93
domains of nursing practice and,
86–87, 96t
external case manager, nurse acting
as, 99
family's daily life and routines,
importance of assessing, 94
health pattern responses of nurses,
86–87
information gathering, 90–92, 100
informed clinical decision making,
87–98
instruments used, 89, 90t–91t
integration of biophysical and
psychosocial data, 92–93
internal case manager, nurse acting
as, 99
intervention plan, 97–98, 100

knowledge deficit as diagnosis, 87
of child with Prader-Willi syndrome
(PWS), case study, 335–336
preassessment phase, 88
program development and evaluation,
100–101
protocols of care used by nurses, 89
purpose of assessment, 86
recommendations, 93–95, 97–98
screening process, 88, 95
service coordinator, nurse acting as,
86, 89, 98–100
sources of data for information
gathering, 91–92
time points and patterns in data
collection, 90–91
treatment utility of assessment, 93
Nursing Child Assessment Feeding
Scales, 90t, 96, 97
Nursing Child Assessment Sleep/Activity
Record 90t, 97
Nursing Child Assessment Teaching
Scales, 90t, 96
*Nursing Standards for Children with Special
Health Care Needs: Guidelines for
Practice,* 89, 91t
Nutrition assessment, 105–128
access of family to nutrition services
and, 125
anthropometry, 110–115, 113t–114t
appropriateness of diet, 107
benefits of, 126
biochemical evaluation, 118, 118t
in case studies of child with, 123–125
Down syndrome, 254–258
phenylketonuria (PKU), 275–276
Prader-Willi syndrome (PWS),
336–339
premature infant follow-up,
231–232, 239, 246–247
challenges to accurate assessment,
108–109
clinical evaluation, 119, 119t
components of, 110–120
dietary history, 116–117
dietary intake, 115–117
Dietary Reference Intakes (DRI) and
Recommended Daily Allowances
(RDA), 108–109
of child with Down syndrome, case
study, 254–258